Perceived Health and Adaptation in Chronic Disease

Chronic diseases have become predominant in Western societies and in many developing countries. They affect quality of life and daily activities and require regular medical care.

This unique monograph will bring readers up to date with chronic disease research, with a focus on health-related quality of life and patient perception of the impact of the diseases and health intervention, as well as psychological adaptation to the disease. It considers the application of concepts and measures in medical and psychological clinical practice and in public health policies. Informed by theory, philosophy, history and empirical research, chapters will indicate how readers might advance their own thinking, learning, practice and research. The book is intended to be provocative and challenging to enhance discussion about theory as a key component of research and practice.

Perceived Health and Adaptation in Chronic Disease will be of interest to researchers and academics alike. It boasts a wide range of contributions from leading international specialists from Australia, Canada, Denmark, France, Germany, the Netherlands, Spain, Sweden, the UK and the USA. This has also allowed the book to provide readers with a multidisciplinary approach.

Francis Guillemin is epidemiologist and rheumatologist, professor of public health, and Director of the APEMAC research unit on chronic diseases, perceived health and adaptation processes, of the University of Lorraine, Nancy, France.

Alain Leplège is professor at Paris Diderot University, France, specializing in health service research and outcome measurement, methodology and epistemology.

Serge Briançon is epidemiologist, professor emeritus of public health, head of the School of Public Health (2001-2016) at the University of Lorraine, Nancy, France.

Elisabeth Spitz is professor of health psychology at the University of Lorraine, Metz, France.

Joël Coste is a rheumatologist, epidemiologist and historian of medicine, and professor at Paris Descartes University and École Pratique des Hautes Études, Paris, France.

Perceived Health and Adaptation in Chronic Disease

Edited by
Francis Guillemin, Alain Leplège,
Serge Briançon, Elisabeth Spitz,
Joël Coste

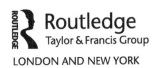

LONDON AND NEW YORK

First published 2018 by Routledge

2 Park Square, Milton Park, Abingdon, Oxfordshire OX14 4RN
52 Vanderbilt Avenue, New York, NY 10017

Routledge is an imprint of the Taylor & Francis Group, an informa business

First issued in paperback 2019

British Library Cataloguing-in-Publication Data

A catalogue record for this book is available from the British Library

---

Library of Congress Cataloging-in-Publication Data

Names: Guillemin, Francis, editor. | Leplège, Alain, editor. | Briançon,
Serge, editor. | Spitz, Elisabeth, editor. | Coste, Joël, editor.
Title: Perceived health and adaptation in chronic disease / [edited by]
Francis Guillemin, Alain Leplège, Serge Briançon, Elisabeth Spitz, Joël Coste.
Description: Abingdon, Oxon ; New York, NY : Routledge, 2017. | Includes
bibliographical references and index.
Identifiers: LCCN 2016050170| ISBN 9781498778985 (hbk.) | ISBN 9781498778992 (ebk.)
Subjects: | MESH: Chronic Disease--epidemiology | Sickness Impact Profile |
Health Status | Quality of Life | Adaptation, Physiological
Classification: LCC RC48 | NLM WT 30 | DDC 616--dc23
LC record available at https://lccn.loc.gov/2016050170

ISBN: 978-1-4987-7898-5 (hbk)
ISBN: 978-0-367-22445-5 (pbk)

Typeset in Goudy
by diacriTech

Table of contents

Acknowledgments

Most of the contributions to this book were previously presented as oral communications at the APEMAC conference on "Chronic Diseases, Perceived Health and Adaptation: Stakes and Future" held on 3–6 June 2014 at the Faculty of Medicine, University of Lorraine, Nancy, France.

The editors are extremely grateful to a number of other scientists, namely Dorcas Beaton (University of Toronto, Canada), Lennart Nordenfeldt (University of Linköping, Sweden), and Annette L. Stanton and Michael A. Hoyt (University of California, Los Angeles, California), who agreed to share their thoughts and knowledge, and to give their viewpoints in additional chapters.

The editors are also very grateful to external scientists who devoted time to reviewing and commenting on several chapters for their thoughtful and fruitful suggestions on content and presentation, which have contributed to improving the overall consistency of this book. In particular, they wish to acknowledge the contributions of Karl Bang Christensen (University of Copenhagen, Denmark), Maël Lemoine (University of Tours, France), Olivier Luminet (Catholic University of Louvain, Belgium), Mariette Mercier (University of Besançon, France), Silke Schmidt (University of Greifswald, Germany), and Cyril Tarquinio (University of Lorraine, France) and the anonymous reviewers invited by the publisher.

The editors are indebted to Angela Verdier for expert English editing and Veronique Baron for secretarial assistance.

Editors

Francis Guillemin, MD, PhD, is an epidemiologist and rheumatologist, a professor at the School of Public Health, the Director of the EA 4360 APEMAC Research Unit on "Chronic diseases, perceived health, and adaptation processes" of the University of Lorraine, Nancy, and the head of the INSERM Clinical Epidemiology Center at Nancy University Hospital, France. He has implemented teaching programs on clinical epidemiology, health measurement, and health economics. He is the director of the Master e-learning program: "Public Health and Environment" with one specialty on "Epidemiology, Clinical research and Evaluation."

His area of research is in outcome measurement for patient-reported outcomes in chronic conditions, with particular interest in rheumatic disorders.

Alain Leplège, MD, PhD, is a health service researcher, specializing in outcome measurement, methodology, and epistemology. A psychiatrist by training, he earned a PhD in philosophy (Paris 1 Panthéon-Sorbonne) with a postdoc in health service research from Johns Hopkins University. He is currently a professor in the Department of History and Philosophy of Sciences, Faculty of Life Sciences, Université Paris Diderot, Paris, France, and the head of the Ville Evrard Mental Health and Disability Research Centre. He is an associate researcher in EA 4360 APEMAC Research Unit on "Chronic diseases, perceived health, and adaptation processes" and an adjunct professor at the Person Centred Research Centre, Division of Rehabilitation and Occupation Studies, Health and Rehabilitation Research Institute, Auckland University of Technology, New Zealand. Since 2012, he has been an adjunct professor at the University of the Sunshine Coast, Faculty of Science, Health, Education and Engineering, Sippy Downs, Queensland, Australia.

Serge Briançon, MD, is an epidemiologist, a professor of public health, and the head of the School of Public Health at Lorraine University, Nancy, France. He is the manager of the epidemiology team of the EA 4360 APEMAC Research Unit on "Chronic diseases, perceived health, and adaptation processes." He has created and headed the Clinical Epidemiology and Evaluation ward at Nancy University Hospital for 17 years. He is a member of the Haut Conseil de la Santé Publique and of the Scientific Committee of the Institut de Veille Sanitaire.

His research area is evaluation of care and prevention in chronic diseases with a particular interest in nephrology disorders and nutrition, using patient-reported outcomes of measure as a main judgment criteria.

Elisabeth Spitz, PhD, is a professor of health psychology at the University of Lorraine, Metz, France. She was the manager of the Health Psychology Research Team in EA 4360 APEMAC Research Unit on "Chronic diseases, perceived health, and adaptation processes" for 10 years. She coordinates the axis "Quality of life, Health, and Handicap" of the Human Science Center of Lorraine (MSHL), and is a past president of the French Association of Health Psychology. She is a co-director of the Master program: Health Psychology and Clinic Psychology.

Her area of research is in the health-related risk management and behavioral self-regulation.

Joël Coste, MD, PhD, is a rheumatologist, an epidemiologist, and a historian of medicine, as well as a professor of public health at the Paris Descartes University, where he leads the Hôtel Dieu Unit of Biostatistics and Epidemiology and Directeur d'Études at the École Pratique des Hautes Etudes (Sciences historiques et philologiques), Paris, France. He is also the manager of the Measurement and chronic diseases team in EA 4360 APEMAC Research Unit on "Chronic diseases, perceived health, and adaptation processes."

His main areas of research interest are measurement in the field of medicine, past and present conceptions of disease and illness, and medical epistemology.

Introduction

Chronic diseases have become predominant in Western societies and in many developing countries. Their causes and pathophysiological mechanisms are often unknown or complex and their impact on mortality is delayed. Nevertheless, they mostly affect quality of life and daily activities, and require regular medical care. Patients with diseases of this type need to adapt to their condition and they have to deploy numerous strategies to do so.

A number of important research developments have surfaced in the last 30 years in the field of health-related quality of life, focusing on the perception by patients of the impact of their diseases, on health interventions, and on psychological adaptation to the disease. The contributions of this research have been the renewal of conceptualizations of handicap integrating the complex interactions among somatic, psychological, sociological, and environmental approaches found in the bio-psycho-social model (Engel) or in the International Classification of Functioning, Disability and Health (ICF) proposed by the World Health Organization (WHO) in 2001. This book focuses on the current state of this research as applied to chronic diseases and sets out to identify the associated challenges and future developments.

The patient perspective is central to this area of research, and it is also central to the concept of perceived health. The implication and empowerment of the patient are the ultimate aims of promoting measures of these parameters and this approach.

The perception of health by the patient with chronic disease changes over time. Health-related quality of life resulting from health interventions strongly depends on heath perceptions. The coevolution of health, its perception, and adaptation triggers the dynamics of the patient's behavior, the relationship with professionals, and the use of health-care resources. The adaptation process is a major phenomenon. It needs time to unfold and is particularly important to consider in chronic diseases. The contribution of health psychology is essential to generate hypotheses within the framework of relevant theories and to test them using appropriate or innovative measurement models. One of the objectives of this book is to link the fields of perception and adaptation.

Specialists from various disciplines, such as clinicians, epidemiologists, philosophers, psychologists, public health professionals, sociologists, and statisticians, have contributed to this comprehensive approach to chronic diseases by the definition of concepts, the clarification of theory, the construction of models, and the development of measures. Usually, the independent contributions of various disciplines in these fields raise epistemic problems. Here, the merging of the different contributions is intended to clarify the common challenges and to increase their coherence.

It can be hoped that a wide audience will appreciate these contributions: researchers, teachers, experts, students in the domains of health psychology, epidemiology, health service research, and health policy as well as professionals in the area of chronic diseases, or patient leaders. The research should contribute to the empowerment of patient partners for research and care.

The benefits of the book's contributions will be substantial in stimulating reflection among researchers. They will show what has been gained in these domains and favor the transfer of these gains into practice by modifying patient and health professional behaviors and influencing health policymakers.

The book will show readers how leading researchers are rethinking chronic disease research and treatment practices and exploring current and future challenges in a wide array of topics.

The book comprises 20 chapters organized in four sections:

- Concepts and Models
- Measurement
- Interpretation of Perceived Health Data
- Knowledge and Decision Making

The authors of the different chapters suggest ways of thinking that are informed by theory, philosophy, history, or empirical research. Each chapter indicates how readers might advance their own thinking, learning, practice, and research. This book is intended to be challenging to enhance discussion on theories as a key element in scientific research and clinical practice.

Concepts and models

Section 1 of this book is devoted to the conceptual issues related to perceived health, quality of life, disablement, adaptation, and chronic disease itself. Because of variations and different usages of all these key concepts, and even controversies on their definitions, clarification and overview were called for from the outset.

Joël Coste shows in Chapter 2 that the very concept of chronic disease has a long and controversial history in medicine (as long as learned medicine itself). However, it received wider attention only in the 1950s. At that time, acute infectious diseases were superseded in the public health agendas of developed countries by long-term noncommunicable diseases. At the same time, scholars from disciplines other than medicine, including psychology and sociology, addressed serious issues such as suffering, distress, disability, and the social consequences of chronic ailments. Carefully considering historical processes, continuities, and dynamics, Coste also sets out to refine and reformulate the issues of coherence, relevance, and usefulness of the concept of chronic disease, both currently and for the near future. Calling for more empirical research within the framework of the bio-psycho-social model to disentangle the effects of *temporality* from those of *irreversibility, incurability, disease activity,* and *disability* in the most prevalent chronic diseases, he proposes, for the time being, to define chronic diseases only in terms of duration. Regarding the usefulness of knowing, saying, or predicting that a disease is or will be long lasting, Coste distinguishes "medicine as a science and medicine as a practice." He recommends that the concept of chronic disease should be at least temporarily used to facilitate the investigation of the long-term direct and indirect components of suffering, disability, and the social consequences of diseases, and scrutiny of health service responses to patients' suffering. Coste considers that the concept and the category "chronic" are more useful in clinical practice (than in "science"), because caregivers obviously need to take the various forms of suffering of the patients and the ethical issues associated with their care into consideration, and above all they need to build a good therapeutic alliance.

In Chapter 3, Donald L. Patrick reviews the conceptual approaches to *perceived quality of life*, defined as a "subjective evaluation of one's life" in relation to the culture in which one lives and to one's values, goals, and concerns. This broad concept is distinct from that of *perceived heath* because quality of life *also* encompasses other aspects of life such as freedom, respect, income security, and happiness. However, because, according to Patrick, it is "near impossible to determine where health and nonhealth aspects begin and end" and because "distinction between objective circumstances and perception of these circumstances is also occasionally blurred," four conceptual approaches to defining and measuring perceived quality of life are considered: theories of need, theories of positive well-being, value approaches, and Sen's capability theory. As Nordenfelt points out in his overview in Chapter 1, two of these define objective rather than subjective quality of life (the theories of need and capability). All approaches except Sen's have been operationalized, and procedures or instruments exist enabling individual measures and empirical studies to compare quality of life across time and groups. The divergence of approaches and the inconsistencies between, and sometimes within, the measurement instruments are clearly evidenced by Patrick, who finally proposes to systematically compare the operationalization of concepts and/or to synthesize the approaches and deconstruct their commonalities. As Patrick reminds us, "perceived quality of life is at the heart of the patient-centered outcomes movement" increasingly endorsed in chronic disease research and practice, and this requires clarity and transparency regarding the conceptual implications of measurement processes.

In Chapter 4, Elisabeth M. Badley reviews the conceptual models of disablement that contributed to the development of the ICF, the current international reference standard for disablement assessment published in 2001. The Nagi model (1965), the International Classification of Impairments, Disabilities, and Handicaps (ICIDH, 1980), and the Disability Creation Process (DCP, 1995) variously consider that disablement results from an interaction between some characteristic(s) of the person's functioning, for example, impairment or disability, and contextual factors. Among these, a person's social and physical environments have long been stressed and investigated as facilitators or barriers in the process leading to restriction in societal participation. Conversely, personal factors, which are recognized as a separate category of contextual factors in the ICF, have been inadequately thought out and are not yet classified. Badley argues convincingly that personal factors may act as facilitators or barriers in the disablement process but can also be what she calls "scene-setters," in the sense that they determine a "repertoires of tasks" a person may perform in the environment and culture in which he or she lives, which in turn determines forms of social participation. Potentially, scene-setting factors include age, gender, educational status, religion, etc. This notion of scene-setters finds echoes in Lennart Nordenfelt's earlier work in which he distinguished two ways in which the environment can affect a person's ability to perform certain actions: a causal way, where an external factor causes an ailment that restricts the person's ability, and another way whereby the environment, together with personal factors, determines actions that can be performed by a given person at a given time: the "platform for action" for this person, as Nordenfelt calls it. In Chapter 1, Nordenfelt further analyzes the relationship between these scene-setters and a person's disability. He also stresses the conceptual regression of the ICF compared with the ICIDH for the distinction between activity and participation, and the confusion it caused in the application of the ICF manual.

Finally, Annette L. Stanton and Michael A. Hoyt address in Chapter 5 the key phenomenon of psychological adjustment to chronic disease and review the conceptualizations of this dynamic and multidimensional process, which definitely cannot be reduced to the mere absence of any psychological disorder. They also review theories concerning the "contributors" to adjustment to chronic disease, namely the theories of stress and coping, self-regulation, and personal growth, and the various factors (socioeconomic, interpersonal, or intrapersonal) that have been shown to contribute to adjustment across time. However, Stanton and Hoyt regret that too few studies have investigated psychological adjustment in longitudinal settings and plead for further and better research on trajectories of psychological distress in the course of chronic diseases. Indeed, to quote them, "greater translation of theory and research on adjustment to chronic disease into evidence-based clinical intervention is a vital goal."

Measurement

The aim of Section 2 is to identify, discuss, and contextualize the new perspectives offered by modern psychometric methods for the validation and calibration of measurement. It also presents two innovative empirical projects that illustrate how these methods can contribute to the actual development of specific instruments consistent with the concepts and domains of investigation identified in the previous chapter.

In Chapter 6, Alain Leplège first recalls the epistemological scene. As is well known, some doubts and criticisms have been raised concerning the scientific claims of the human and social sciences. In particular, they have been accused of not being sufficiently mathematical, experimental, or predictive, especially when compared with natural sciences such as physics. Against these criticisms, several lines of defense have been raised. The development of sound measurements is an essential step, inasmuch as the validity of the conclusions of any experiment that tests hypotheses by comparing empirical consequences to selected observations, is dependent on the validity and precision of the observations and measures performed. This being said, the general epistemological question addressed by this section is whether we can apprehend measurement in the social sciences in the same way as measurement in the natural sciences. More specifically, this question could be: Should measurements developed in the social sciences for the purpose of aggregating or comparing subjects and groups meet the same kind of invariance requirements as those used in the natural sciences? By invariance what is meant here is the absence of item bias. For instance, subjects belonging to different groups (e.g., men and women) should understand a given question in the same way (i.e., invariantly) if the responses to this question are to be used to compare these two groups.

In Chapter 7, David Andrich argues convincingly that the contribution and significance of the work of the Danish mathematician Georg Rasch for the understanding and practice of social measurement reside in (1) an a priori criterion of invariance of comparisons within a specified frame of reference; (2) rendering this criterion in the form of a class of probabilistic models that have sufficient statistics for all parameters, together with a body of knowledge of statistical inferences; and (3) anchoring the models in an empirical paradigm for item and test construction. The chapter makes some brief comparisons with classical test theory and item response theory, and suggests that distinguishing these two types of theories could not only reduce confusion in social measurement but also encourage greater exploitation of the full contribution of Rasch theory to the development of meaningful measures in the social sciences.

Alan Tennant, in Chapter 8, provides historical context for the discovery by Georg Rasch and shows its potential for developing and improving scientific research in the human, social, and medical sciences. He starts from a review of the recent development of Patient-Reported Outcome Measures (PROMs) covering a wide range of constructs (theoretical perspective) consistent with the bio-psycho-social model as defined in the ICF. These range from fatigue (Impairment of Function) and job limitations or restrictions (Activity and Participation) to the availability of services (Environmental) (WHO, 2001) to assess the efficacy of a particular intervention in improving (or restoring) individual and population health.

He provides a precisely documented history of psychometric concepts and methods, and of the main methodological and conceptual debates that have developed within this discipline, for example, the importance of the concept of unidimensionality for the measurement of psychological attributes, the crucial importance of a clear understanding of the concept of invariance, and the need for fundamental measurement. He recalls the progressive development of quality indicators for this type of measurement and their methodological importance beyond the measurement of psychological traits. In his own words, "the ubiquitous questionnaire applied to health outcomes can comprise a wide range of concepts, not just psychological attributes such as self-esteem, but all aspects of functioning as defined by the ICF, as well as quality of life. Items from scales of this type are summed to ascertain the magnitude of a hypothesized latent [underlying] construct."

Tennant contrasts what, like many others, he calls the classical test theory (Spearman, Nunnally, etc.) with the more recent "modern test theory," which, from a methodological viewpoint, focuses on what is known in general as item response theory (IRT). IRT is a general statistical theory about item [question] and scale performance, and how that performance relates to the underlying (or latent) abilities that are measured by the items in the scale. IRT includes a family of different models with different attributes and features, although many share the same underlying assumptions, such as unidimensionality. He notes that in IRT, in general, there are two distinct, and for some incompatible, approaches, the approach belonging to the Rasch family of models and that belonging to all other IRT models. The former, it is argued, is consistent with the principles of fundamental invariant measurement, whereas the latter is concerned with finding the model that best explains the data. He discusses the practical importance, from the end-user perspectives, of the various theoretical and methodological differences and contrasts.

The two following chapters aim to illustrate how these epistemological issues and methodological perspectives are operationalized and how they can contribute to the development of concrete contemporary research projects. As we have already noted, given that most medical interventions today seek to prevent further morbidity and to improve patient functioning as well as their perceived health status, a precise, reliable, and valid, that is, objective empirical assessment of patient-reported subjective health status is warranted. Patient self-reported health measures are used (1) to monitor treatment success, (2) to predict other health outcomes, (3) to screen for health disorders, or (4) to allocate resources. There is a plethora of instruments available today that can assess a wide range of health constructs with excellent psychometric properties. For practical, economic, and scientific reasons it is generally recommended to use one of the instruments available. New research questions are however appearing, and new tools will need to be developed. Several federal institutions in the United States have issued guidance documents for the development of self-assessment instruments.

In Chapter 9, Nina Tamm, Janine Devine, and Matthias Rose provide an update on these methodological recommendations for the development of instruments today, such as the Patient-Reported Outcomes Measurement Information System (PROMIS) which is currently one the most comprehensive efforts worldwide for the development of tools for the assessment of patients' subjective health status (www.nihpromis.org).

In Chapter 10, Wilfred F. Peter, Francis Guillemin, and Caroline B. Terwee describe a novel method of interacting with respondents to better measure performances in daily life, as opposed to capacities evaluated in laboratory conditions, at the same time drawing on modern psychometric methodologies to assess the properties of an experimental design of this sort. The computerized Animated Activity Questionnaire (AAQ) was developed to assess activity limitations in hip and knee *osteoarthritis* (OA) patients. It combines the advantages of PROMs and performance-based tests, without many of their limitations.

It can be noted that in ongoing research and development, item response theory (IRT) analyses are underway to estimate the quality of the individual items in the AAQ to see how well they measure activity limitations and how appropriate they are for respondents. These analyses can also be used to examine whether the AAQ can be shortened for use in daily clinical practice and whether its items are suitable for the development of a computer adaptive test (CAT) version in the future. In a CAT version, items are administered in a sequence determined by a computer on the basis of responses to previous questions. With a CAT version, patients do not need to complete all items since its length is similarly determined by the computer as well, and the items are tailored to the patient. The field of measurement for CATs is drawing increasing attention. Another important next step is to make the AAQ ready for large-scale use in clinical practice and research. For this purpose, a web-based application is to be developed through which the AAQ can be administered in all kinds of clinical and research settings. The aim of this application is to enable the AAQ to be downloaded in a local computer or to be provided as an online service.

Overall, these conceptual, methodological, and application perspectives are the subject of a large body of research across the world and a crucial element in the current development of e-health technology. An important condition for the validity of these applications is the precision and validity of the measures. The standardization of the measurement system, the ability to compare and even equate the results of different tests, is also currently the subject of much attention.

Interpretation of perceived health data

Section 3, introduced by Dorcas Beaton in Chapter 11, addresses the difficult problem of interpretating perceived health and quality of life data. More specifically, it discusses cross-sectional and longitudinal data interpretation, using empirical studies that illustrate the implementation of data collection methods of this type in the context of clinical and public health research. Although the two types of research appear quite different, they are in fact conceptually and methodologically very close, and their apparent dissimilarity arises mainly from differences in their implementation settings and logistic constraints. In clinical research, the aim is to describe, explain, or improve a situation, a condition, or an event among "patients," namely persons affected by a clinically defined condition, mainly focusing on the consequences of the condition in question. In public health research, the task is similar, but applied to a general population or subpopulation, that is to say to persons who are presumably healthy, thus mainly focusing on the causes of a condition. The data collected, the indicators used, the design chosen, and the parameters estimated are close. This section is thus devoted to two approaches, in the general population and in a patient population, and to two methodologies: quantitative and qualitative.

In Chapter 12, Jordi Alonso et al. review the Wilson and Cleary model of quality of life in the light of empirical data exploring the pathway from chronic mental and physical conditions to perceived health through disability. International data and the use of the relevant structural modeling equations to identify the pathways of interest, provide evidence about the indirect role of disability. The implications of this resurface at the interface between clinical practice and public health: Health professionals need to address the issues of disability to increase perceived health status among individuals with chronic conditions, whereas public health stakeholders need to gain knowledge by monitoring disability and its contextual factors in the general population. Alonso et al. acknowledge that the model implemented is not complete with respect to the proposal by Wilson and Cleary, and suggest further developments to include other mediating factors such as personal, economic, social, and environmental factors and also the need to start from biological factors. The chapter echoes the preoccupations of Patrick in Section 1 and provides a two-way ticket from theory to empirical data.

In Chapter 13, Florence Jusot et al. discuss the place of perceived health indicators for monitoring the scale of health inequalities according to socioeconomic and educational levels, a major public health issue. The challenge is to know whether or not perception-based health indicators are relevant for this purpose. For certain authors, perception-based indicators are obviously less satisfactory than others because they are subject not only to greater measurement errors but also to a systematic underestimation of inequalities because of the different expectations in privileged and underprivileged populations. F. Jusot et al. explore four health indicators—reported chronic diseases, activity limitations, self-assessed health, and the SF-36 mental health score. These cover the different health dimensions collected in a French representative national survey. The authors generate a continuous health score using a factor analysis and then implement a simultaneous equation model enabling the estimation of reporting heterogeneity for the four indicators. Despite the limitations of the approach, which they clearly set out, they provide a convincing demonstration that perceived health indicators are to be preferred to reported chronic diseases.

In Chapter 14, Thierry Lang et al. address the same question and suggest that perceived health indicators tend to underestimate social inequalities and should be avoided in public health. They consider reported chronic diseases to be the objective and to provide a gold standard with which to compare perceived health indicators, and their results are in line with this. Confronting the approach proposed by Lang et al. to that proposed by Jusot et al. will be a very stimulating reflection for readers—beginners or advanced—on the difficulties of bridging the gap between research results and their utilization in public health policies. It will also offer them the opportunity to try to bring their own answers to the following questions:

- Do perceived health indicators, when available before the onset of disease, enable better assessment of the health advantages of the upper classes?
- Is the subject the most competent person to estimate his or her level of health, irrespective of social class, or should this ability be considered diminished in underprivileged populations?
- Can self-reported morbidity be viewed as "objective," or is it the result of a long selection process that begins with access to care, which itself differs according to social class?
- Because health inequalities are evidenced using classic morbidity indicators, is there any reason for using perceived health indicators within a pathological group to define health policies?

In Chapter 15, Antoine Vanier et al. review the concept of response shift, overhyped in the last 20 years in longitudinal and efficacy clinical studies using perceived health criteria. Transposed from the education sciences, its application in this context led to refinements in hypotheses on the mechanisms, to the development of strategies for collecting appropriate data (e.g., then-test), and to the development of statistical models, such as the structural models using Schmitt's technique and Oort's procedure, or longitudinal modeling analysis and latent trajectory analysis. This chapter offers a didactic approach to response shift, which can suit both casual and seasoned readers; fundamental questions are raised about the relevance of the concept and its interpretation in efficacy studies where a change in perceived health is to be explained.

In Chapter 16, Anne-Christine Rat and Jacques Pouchot pursue the interpretation of perceived health change over time and also consider the interpretation of cross-sectional data applied to the field of osteoarthritis; their interpretation is supported by empirical data. Cross-sectional data on perceived health are subject to complex problems of interpretation, and these problems are not very different from those observed with indicators that are supposed to be more objective. The advantages of generic instruments, which make it possible to compare a specific condition with other conditions in the general population and contribute to the evaluation of the burden of disease, are pointed out. The "patient-acceptable symptom state" can be useful to complete the patient's assessment of his or her state of health using his or her own frame of reference. Is the patient's point of view finally captured using these criteria? For longitudinal data interpretation, the authors call on other concepts and indicators developed in the literature, namely the concepts of "responder" and "minimum important difference." We are here at the confluence between methodological and clinical issues, resolvable neither by methodologists alone nor by clinicians alone. Lines of approach are proposed to interpret categorical changes (binary definition of a treatment responder and attempt to appraise the expected number of responders) and continuous changes (defined by a mean change assumed to reflect a common lag by all patients, which is required to reach sufficient level). A minimum important difference would be that which could be detected clinically—that is, detected by a physician during a medical interview—as being an improvement or a deterioration.

Knowledge and decision making

The purpose of Section 4 is to present and discuss the impact of perceived health and chronic diseases from the viewpoint of complementary approaches in the philosophy of welfare economics, in health psychology, and in public health. This section mainly addresses three questions: (1) how to promote welfare economics as a branch of economics that focuses on the optimal allocation of resources and how this affects social welfare; (2) how to promote the transfer of quality of life indicators and perceived health indicators into practice in various chronic diseases, such as multiple sclerosis, cancer pain, diabetes mellitus, rheumatic disorders, or hemophilia; and (3) how to favor the use of perceived health data as decision markers in health policies.

Emmanuel Picavet, in Chapter 17, *Perceived Individual Freedom and Collectively Provided Care*, raises the question of whether we should prioritize patient freedom despite the fact that this may involve health risks, follow health-care recommendations, or find a compromise between the two. In situations of loss of independence, attested by medical indicators, does care that appears adapted according to collective consensus, such as "good practice" guidelines, enable the people concerned to preserve their individual perception of freedom? The patient who is physically or intellectually affected or disabled still needs to retain his or her freedom as determined by the professional knowledge derived from good practice guidelines to decide on what is good or not good for himself or herself. This may not always be compatible with the patient's wishes. In the future, a wise strategy could be to reach an agreement on a balance between independent initiative and risk prevention.

The two following chapters are intended to illustrate how Patient-Reported Outcomes (PROs) and Patient-Reported Outcome Measures (PROMs) can be used in clinical practice and how they can help in decision making.

In Chapter 18, James Elander and Elisabeth Spitz illustrate the advantages of using PROMs in research, but they also show that PROMs can be used effectively in routine clinical practice. They illustrate this by the use of PROMs in the field of chronic pain management among people with rheumatic disorders and hemophilia. They discuss the obstacles to the use of PROMs, and also situations that promote the use of PROMs, for example, how PROMs can be used effectively at different times in chronic pain self-management programs. They present evidence about pain acceptance and pain coping and the way this influences patient-reported quality of life. The advantages of using PROMs in pain self-management programs are detailed, and the authors report an experiment on the use of a DVD enabling the patients to become actors. They make certain recommendations for the use of PROMs in clinical practice and clinical interventions.

In Chapter 19, Emmanuelle Busch and Marc Debouverie set out three examples of application of PROMs to evidence-based practice: fatigue in multiple sclerosis, cancer pain, and quality of life in diabetes. They show that PROMs can be used in clinical practice to help patients to "legitimize" their symptoms, guide the clinician in shared decision making in everyday clinical practice, and facilitate decision making for a change of treatment. They also address the issue of different approaches to the measurement of patient-reported health outcomes that need to be taken into account: generic instruments, disease-specific instruments, and situation-specific instruments.

Finally, in Chapter 20, Serge Briançon recalls the utility of PROMs, in particular, quality of life measures, in the context of chronic disease. He reports that the assessment of perceived health is very unevenly conducted and taken into account in different countries, different cultures, different care settings, and different pathologies. From 1991, when the WHO initiated the World Health Organization Quality of Life (WHOQOL) project, to 25 years later, when quality of life indicators are—albeit too rarely—used as an aid in public health decisions, the author presents the interest of policymakers in perceived health indicators, alongside the failures in the formalization of systematic assessment of perceived health indicators in the general population.

Should health appraisal become entrenched in the biomedical approach, or should it be rejuvenated through the innovative bio-psychosocial approach? What are the challenges for planning in public health?

Section 1
Concepts and models

1 Introduction

Lennart Nordenfelt

For centuries, chronic illness and disablement are the areas that have been neglected by the representatives of health care and even more by the medical scientists. As Joël Coste describes in great detail in Chapter 2, during Antiquity and the Middle Ages, there was a considerable indifference and even intolerance toward the chronically ill. For a long time, doctors consistently denied that chronic illness was a special problem. Many doctors saw chronic disease just as a long-lasting disease. Coste informs us that even as late as the 18th century, experts could dismiss the category of chronic diseases as being of no help during the first phase of a disease. This indifference is partly understandable. In the early days, the majority of the population never reached old age. The major health problems were due to acute infectious diseases, which were often fatal. Today, on the other hand, the population of elderly people is growing at a high speed. And the elderly tend to attract various chronic diseases. (In the United States, for instance, approximately half of the adult population has some chronic disease.) Partly as a consequence of this tragic fact, many people also become more or less disabled. Some of these disabilities are devastating not only for the individuals affected but also for the society as a whole.

This situation calls for a mobilization of effort, that is, directly caring effort and also intellectual effort. This is to reach a greater understanding of the phenomena of chronic illness and disability. The content of this section of the present volume provides excellent examples of the intellectual endeavor needed.

Annette Stanton and Michael Hoyt, for instance, provide a very helpful overview of the vast existing literature on the psychological consequences of chronic diseases, in particular, such consequences that are adjustments to the diseases in question. The authors present a model of psychological adjustment to chronic disease, as well as make substantial recommendations to further the research in this area. For example, they call for a deeper examination of the links between patient-reported psychosocial outcomes and chronic disease morbidities, and mortality. The authors further note that there are relatively few studies that have tested comprehensive models of adjustment in longitudinal designs. Therefore, they emphasize that there should be research on temporal trajectories and adaptive outcomes.

The other authors in this section of this volume focus, in their various ways, on conceptual issues related to chronic illness and disability: Elizabeth Badley is concerned with the classification of disabilities, Donald Patrick with the notion of perceived quality of life, and Joël Coste with the historical development of the concept of chronic disease. These authors illustrate extremely well the profound difficulty attached to the performance of conceptual analysis in the area of illness and disability. One fundamental reason for this is that the concepts of illness and disability, as well as all their subspecies, are mixtures of facts and values. When a person is ill or has a disability there is of course a certain factual state of affairs. For instance, the person cannot move his or her leg in a particular environment. But for this state of affairs to be designated an illness or a disability, it has to be evaluated in relation to a norm that has been set by society or by individual people. Often, however, the norm is not made explicit and can be invisible to an ordinary spectator. A clarifying conceptual analysis is then called for.

In a very rich review of various conceptual models of disability, including the modern International Classification of Functioning, Disability, and Health (ICF), Elizabeth Badley pays particular attention to the contextual factors concerning disability. These factors can be both environmental and personal, that is, they can exist both outside and inside the person. As Badley notes, the existing conceptual models tend to focus on such factors that act as barriers causing disablement or act as facilitators mitigating the impact of a health condition. Badley discovers, however, a further role that a contextual factor can have in relation to disability. She introduces the notion of a *scene-setter*. "These are the environmental and personal characteristics which determine the repertoires of tasks an individual might undertake, and the manner in which they are carried out, and which define available options and opportunities for societal participation" (p. 13). Personal factors that are potentially scene-setters include age, gender, and educational status, she says.

Badley's notion of a scene-setter is similar to one that I proposed in a different context and with a different mode of distinction (Nordenfelt, 1995, postscript). I distinguished between two salient different ways in which the environment can affect a person's ability to perform certain actions. The first is the clearly causal way, whereby an external factor—for instance, the presence of a certain pathogen—can cause a disease in a person and thereby indirectly restrict his or her ability. The second is the very different way whereby the environment influences this person's abilities as a *platform for action*. A physical and cultural environment (as well as, of course, personal factors) can define the range of actions performable by a particular person at a particular time. These factors, taken together, define the platform for action for this person. The relation between the scene-setter or the platform of action, on the one hand, and a person's ability or disability, on the other, is very different from the causal relation between the environment and the person, where the environment causes a disease or an impairment and as a result limits the person's range of activities. Likewise, it is different from the case where a part of the environment, for instance, air pollution, worsens the health condition of the person and indirectly limits the range of the person's activities.

I agree with Badley that the issue of contextual factors, as defined by the ICF, is in need of further investigation. An equally acute issue, which is mentioned but not developed in Badley's chapter and which has preoccupied several scholars, including Badley (2008), Whiteneck et al. (2009), Thyberg et al. (2015), and Nordenfelt (2003), concerns the major distinction between the concepts of activity and participation. In the ICF, in contradistinction to its forerunner, the International Classification of Impairments, Disabilities, and Handicaps (ICIDH), the distinction between the two categories is made at best in a half-hearted way. The categories are divided in principle, but their subcategories are referred to by identical labels. This has caused a lot of confusion in the application of the manual.

Donald Patrick, in his chapter, gives a wide overview of four conceptual approaches to defining and measuring perceived quality of life: the theories of human needs, the theories of positive well-being, the theories of capabilities, and the value approaches. He declares "The purpose of this review is to inform understanding of chronic diseases and their impact, including measurement, and to outline possible ways forward in providing sound and explicit conceptual bases for measurement" (p. 4). The last words in this quotation are crucial. Measurement of quality of life will become pointless if the basic concept of quality of life to be employed is not made explicit. Many of the instruments that have been used for the measurement of quality of life have no clear conceptual basis and can therefore give no useful information (consequently, their results can be used in comparisons between the results of different instruments). Thus, Patrick's mission, to identify various different conceptual backgrounds to the contemporary uses of the concept of quality of life, is very laudable.

Patrick very explicitly focuses on *perceived* quality of life, which he defines as a subjective evaluation of one's life in relation to the culture in which one lives one's values, goals, and concerns. Patrick thus discusses a concept of *subjective* quality of life, in contrast to possible concepts of *objective* quality of life, the most celebrated of which is Aristotle's idea of *eudaimonia* (1976). Given this premise it is noteworthy that Patrick pays so much attention to certain theories that, at least on the face of it, define a concept of objective quality of life, viz. the theories of need and capability. Needs and capabilities are certainly often acknowledged by their subjects but they need not always be. Clearly, Patrick only has in mind the cases where the subjects are aware of their needs and capabilities and subjectively evaluate their life situation as they see it. However, other theorists, with an inclination toward a notion of subjective quality of life, might instead head directly toward the person's subjective evaluation of his or her life, skipping the detour via needs and capabilities. This can be done without denying the importance of the latter concepts for other purposes (Nordenfelt, 1994).

As mentioned above, Joël Coste gives a very illuminating historical exposition of the development of chronic diseases over time—but very interestingly he also gives an exposition of the development of the *concept* of chronic disease. Coste informs us about the slow evolution of a reasonable concept of chronic disease. Mainstream doctors during the last couple of hundred years have been influenced by traditional ontological conceptions of disease and have been looking for "the germ" or, nowadays, "the particular gene" that can account for disease specificity in the area of chronic diseases. Coste emphasizes that this quest for criteria of identification is illusory. Therefore, it is rather scholars and researchers from other disciplines than medicine (e.g., psychology and sociology) who have addressed issues concerning the identification of chronic diseases in a fruitful way. These scholars point to and analyze psychological and sociological facts about chronic diseases, such as suffering and disability, thereby constructing more complex concepts of chronic *illnesses* rather than chronic *diseases*.

It is significant, and it proves Coste's point, that the four chapters forming this section, which, in their different ways, are excellent examples of high-quality contemporary research in the area of chronic illness and disability, have all been written by scholars from outside mainstream medicine.

References

Aristotle. (1976). *The Nicomachean Ethics*, transl. by J.A.K. Thomson. London: Penguin Books.

Badley, E. M. (2008). Enhancing the conceptual clarity of the activity and participation components of the International Classification of Functioning, Disability and Health. *Soc. Sci. Med.*, 66(11), 2335–2345.

Nordenfelt, L., ed. (1994). *Concepts and Measurements of Quality of Life in Healthcare.* Dordrecht, the Netherlands: Kluwer Academic Publishers.

Nordenfelt, L. (1995). *On the Nature of Health: An Action-Theoretic Approach* (2nd Revised Edition). Dordrecht, the Netherlands: Kluwer Academic Publishers.

Nordenfelt, L. (2003). Action theory, disability and ICF. *Disabil. Rehabil.*, 25(18), 1075–1079.

Thyberg, M., Arvidsson, P., Thyberg, I., and Nordenfelt, L. (2015). Simplified bipartite concepts of functioning and disability recommended for interdisciplinary use of the ICF. *Disabil. Rehabil.*, 37(19), 1783–1792.

Whiteneck, G., and Dijkers, M.P. (2009). Difficult to measure constructs: Conceptual and methodological issues concerning participation and environmental factors. *Arch. Phys. Med. Rehabil.*, 90 (11 Suppl.), S22–S35.

2 Chronic disease in medicine: Past, present, and possible future of a problematic concept

Joël Coste

The concept of chronic disease has a long and controversial history in medicine, dating back to the first century BC, and its history is punctuated by repeated and lively debates over the usefulness, consistency, and relevance of the concept for both the practice and science of medicine. As for many complicated problems, adopting a historical perspective allows both continuities and changes to be considered, revealing the dynamics of ideas and practices. By facing in both directions, like a "Janus head" (Temkin, 1977) looking forward and back, we can infer something of the future, at least the near future, of these ideas and practices. This is the approach I will adopt here: After presenting a short history of the concept of chronic disease, I will consider historical processes, continuities, and dynamics to refine and reformulate the questions about the consistency, the relevance, and finally the very usefulness of the concept of chronic disease in medicine in both the current and the near future.

A short history of the concept

Hippocratic doctors, the founders of rational medicine, recognized that certain diseases were long lasting but did not make a clear distinction between chronic and acute diseases (Jouanna, 1992). Hippocratic medicine emerged in an environment where infectious diseases were ubiquitous, and indeed malaria was very prevalent in ancient Greece (Grmek Mirko, 1983); consequently, there was considerable attention given to acute diseases, to their prognosis, to the regimen that should be applied during their course, and also to their rhythms and critical times, especially to the *kairos*, the time to judge and to act against them. This led to the development of a complex "arithmology" of good and dangerous days during the course of the disease, influenced by Pythagorean theorem. Classical Greek society was not very tolerant of the people who were ill, as reflected by Plato's opinion in the third book of *The Republic*:

> . . . to require the help of medicine, not when a wound has to be cured, or on occasion of an epidemic, but just because, by indolence and a habit of

life such as we have been describing, men fill themselves with waters and winds, as if their bodies were a marsh, compelling the ingenious sons of Asclepius to find more names for diseases, such as flatulence and catarrh; is not this, too, a disgrace?

(Plato, n.d.)

The late Hellenistic and Roman societies were probably less intolerant to the chronically ill and disabled. Indeed, the category "chronic disease" emerged and gained popularity in the first century BC; this was probably due to the diffusion of Methodism, a doctrine for which the distinction between acute and chronic was one of the three major criteria defining therapeutic indications (Nutton, 2004). This distinction was further used by Celse and also by Pneumatists including Archigenus and Aretaeus of Cappadocia. All these authors produced lists of acute diseases and lists of chronic diseases (not always agreeing with each other) but some of them clearly understood the common consequences of these diseases for the patient, the doctor, and the patient–doctor relationship. Aretaeus of Cappadocia was a physician who lived in the second century AD; the introductory chapter of his book entitled *Causes and Symptoms of Chronic Diseases* is exemplary of this understanding and is illuminating. It states:

Of chronic diseases the pain is great, the period of wasting long, and the recovery uncertain; for either they are not dispelled at all, or the diseases relapse upon any slight error; for neither have the patients resolution to persevere to the end; or, if they do persevere, they commit blunders in a prolonged regimen. And if there also be the suffering from a painful system of cure, – of thirst, of hunger, of bitter and harsh medicines, of cutting or burning, – of all which there is sometimes need in protracted diseases, the patients resile as truly preferring even death itself. Hence, indeed, is developed the talent of the medical man, his perseverance, his skill in diversifying the treatment, and conceding such pleasant things as will do no harm, and in giving encouragement. But the patient also ought to be courageous, and co-operate with the physician against the disease. For, taking a firm grasp of the body, the disease not only wastes and corrodes it quickly, but frequently disorders the senses, nay, even deranges the soul by intemperament of the body. (Aretaeus, 1856)

Despite its insights into the consequences of chronic diseases in general in terms of patient suffering and psychological distress, and of the patient–doctor relationship, Aretaeus' text was lost until it was rediscovered in the sixteenth century when it became available again to mainstream medicine. One reason for the long eclipse of the category of chronic disease in the history of medicine may be found in the hostility of Galen (AD 129–199), the most influential physician of Antiquity. Galen repeated several times that the duration of disease was irrelevant to medical practice, and especially to therapeutics; he believed that *speed*, that is, speed to the critical events, was more relevant than *duration* of disease. In the Middle Ages, almost all physicians were followers of Galen, and very few were interested in or even mentioned chronicity of diseases in their texts. Among the exceptions were the *Poem of Medicine* by Avicenna (980–1037), a relatively minor text, in which he acknowledged the existence of diseases of long duration, usually "cold" and less severe. The *Treatise on the Prognosis of Acute and Chronic Diseases* by Gentile da Faligno (d. 1348) similarly reported the cold nature of chronic diseases, and also the difficulty of "coction" of humors and consequently of "crisis" in such diseases.

Between 1675 and 1710, Thomas Sydenham (1624–1689) and Hermann Boerhaave (1668–1738) thought about chronic diseases and their ideas were brought together and rendered more coherent in the 1750s by Gerard Van Swieten (1700–1772), a disciple of Boerhaave. These conceptions of chronic diseases, which were far from forming a fully elaborated doctrine, were developed within the framework of humoral theory, and used as the Hippocratic and Galenic concepts of "crisis," "coction" of humors, and "diathesis" (disposition to disease). However, they also incorporated "modern" pathophysiological explanations based on Sydenham's iatromechanism (Sydenham, 1683) or Boerhaave's iatrochemistry (Boerhaave, 1709) and their therapeutic counterparts such as thermal waters and baths or body movement and exercise, for example, frictions and horse riding. These conceptions were paradigmatically applied to gout by Sydenham or to chronic suppurations such as phthisis by Boerhaave. These authors insisted that the patient was responsible for the development of disease ("acutos dico, qui ut plurimum habet authorem, sicut chronici ipsos nos" said Sydenham) (Sydenham, 1682), usually incriminating some error or "indulgence" (Cadogan, 1771) in the diet or regimen. Thus, they put psychological pressure on the patient to be cooperative and "observant" of the treatments, which were necessarily long and sometimes unpleasant (they also put pressure on the doctor to avoid sentimentalism). In the following decades, thinking continued to develop, with a more clinical leaning in Austria with Van Swieten and Joseph von Quarin (1733–1814), a more hygiene-based attitude in Britain with George Cheyne (1671–1743) and William Cadogan (1711–1797), and a more theoretical approach in France with two prominent physicians from the Vitalist school of medicine of Montpellier, Théophile de Bordeu (1722–1776) and Charles-Louis Dumas (1765–1813). Théophile de Bordeu was involved in the family business of spa treatments in Barèges and favored a tight link between chronic diseases and thermalism; belief in this link strengthened in the nineteenth century, illustrated by a dedicated medical literary genre boasting the merits of spa "stations" for some, or sometimes for all, chronic diseases (thermalism became increasingly popular in Europe in the nineteenth century and many medical doctors became involved).

In 1812, Charles-Louis Dumas presented the most comprehensive theory of chronic disease ever developed in a voluminous treatise of 780 pages entitled *General Doctrine of Chronic Diseases to Serve as a Foundation for the Theoretical and Practical Knowledge of These Diseases* (Dumas, 1812). Dumas viewed chronic diseases as the continuity of acute diseases and explained their duration by the slowness of the pathological process: slowness of the beginnings and slowness of the progress to crisis, delayed due to depressed vital forces, bad constitution, and passions of the soul. Dumas also thoroughly analyzed the role of what we now call "psychological factors" as predisposing or precipitating factors in the causal chains leading to disease or its flares.

However, although the category of chronic diseases reemerged into medical thinking during the eighteenth century, there remained strong opposition and resistance. In particular, the first nosologists, including Boissier de Sauvages and Pinel, criticized the category for being of no help on "day 1 of the disease" and for the absence of any natural (nonarbitrary) limit in duration to define chronicity (François Boissier de Sauvages de Lacroix, 1771). In the nineteenth century, there were many, especially in the medical élite practicing in hospitals, who defended an ontological conception of disease; they wanted to identify *species of diseases like species of flowers* on the basis of the anatomo-clinical method. Indeed, the category of chronic disease was increasingly rejected as unhelpful or even counterproductive. The return of major epidemics, such as cholera in the middle of the century, and the development of industrialism, which focused on public health concerns and efforts on acute diseases and external or environmental factors did not encourage reflection on chronic disease.

Another category that was used only briefly in medicine but persisted longer in the hospital community deserves a few words: that of "incurable." Doctors have never appreciated this heterogeneous category, which refers to their limitations, or at least, the limitations of medicine. However, hospitals for "incurables" were founded in many towns in Europe from the beginning of the sixteenth century onwards, to receive and care for poor and often old patients with inveterate diseases and disabilities, and sometimes insanity. This blanket appellation (and the segregation of patients it covered) was progressively abandoned at the end of the nineteenth and the beginning of the twentieth century and the hospitals and wards described in this way metamorphosed into long-stay units or geriatric hospitals.

Despite being promoted by Ernst Philip Boas (1891–1955), who experimented with Montefiore in the Bronx in the twenties, "hospitals for chronic diseases" did not really succeed and did not spread, even in the United States; this was despite the well-thought-out organization, including medical care and nursing as well as social services, entertainment, and welfare, and occupational therapy facilities. The model of the sanatorium for tuberculosis patients, upon which Boas drew his inspiration to design his hospital for chronic diseases, was probably too unattractive and soon became obsolete when tuberculosis could be cured with antibiotics after the World War II.

In the fifties, pathocenosis was changing, with infectious diseases, including chronic diseases such as tuberculosis and syphilis, declining even faster, and the continuous increase of cardiovascular diseases and cancers, especially those due to smoking. These trends prompted reflections on public health policies to tackle the newly epidemic chronic diseases (Coste, 2014). In the United States, a

Commission on Chronic Illness was assembled between 1950 and 1956 to "help define, identify and classify the problem of chronic illness" (The Commission on Chronic Illness, 1956). This commission also provided one of the first of a long series of definitions of chronic illness or chronic disease as comprising "all impairments or deviations from normal which have one or more of the following characteristics: are permanent, leave residual disability, are caused by nonreversible pathological alterations, require special training of the patient for rehabilitation, may be expected to require a long period of supervision or care." A new medical journal, the *Journal of Chronic Diseases*, was also launched in 1955 with the aim of publishing research on chronic illness, but rather "in its beginnings than in its endings" (Moore and Seegal, 1955) to quote Joseph Earle and David Seegal, the first editors of the journal. This statement was indeed programmatic and anticipated somewhat the change of the name of the journal in 1988 to *Journal of Clinical Epidemiology*. The foundation of the *Journal of Chronic Diseases* was contemporary to the development of "modern epidemiology," or "epidemiology of risk factors" as some English-speaking authors called it. Early landmark studies of this type were those conducted by Doll and Hill on lung cancer and that of Framingham on cardiovascular diseases. Modern epidemiology focused on individual risk factors and especially on behaviors and often led to public health recommendations of astonishing similarity to those of the hygienist physicians of eighteenth century Britain (particularly "healthy diet" and physical exercise).

"Endings" of chronic diseases, and the consequences of these diseases on the daily life of the subjects, were more slowly and belatedly addressed, and this was done mainly by scholars and researchers in disciplines other than medicine (e.g., sociology, psychology, and economy). This quickly led to the creation of subdisciplines, including health sociology, health psychology, and health economy, addressing health problems, and especially chronic diseases and their manifold consequences. The American psychiatrist George L. Engel (1913–1999) developed a biopsychosocial model in 1977 and it was subsequently endorsed by the World Health Organization through the conceptual framework of the International Classification of Functioning, Disability, and Health (ICF) in 2001. This has certainly facilitated multidisciplinary and interdisciplinary research on chronic diseases and the involvement in such research of mainstream medical doctors and clinicians. However, the so-called mainstream doctors and clinicians remained, and still predominantly remain, influenced by ontological conceptions of disease, with "the gene" replacing "the germ" in the often illusory quest for disease specificity. These doctors have been reluctant to consider nonphysical aspects of illness and they also tend to resist sharing authority over care. However, some important research has been devoted to understanding the psychological effects of, and psychological adjustment to, chronic disease, and to disentangling the cognitive processes involved. Lazarus and Folkman's stress and coping theory (1984) was the foundation for much of the research at the end of the twentieth and the beginning of the twenty-first century into disease-related adjustment. Many important empirical studies, also in this period, addressed the role of social factors, both those supporting and those impeding adjustment to chronic disease. In parallel with these psychological and social studies, much thought was given to the issue of patient "self-management" or "collaborative management" of chronic disease, in which the patient himself or herself or their family is considered to be the primary care giver. Several teams, mainly from the US West Coast, including those of Halsted R. Holman (b. 1925) and Kate R. Lorig (b. 1942) in Palo Alto and of Michael Von Korff in Seattle, defined principles of self-management of chronic illness and carried out pioneering experiments in this area with promising results. Somewhat surprisingly, twentieth-century philosophers have largely stayed away from questions and debate about chronic diseases. Fashionable philosophers and writers such as Illich and Foucault criticized at length "medical power" and its various forms but paid no attention either to people or to people's suffering. Nevertheless, some authors influenced by phenomenology such as Georges Lantéri-Laura (1930–2004) and S. Kay Toombs provided useful contributions to understanding patients' perceptions, and Lennart Nordenfelt (b. 1945) addressed chronic illness in the context of quality of life within the analytic tradition of philosophy (1995). In particular, Nordenfelt offered a conceptual framework and an illuminating systematization of the different sorts of suffering (direct and indirect) in chronic disease that is of immediate use to care givers.

In this short overview of the history of the concept of chronic disease, I have tried to highlight continuities and changes in ideas and practices relevant to chronic disease in medicine over a long period of time. We can identify three groups of continuities and even stubborn continuities. First, the consequences of chronic diseases on the daily life of the patients, involving prolonged periods of suffering and disability. Second, the difficulties of managing chronic suffering by the physicians or care givers, and third, the frustrating patient–doctor relationships. Not one word of Aretaeus' text, quoted above, dealing with these aspects twenty centuries ago needs be changed. However, in addition to continuities, there have also been many changes, particularly during the last 50 years. Above all, chronic diseases are making a massively larger contribution to the overall burden of disease on the population, especially in Western countries where the demographic phenomenon of aging has sharply increased this trend. Medical thinking about chronic disease was underdeveloped for a very long time and further atrophied during the quest for specificity of diseases in the nineteenth and twentieth centuries. Consequently, the intellectual framework was clearly unprepared for the current challenge, which became more and more demanding as health systems remained mainly hospital centered and adapted to acute ailments. Other important trends include the new social demands for health (healthism) (Greenhalgh and Wessely, 2004) and health care, and for shared health management. Despite the large diversity between countries, this has led to supplementary pressure on clinical medicine and its practitioners dealing with chronic diseases. Discarding the possible (and in no way unrealistic) scenario of a new pathocenosis change with the reemergence of infectious diseases and violence, the Janus face looking forward may observe these trends continuing over the coming decades, by virtue of their own momentum. In view of these likely trends, it would be useful to refine and reformulate several currently asked questions regarding consistency, relevance, and usefulness for medicine of the category of chronic disease.

Refining and reformulating questions about consistency, relevance, and usefulness for medicine of the chronic disease category

Consistency

An important, more lasting question is whether one should consider and speak of a patient as having *a chronic disease* or as having *one of a host of chronic diseases* sharing common long-lasting processes. The still variable and unstable definitions recently given to chronic diseases attest to the pertinence of this question (Table 2.1) (Goodman et al., 2013). Reasoning in terms of lists of chronic diseases clearly appears to be medically archaic, but the generic and specific components of suffering and the consequences of chronic diseases remain to be determined for even the most common chronic diseases. Comparative empirical research into the consequences of these diseases is

Table 2.1 Sample of twenty-first century definitions of chronic disease, illness, or condition

Hwang et al. (2001)	We define a person as having a chronic condition if that person's condition has lasted or was expected to last 12 or more months and resulted in functional limitations and/or the need for ongoing medical care.
Bernstein et al. (2003)	A chronic disease or condition has one or more of the following characteristics: it is permanent; it leaves residual disability; it is caused by nonreversible pathological alteration; it requires special training of the patient for rehabilitation; or it may be expected to require a long period of supervision, observation, or care.
Warshaw (2006)	Chronic illnesses are "conditions that last a year or more and require ongoing medical attention and/or limit activities of daily living."
Friedman et al. (2008–2009)	A chronic condition is defined as a condition that lasts 12 months or longer and meets one or both of the following tests: (1) it places limitations on self-care, independent living, or social interactions; and (2) it results in the need for ongoing intervention with medical products, services, or special equipment.

(Continued)

Table 2.1 (Continued) Sample of twenty-first century definitions of chronic disease, illness, or condition

Anderson (2010)	A chronic condition is a general term that includes chronic illnesses and impairments. It includes conditions that are expected to last a year or longer, limit what one can do, and/or may require ongoing medical care. Serious chronic conditions are a subset of chronic conditions that require ongoing medical care and limit what a person can do.
US Department of Health and Human Services (HHS) (2010)	Chronic illnesses are "conditions that last a year or more and require ongoing medical attention and/or limit activities of daily living."
McKenna and Collins (2010)	They are generally characterized by uncertain etiology, multiple risk factors, a long latency period, a prolonged course of illness, noncontagious origin, functional impairment or disability, and incurability.
US Department of Health and Human Services (2011)	A health condition is a departure from a state of physical or mental well-being. In the National Health Interview Survey, each condition reported as a cause of an individual's activity limitation has been classified as chronic, not chronic, or unknown if chronic, based on the nature and duration of the condition. Conditions that are not cured once acquired (such as heart disease, diabetes, and birth defects in the original response categories, and amputee and old age in the ad hoc categories) are considered chronic, whereas conditions related to pregnancy are not considered chronic. Other conditions must have been present for 3 months or longer to be considered chronic. An exception is made for children aged less than 1 year who have had a condition since birth: such conditions are always considered chronic.
World Health Organization (2011)	Chronic diseases are diseases of long duration and generally slow progression.
Florida Department of Health (2011)	Chronic diseases have a long course of illness. They rarely resolve spontaneously, and they are generally not cured by medication or prevented by vaccine.

Source: Adapted from Goodman et al., *Prev. Chronic. Dis.*, 10, 120239, 2013.

therefore needed. The way to consider mental disorders also needs to be discussed, as most of them are chronic and still ill-defined, usually as syndromes in which expressions of suffering are common and poorly specific. Comparative research within the framework of the biopsychosocial model is needed to clarify this issue. In the meantime, it is probably best to define chronic diseases as simply and objectively as possible, that is, only in terms of duration. I agree with Perrin et al. (1993) and like them to suggest a disease be considered chronic if it has lasted or is expected to last more than 3 months, according to the best knowledge of the prognosis of the disease.

Relevance of chronicity relative to competing concepts

The concept of chronicity is now clearly distinguishable from those of irreversibility, incurability, disease activity, disability, and handicap. However, its relevance relative to these "competing" concepts appears to depend heavily on the issue investigated and the focus of attention, for example, the pathological process, the type of suffering, or the consequences for life. The issue of "temporality" of disease deserves further attention as far as the life of a patient with chronic disease is concerned; this should be addressed less simplistically than in terms of duration or "chronology" with time being only one-dimensional and linear. Although medicine should certainly not refer in any way to nonlinear time, as Hippocratic doctors did, the pertinent measures of time have not been defined. Indeed, measures are required to assess empirically "perceived" or "lived" time, which has been suggested to be relevant in chronic diseases (Kay Toombs, 1990). Once again, substantial further empirical research appears to be desirable to evaluate the complex dynamics and interactions of time and disease, their *consequences* for patients, and the *adaptations* of patients to both. Such research might involve many different chronic diseases and cultural contexts and needs to be carefully designed to disentangle the effects of time from those of irreversibility, incurability, disease activity, and disability.

Usefulness of the category of chronic disease for medicine

Finally, the usefulness of knowing, saying, or predicting that a disease is or will be long lasting or chronic should be considered. It is first necessary to consider medicine as a science and as a practice; within the science of medicine, we can distinguish pathology, nosology, clinical research, and health services research. For pathology and nosology, which are, respectively, the science of diseases (including etiology and physiopathology) and the science of their classification, the "chronic" category clearly appears to be insufficient. It should only be considered as provisional and palliative, as were, for example, "chronic gastric ulcer" or "chronic polyarthritis" until they were dismembered or reclassified. The "black box" nature of the "chronic" category, for example in "chronic low back pain" or "chronic fatigue," is a weakness. Indeed, it may even impede biological and epidemiological research into causes and mechanisms, as patients of different subtypes are likely to be brought together into a single but heterogeneous group. For clinical research on diagnosis, prognosis, therapeutics, and rehabilitation, the category may be temporarily useful: it may facilitate investigation of long-term evolution of direct and indirect components of suffering, disability, and social consequences of chronic ailments. The identification and possibly the quantification of generic and specific parts of the components of suffering in most common chronic diseases would be especially useful for therapeutics and rehabilitation. The same may be said for health services research, which should not be limited to cost evaluations, how to make savings and management of flows of patients across health services; it should extend to the responses to patients' suffering. In clinical practice, the category "chronic" may also be useful to indicate the need for care givers to evaluate and appropriately respond to the various forms of suffering, ideally involving a multidisciplinary team. Similarly, it signals the need for both good relationships between patients and care givers and awareness of ethical issues associated with care of patients having chronic ailments, allowing to discard long lasting and unsupported representations of these patients as being feeble or predisposed to disease.

References

Anderson, G. (2010). *Chronic Care: Making the Case for Ongoing Care.* Princeton, NJ: Robert Wood Johnson Foundation.

Aretaeus. (1856). *The Extant Works of Aretaeus, the Cappadocian* (ed. & Transl. Francis Adams). London: Sydenham Society.

Bernstein, A.B., Hing, E., Moss, A.J., Allen, K.F., Siller, A.B., and Tiggle, R.B. (2003). *Health Care in America: Trends in Utilization.* Hyattsville, MD: National Center for Health Statistics.

Boerhaave, H (1709). *Aphorismi De Cognoscendis Et Curandis Morbis.* Leyden: Van der Linden.

Cadogan, W. (1771). *A Dissertation on the Gout, and All Chronic Diseases, Jointly Considered.* London: Dodsley.

Coste, J. (2014). Les maladies dominantes au XXe siècle. In: D.B. Fantini, L. Lambrichs (eds.), *Histoire De La Pensée Médicale Contemporaine, Tome 4* (pp. 259–278). Paris: Le Seuil.

Dumas, C.-L. (1812). *Doctrine Générale Des Maladies Chroniques, Pour Servir De Fondement à La Connaissance Théorique Et Pratique De Ces Maladies.* Paris: Méquignon-Marvis.

Florida Department of Health. (2011). Chronic disease definition. Available at: http://www.doh.state.fl.us/family/chronicdisease/

François Boissier de Sauvages de Lacroix. (1771). *Nosologie Méthodique, Dans Laquelle Les Maladies Sont Rangées Par Classes, Suivant Le Système De Sydenham, & L'ordre Des Botanistes, Tome Premier* (par. 48), Paris: Hérissant.

Friedman, B., Jiang, H.J., and Elixhauser, A. (2008–2009). Costly hospital readmissions and complex chronic illness. *Inquiry, 45*(4), 408–421.

Goodman, R.A., Posner, S.F., Huang, E.S., Parekh, A.K., and Koh, H.K. (2013). Defining and measuring chronic conditions: Imperatives for research, policy, program, and practice. *Prev. Chronic. Dis., 10*, 120239.

Greenhalgh, T., and Wessely, S. (2004). 'Health for me': A sociocultural analysis of healthism in the middle classes. *Br. Med. Bull., 69*, 197–213.

Grmek Mirko, D. (1983). *Les Maladies à l'Aube de la Civilisation Occidentale.* Paris: Payot.

Hwang, W., Weller, W., Ireys, H., and Anderson, G. (2001). Out-of-pocket medical spending for care of chronic conditions. *Health Aff. (Millwood), 20*(6), 267–278.

Jouanna, J. (1992). *Hippocrates* (p. 220). Paris: Fayard.

Kay Toombs, S. (1990). The temporality of illness: Four levels of experience. *Theor. Med., 11*, 227–241.

McKenna, M., and Collins, J. (2010). Current issues and challenges in chronic disease control. In: P.L. Remington, R.C. Brownson, and M.V. Wegner (eds.), *Chronic Disease Epidemiology and Control* (2nd Edition, pp. 1–24). Washington, DC: American Public Health Association.

Moore, J. E., and Seegal, D (1955). Announcement. *J Chronic Dis., 1*, 1–7. 1955.

Nutton, V. (2004). *Ancient Medicine.* London: Routledge.

Perrin, E.C., Newacheck, P., Pless, I.B., Drotar, D., Gortmaker, S.L., Leventhal, J., et al. (1993). Issues involved in the definition and classification of chronic health conditions. *Pediatrics, 91,* 787–793.

Plato (n.d.), *Republic, Book III* (pp. 405–406).

Sydenham, T. (1682). *Dissertatio Epistolaris.* London: Kettilby.

Sydenham, T. (1683). *Tractatus De Podagra Et Hydrope.* London: Kettilby.

Temkin, O. (1977). *The Double Face of Janus and Other Essays in the History* (pp. 3–37). Baltimore, MD: The Johns Hopkins University Press.

The Commission of Chronic Illness. (1956). *Public Health Reports, 71,* 678.

US Department of Health and Human Services. (2010). *Multiple Chronic Conditions—A Strategic Framework: Optimum Health and Quality of Life for Individuals with Multiple Chronic Conditions.* Washington, DC: US Department of Health and Human Services. Available at: http://www.hhs.gov/ash/initiatives/mcc/mcc_framework.pdf (accessed on 21 February 2013).

US Department of Health and Human Services. (2011). *Health, United States, 2010: With Special Feature on Death and Dying* (pp. 486–487). Hyattsville, MD: Centers for Disease Control and Prevention, National Center for Health Statistics. Appendix, definition of "condition."

Warshaw, G. (2006). Introduction: Advances and challenges in care of older people with chronic illness. *Generations, 30*(3), 5–10.

World Health Organization. (2011). Chronic diseases. Available at: http://www.who.int/topics/chronic_diseases/en/.

3 Conceptual approaches to perceived quality of life

Donald L. Patrick

Introduction

Several decades ago, my colleague Dick Joyce, in response to my question, "what is quality of life?" answered, "it is what the person says it is" (Joyce CRB, personal communication). Both my question and Dick's answer illustrate the essential challenge in defining and measuring the perceived quality of life (QoL). It is simple in conception but difficult in operationalization. The perception of QoL can be an attribute of the individual, an attitude, a personality trait, a situational response, a feeling state, and/or a rational judgment (Bullinger, 1999). The challenge in defining the perceived QoL is related to the duality notions of Aristotle (Nagel, 1961), and more recently to the notions of neo-Kantian philosopher Wilhem Windelband (Windelband and Oakes, 1980) who described the tension between two forms of explanation in the social sciences—nomothetic and idiographic. In the nomothetic, we are striving for generalization and objective phenomena, such as those of the natural sciences, whereas in the idiographic we seek knowledge of unique, subjective phenomena. These two kinds of explanations embody major differences in scientific logic, research methods, and further understanding of the notion of QoL as a perception.

Adding further complexity to this tension is the extent to which the perceived QoL is viewed from within the context of health and health care. Often this context is assumed, particularly from authors focusing on health aspects. Subjective QoL, however, can be viewed as encompassing freedom, respect, income security, happiness, or other important values and life aspects, in addition to health. When disease and illness occur, often a person changes his or her mind. Aristotle recognized this in defining happiness in the *Nichomachean Ethics*: "When it comes to saying in what happiness consists, opinions differ, and the account given by the generality of mankind is not at all like that of the wise. The former take it to be something obvious and familiar, like pleasure or money or eminence, and there are various other views, and often the same person actually changes his opinion. When he falls ill, he says that it is his health, and when he is hard up he says that it is money" (Aristotle, 1976). Indeed, how people view QoL during dying and death in contemporary American culture is inextricably connected to health, as health and health care are prominent foci (Patrick et al., 2003; Stewart et al., 1999).

This chapter reviews conceptual approaches to the perceived QoL. Because it is near impossible to separate out where health and nonhealth aspects begin and end, and the duality of the nomothetic and idiographic is forbidding, this chapter reviews both approaches and blurs the distinction between health and nonhealth. The distinction between objective circumstances and perception of these circumstances is also occasionally blurred, because some approaches incorporate both. The purpose of this review is to inform the understanding of chronic diseases and their impact, including measurement, and to outline possible ways forward in providing sound and explicit conceptual bases for measurement.

The nature of measurement

All measurements include assumptions about the nature and value of the constructs used in the measurement process; yet the role of theory in developing and interpreting QoL measures is often neglected. Theory, in fact, guides implicitly or explicitly the selection of content, the measurement process, and the interpretation of results. Even though developers and users may not identify a particular theory or set of theories in selecting the concepts and domains to be included in the measurement, the measures themselves reflect the investigator's ideology and values as well as the culture of the society in which he or she lives.

The measurement operations used to assign numbers to concepts and domains of QoL also reflect theoretical assumptions. Measurement theories differ on how the nature of the phenomena under investigation is perceived and on how numbers are assigned to constructs using specific rules. Because of these theoretical differences in conceptualization and measurement, different measurement strategies and instruments may yield different data and conclusions, thereby sending patients and providers as well as analysts and decision makers down different paths.

Two major problems arise with the supposedly "atheoretical" use of measures in collecting and analyzing health status and quality of data. First, unless the investigator considers the possible determinants of the perceived QoL, it is difficult to interpret results. This is particularly true in nonrandom research designs. Many cultural, political, and social processes influence the meaning and measurement of QoL. The analyst must consider these influences to understand how respondents react to QoL questions and to analyze data in a manner consistent with measurement assumptions and the particular study design.

The second difficulty arises in interpreting relationships among different objective circumstances or measures of health status and the perceived QoL concepts. Descriptors, such as income, housing, marital status, and clinical indicators, such as blood pressure or psychiatric diagnosis, may be associated with physical, psychological, or social functioning, which in turn may be associated with satisfaction with health. When the concepts are contained in a theory of biological, psychological, and social processes that specifies the system of relationships connecting the concepts, the investigator can analyze the change in one measure as related to change in another measure (Wilson and Cleary, 1995). For example, when blood pressure changes or walking improves, what is observed in perceptions? Or at a more social level, when access to health care improves, what changes in the perceived QoL are seen or can be expected?

Overview of conceptual approaches

Theoretical relationships among disease, its indicators, and functional status are sometimes possible to specify; however, relationships among measures of function and feelings of positive well-being are often difficult to predict with any precision. For example, emotional well-being might well improve with advancing age or diagnosis of a life-threatening illness may improve reports of QoL. A variety of theories or conceptual approaches have been invoked to help define and specify the perceived QoL and its determinants, although no single grand theoretical approach has emerged.

Four major conceptual approaches are reviewed here: (1) theories of human need, (2) theories of positive well-being or happiness, (3) value-based approaches, and (4) Sen's capability approach. The last one, based on Amartya Sen's thinking, is often not included as a measure of perception, though there are aspects that are clearly subjective. These conceptualizations have influenced how we approach defining, measuring, and using the perceived QoL. They derive from anthropology, economics, philosophy, psychology, sociology, and related fields. Classical psychometric theory, modern test theory, utility theory, and psychophysics are the underpinnings for the assignment of numbers of different measurement theories. Again, no single theory appears sufficient to encompass the myriad concepts or operations involved in defining and measuring the perceived QoL.

Theories of human need

The concept of "need" has been used by many analysts, most notably Abraham Maslow (1943), to denote a drive or some inner state. Maslow outlined five needs, organized in a pyramid or hierarchy of "prepotency"—physiological needs, safety needs, belongingness and love needs, esteem needs, and the need for self-actualization (Maslow, 1943). The theory proposes that one's needs at base, for example, food and water or physiological needs, must be satisfied before safety needs become prominent. In turn, the need for belongingness and love is a necessary building block for self-esteem. At the top is a "self-actualized" person or in Maslow's terms, "what a man can be, he must be." Maslow had a different purpose for delineating these levels of need, nonetheless the concept has influenced thinkers and researchers for many decades, because of its centrality to the QoL concept.

Needs can be seen as goals that are universal and it is here that theories of human need have influenced item generation in health status and QoL questionnaires. The goals of individuals have been captured in the items in questionnaires. Once the fundamental needs of different populations have been identified, measurement becomes a process of determining the extent to which these needs have been satisfied. Most life satisfaction measures are derived, knowingly or unknowingly, from these origins according to needs-based theory.

Needs-based models of QoL have been used in assessing the QoL of persons with chronic health conditions or disabilities. Many persons with disabilities, lasting a lifetime or with onset later in life, have little room for improvement in some aspects of functional status, such as ambulation, mobility, or physical function in general. Performance of activities, that is, actual behavior or capacity to behave, is therefore constrained in comparison with persons without these limitations. The perceived QoL, however, is another matter when viewed as people's "perceptions of their position in life in the context of their particular culture and value systems and in relation to their personal goals, expectations, standards, and concerns" (WHOQOL Group, 1993). The perceived QoL can only be known to the individuals concerned and reflects an evaluation of circumstances both intrinsic and extrinsic.

QoL for people with disabilities is an outcome that reflects the influence and interaction of environmental factors, the life course of an individual or group, the disabling process, and opportunity (Patrick, 1997). All aspects of the total environment may influence these perceptions, along with the values and preferences, the impacts of the disabling process, and the level of opportunity afforded the individual.

Measures have been developed based on the theoretical orientation of human needs. Hunt and McKenna (1992) championed this approach using their needs-based model in developing a measure of depression (Hunt and McKenna, 1992). The needs-based model has been used to develop other disease-specific measures, including those for irritable bowel syndrome and urinary incontinence, and for developing a measure of the perceived QoL for adolescent self-report (Edwards et al., 2002; Patrick et al., 1998; Patrick et al., 1999). The perceived quality of life (PQoL) scale was developed by Patrick et al. (1988) to evaluate outcomes of intensive care treatment. This measure was based on the concept of "critical need satisfaction" as a core concept reflecting subjective evaluation of QoL. Items were generated using theories of human need in addition to in-depth interviews with different populations of older adults, well persons, and persons with *disabilities*. Cognitive debriefing of persons with varying levels of functional status who completed the instrument led to additional items on satisfaction with functional status (Patrick, 2014).

The World Health Organization Quality of Life (WHOQOL) Group also defined QoL based on a concept highly related to need satisfaction (WHOQOL Group, 1993, 1995). The WHOQOL group defined QoL as an individual's perception of their position in life in the context of the culture and value systems in which they live, and in relation to their goals, expectations, standards, and concerns. The language of goals and standards is need based. The WHO Group went on, however, to relate the definition to the person's physical health, psychological state, level of independence, social relationships, and their relationship to salient features of their environment. This is where the distinction between health and nonhealth is blurred, but the idea was definitely related to the disease, as the original conception of the WHOQOL in the Mental Health Division of WHO was as an extension of the International Classification of Disease 1, International Classification of Impairments, Disabilities, and Handicaps (Norman Satorius, personal communication).

Theories of positive well-being and happiness

A large number of theorists and investigators, primarily from psychology, have attempted to define positive health and QoL, often viewed as concepts and domains located on the upper end of the health–illness continuum. Many of these attempts have been in the mental health field, because mental or psychological well-being constructs are central to our notions of positive health (Jahoda, 1958). Models of psychological well-being guide the assessment of QoL by exploring subjective reactions to life experiences (Diener, 1984). These models are numerous, ranging from personality-type theories, social learning theory, and theories of personal control to theories of specific subjective phenomena such as happiness, elation, or optimism.

Zautra and Goodhart (1979) reviewed four psychological models that have contributed concepts to health status and QoL: (1) the epidemiologic model of stressful life events, (2) the crisis-management model of coping, (3) the competency model emphasizing self-mastery, and (4) the adaptation-level model (Zautra and Goodhart, 1979). Together these four models suggest two sets of human needs, similar to the needs-based conceptual approaches: (1) to avoid and/or adjust to painful life experiences and (2) to develop and sustain life satisfaction by increasing competence, skills, and mastery over the environment. QoL is viewed as enhanced to the degree that both adjustment and competence needs are fulfilled. Thus a person *with* a chronic disease or impairment *might* have a high QoL, avoiding depression and mastering independence or use of personal assistance, and a person without disease or impairment might have a low QoL, being depressed and dissatisfied with his or her situation.

The linkage of personality types and emotional reactions to health and illness derives from the Greek notions of the four humors within the body. These humors correspond to physical states. Freud and Fromm made major contributions to this theory with the concepts of neurosis and egoreceptive states. Alexander (1950), another psychoanalytic therapist, was influential in trying to link physical symptoms with constellations of personality traits (e.g., asthma with repression and peptic ulcers with oral dependency needs).

He failed to support this link because symptom patterns and a specific disease could not be matched with a specific personality type, because there were many individuals with a particular disease who had a personality type that did not match. Strickland (1984) notes that the assumed relationships between emotional states and physical health or disease have not been clearly demonstrated. Furthermore, other concepts and ideas, including physical, psychological, and social paradigms, are necessary to explain individual reactions and their concomitants.

Another conceptual focus for positive health research centers on concepts of the self: the unique attitudes and cognitive characteristics of individuals. Numerous attempts have been made to define and measure self-esteem (Pyszczynski et al., 2004; Rosenberg, 1979). However, there is little consensus on a definition of self-esteem, and the measurement techniques often do not yield comparable findings. Another more promising direction of investigation concerns self-efficacy, the perception of oneself as effective and competent (Bandura, 1982). Although self-efficacy usually refers to behaviors and not health states, Kobasa (1979) put this concept into an existential framework by describing characteristics of commitment, control, and response to challenge. In her study of middle-management executives under high stress, Kobasa found that the executives who did not fall ill had a strong sense of values, goals, and capabilities—a hardiness that functioned as a resistance-to-illness resource in the event of stress. This focus on hardiness has extended to this day in different measures used widely in clinical psychology research.

Theories of happiness or subjective well-being have existed since the ancient Greeks. Diener and colleagues review telic, activity, top-down and bottom-up, associationistic, and judgment theories of happiness, all of which link happiness to different levels of human experience (Diener, 1984, 1994; Diener and Biswas-Diener, 2008; Diener and Diener, 1996; Diener and Seligman, 2002). Maslow's telic or end-point theory related the states of well-being to environmental or ecological systems. In this theory, subjective well-being results when individuals fulfill the needs at their particular levels such as physiological needs, safety needs, love needs, esteem needs, and self-actualization needs (Maslow, 1943). Even though need theory is often cited in relation to QoL research, little empirical evidence exists linking the constructs derived from this theory to health and QoL.

Andrews and Withey (1974) invoked a top-down or personality-based approach to happiness; they amass data to suggest that the accumulation of positive experiences (from the bottom up) does not necessarily predict global life satisfaction (Andrews and Withey, 1974). Other psychological theories of subjective well-being have seldom been used in developing health status and QoL indicators, although judgment-based theory bears a striking relationship to the utility theory reviewed below. Psychological theories of subjective well-being differ substantially in their treatment of happiness or QoL as a personality trait versus a psychological state and in the different constructs employed. Constructs of happiness have been neither rigorously defined nor subjected to a hypothetico-deductive process where theory and data interplay in repeated studies.

Adaptation theory stresses the satisfaction derived from experiences and people (Diener et al., 2006). Satisfaction is a pivotal concept in QoL. Although wide agreement exists about the major categories of fundamental life needs, satisfaction is experienced only by the person with that need. Nevertheless, the concepts of satisfaction are often involved in normative measures of health status and QoL. Along the lines of Maslow's theories, important needs include material, physical, psychological, social, and spiritual well-being as well as a sense of satisfaction with one's opportunity for access to the total environment, education and training, and employment. Little is known about the relationship of need satisfaction to other health status and QoL outcomes. In some populations, functional status correlates only moderately with satisfaction with health or the perceived QoL (Patrick et al., 2000). This lack of correlation suggests that satisfaction must be considered separately from behaviors often contained in functional status measures.

Sen's capability approach

The capability approach is defined by its focus upon the moral significance of individuals' capability of achieving the kind of lives they have reason to value. This distinguishes it from more established approaches to ethical evaluation, such as utilitarianism or resourcism, which focus exclusively on subjective well-being or the availability of means to the good life, respectively. A person's capability to live a good life is defined in terms of the set of valuable "beings and doings" such as being in good health or having loving relationships with others to which they have real access. The capability approach was first articulated by the Indian economist and philosopher Amartya Sen in the 1980s and remains most closely associated with him (Nussbaum and Sen, 1993). It has been employed extensively in the context of human development, for example, by the United Nations Development Programme, as a broader, deeper alternative to narrowly economic metrics such as growth in gross domestic product (GDP) per capita. Here "poverty" is understood as deprivation of the capability to live a good life, and the "development" is understood as capability expansion. Whether or not people take up the options they have, the fact that they do have valuable options is significant and is the perceptual content in the capability approach. For example, even if the nutritional state of people who are fasting and starving is the same, the fact that fasting is a choice not to eat should be recognized. The choice is defined by both the function and the perception of freedom.

Sen's capability approach has criticized the form of utilitarianism behind welfare economics and rejects each of its three pillars: (1) act consequentialism, (2) welfarism, and (3) sum-ranking. How people *feel* about their lives, psychological states, are central and not reflective valuations. The capability approach in principle allows a very wide range of dimensions of advantage to be positively evaluated ("what capabilities does this person have?"). This allows an open diagnostic approach to what is going well or badly in people's lives that can be used to reveal unexpected shortfalls or successes in different dimensions, without aggregating them all together into one number.

Sen (1985) has identified the features, scope, advantages, and considerations of the capability approach in relation to measures of QoL. Sharing much in common with many other philosophers, the capability approach argues that the QoL should be conceived and measured directly in terms of functionings and capabilities instead of resources or utility. The central feature of well-being is the ability to achieve valuable functionings. The need for identification and valuation of the important functionings cannot be avoided by looking at something else, such as happiness, desire fulfillment, opulence, or command over primary goods. *Functionings* are beings and doings that people value and have reason to value such as being safe, well-nourished and literate, or quite complex such as expressing oneself in a painting, exquisitely. Note that by definition functionings are valuable both objectively and to the person. The capability approach recognizes genuinely distinct, plural and incommensurable kinds of human achievements. They are incommensurable in the sense that no permanent priority or relative weight can be associated with them. The weights QoL measures applied to different functionings are, therefore, value judgements that reflect the relative *importance* of each functioning.

Capability refers to "the various combinations of functionings (beings and doings) that the person can achieve." Capability is, thus, a set of vectors (or *n*-tuples) of functionings, reflecting the person's freedom to lead one type of life or another... to choose from possible livings. Each of our capability set represents "the *real opportunity* that we have to accomplish what we value" (Sen, 1992). Capability thus captures not only achievements but also unchosen alternatives; it scans the horizon to notice roads not taken. It checks "whether one person did have the opportunity." Thus, capability is a particularly rich kind of opportunity freedom, and functionings are a wide and flexible category.

The proposal is that QoL should be considered in the space of capability and functionings. Most measurements reflect achieved functionings rather than capabilities, as opportunity is notoriously difficult to measure outside of perceptions of the individual. Information on capabilities may be obtained directly from household surveys, for example, in questions such as "do you have/do x"—if you do not is that because you do not want x or because you are not able to obtain/do x?

Operationalization of the capability approach is inherently difficult without consensus on the functionings (nomothetic approach) or individual identification (idiographic). The notion of opportunity has been central to QoL thinking for many decades (Patrick and Erickson, 1993). Opportunity is a core concept for people with disabilities and has been defined as the end result of health promotion for this important population group (Patrick, 1997). Although actual measures may be difficult to construct based on Sen's theory, the concepts of capability and functioning will continue to influence philosophers and research-ers alike when considering definitions and measurement.

Value approaches and utility theory

Values, and specifically preferences for health, play a central role in definitions and measurement of the perceived QoL. Health, itself, is a value in relation to other primary aspects of life. What is important to people has been used broadly in creating measures of PQOL. Value terminology and preference measurement have become prevalent in a broad range of social and behavioral sciences. In economics, efforts to develop measures of utility go back to the eighteenth cen-tury, as in "indifference curve" analysis, and to define various types of value, such as value-in-use and value-in-exchange. Anthropologists developed the concept of values within the context of dominant cultural patterns. Finally, psychologists have explored value concepts in relation to attitudes, beliefs, opinions, and decision making.

There are considerable confusion and controversy surrounding the pre-cise placement of values in the sociopsychological domain of attitudes, needs, beliefs, cognitive orientations, lifestyles, norms, motives, sentiments, and pref-erences. The measurement of health-state preferences follows in the tradition of treating *values* as standards of the desirable, which influence selective behav-ior. In this view, "a value is a conception, explicit or implicit, distinctive of an individual or characteristic of a group, of the desirable, which influences the selection from available modes, means and ends of action." This definition focuses on the relationship between values (conceptions of the desirable) and selective behavior (the choice between alternatives).

Values are presumed to exist in advance of and independent from the context in which they are studied and measured. At this more abstract level, values are identified as attitudes, orientations, or belief systems that are organizing concep-tions of a person's world. In studying behavior, however, values can be narrowly conceived as preferential judgments, responses, or choices that arise from human experience and may be influenced by anything that affects experiences. Thus values are synonymous with judgments of the desirability of a particular set of outcomes or situations that describe what is labeled "good" or "bad." The term *preference* is used to connote the exact meaning of value, desirability, or utility.

Utility measures. Measures of health status and QoL that incorporate explicit values in the ordering of health states are referred to as utility-weighted or preference-weighted measures. These measures contrast with those that use statistical weighting to define the magnitude of dysfunction or health of individuals and groups. Assignment of weights explicitly requires that rep-resentative individuals, sometimes referred to as judges, be confronted with options incorporating concepts based on functionalist, positive health, and QoL theories. The developers of health status and QoL measures have assumed that health states can be ranked; that is, if presented with health states *A* and *B*, people can meaningfully say whether they prefer *A* to *B* or *B* to *A*, or whether they are indifferent. To satisfy this criterion, the analyst must clearly define the states and their operational components so that between any two function levels the individual can clearly express a preference for one level over the other or can clearly recognize his or her indifference between any two function levels. Researchers have borrowed theoretical constructs and the resulting techniques developed by economists, psychologists, and other decision scientists to explain how individuals select between different options.

One widely used approach for obtaining weights for health status and QoL measures is utility theory. The classical theory of utility was derived from the eighteenth-century work of Jeremy Bentham. He formulated the utility principle that all individuals and society, as an aggregate of individuals, are directed toward a single end to increase pleasure and decrease pain (Bentham, 1948). Bentham asserted that people choose actions that increase pleasure. According to this utilitarian philosophy, preferences can be cardinally measured, that is, measured on an interval or a ratio scale. In measuring utility up to a cardinal scale, economists in the early twentieth century developed the notion of ordinal utility. With this type of utility, people report how much of one commodity is equal to standard amounts of a second commodity. This method of ranking preferences differs from classical utility in the point of origin and the arbitrary units of scale. It obtains many of the same results, however, as the classical theory while overcoming the difficulty of measurement. Louis Leon Thurstone, a psychologist, measured ordinal utility indirectly by plotting indifference curves (Thurstone, 1959).

Utility theory, whether classical or ordinal, assumes that choices can be made with certainty. John von Neumann and Oskar Morgenstern (1944) developed the notion of expected utility as a way of incorporating uncertainty into preference judgments. As von Neumann and Morgenstern showed, if *A* and *B* states (health) are presented as gambles, and if certain axioms are satisfied for expressions of preference, then such preferences can represent the underlying mental structure as a cardinal utility function. Gambles lead to utility functions in contrast to value functions, and utility functions are seen as necessary in prescribing behavior with respect to risky options. Expected utility theory, appropriate for decisions with uncertain prospects, is a normative or prescriptive model for rational decision making, a theory of "ought," not a theory of "is." The von Neumann and Morgenstern theory does not describe how persons actually make decisions or behave under uncertainty. Rather, the theory describes how persons ought to make decisions under rationality.

Game theory, as von Neumann and Morgenstern described their theory, centers on the assumption that the utility of two objects or outcomes is reflected by the relative expectations for the occurrence or acquisition of the two outcomes. Thus, the issue of assigning utilities to outcomes expands to the problem of assigning values to *gambles,* which are choices about outcomes that are not a sure thing. By constructing various game situations, the investigator can determine the value or expected utility of gambles and outcomes. The concepts of game theory have suggested many new directions for experimentation in utility measurement.

However, these methods of measurement, although appealing because of their logic and mathematical rigor, are difficult to apply to preference measurement studies concerned with outcomes not usually associated with gambles or risks.

Two examples of individualized measures are based on values or goals.

Goal attainment scaling (GAS). Measurement through GAS was first introduced in the 1960s by Kiresuk and Sherman for assessing outcomes in mental health settings (Kiresuk and Sherman, 1968). Since then it has been modified and applied in many other areas. GAS is a method of scoring the extent to which a patient's individual goals are achieved in the course of intervention. In effect, each patient has their own outcome measure, but this is scored in a standardized way as to allow statistical analysis. Traditional standardized measures include a standard set of tasks (items) each rated on a standard level. In GAS, tasks are individually identified to suit the patient, and the levels are individually set around their current and expected levels of performance. Patients or caregivers define and agree on expected levels of what the patient does or feels. As an outcome measure, there is growing evidence for the sensitivity of GAS (Rockwood et al., 1993, 1997). GAS potentially avoids some of the problems of standardized measures including floor and ceiling effects and lack of sensitivity.

The individual schedule for evaluating quality of life (SEIQoL) method samples the individual's most important elements of his or her QoL (McGee et al., 1991). The objective is to clarify the concept of QoL for the respondent and to elicit elements (cues) that the subject considers contribute to his own QoL. As few as three or as many as eight can be accommodated, but if the number is small, he is encouraged to nominate more. Usually one element will fall in each of the generally agreed QoL domains—cognitive, affective, social, physical, ecological, and religious. Two kinds of information about each cue are then sought: first, the subject's satisfaction with its current functioning. He or she marks this on a 10 cm visual analog scale, anchored at 0 as "Worst Possible" and at 10 as "Best Possible." Because of the relative importance attributed to each cue, their weights must also play a part in determining QoL. These are elicited by estimation of the importance of different cues contained in sample cases. Each case profile is based on the cues chosen by the respondent and random, computer-generated values of these. The cue weights are extracted by multiple regression analysis. The respondent's overall IQoL score is obtained from the summed products of each cue's rating and weight. The variance accounted for by the regression of the judgments of QoL upon the cues, R^2, is the measure of internal validity. Replicates are usually included in the set of profiles to examine the robustness, r, of the individual judgment "policy" or model.

The SEIQoL approach has been used in a wide variety of applications, including, for example, radiation therapy, advanced cancer, and chronic obstructive pulmonary disease (Becker et al., 2014; Farquhar et al., 2010; Wettergren et al., 2011). The SEIQoL can be adapted for most clinical conditions and populations that can report for themselves and has proven useful particularly in clinical contexts and clinical practice. It is a systematic approach for providing individualized assessment of what people consider to be important about health and living.

The way forward

This brief review of different conceptual approaches raises the question of how might the field move forward and possibly synthesize the approaches. Clearly there are overlapping concepts and constructs contained in the individual approaches. It would be possible to deconstruct the commonalities. The approach of conceptual mapping might be useful in identifying the overlap (Bullinger, 1999; van Bon-Martens et al., 2014). The goal is literature synthesis at least at the conceptual level.

The second possibility is to compare systematically the operationalizations of hypothesized concepts, such as satisfaction and happiness. Measures may be labeled as happiness, whereas the concept measured is satisfaction. Recording the concept being tapped by each instrument is a basic foundation in cultural adaptation and translation of patient-reported outcome (PRO) instruments. Using this approach to compare concepts of different instruments would be a useful exercise in many QoL fields.

At minimum, developers of outcome instruments and users of these instruments in application to chronic disease and treatment need to recognize that all items and all measurement processes have conceptual implications. Thus, being transparent in what the content of an instrument is intended to measure is recommended. This is particularly important in using concepts and measures in regulatory practice (Patrick et al., 2007). Using items and labels consistent with the concepts being measured makes the selection and use of measures more straightforward.

The perceived QoL is at the heart of the patient-centered outcomes movement, the approach that is increasingly used in chronic disease research and practice. Deepening our understanding of what patients think of their QoL with different health conditions and using different treatments brings out the "person" in personalized medicine and health care. Many of the conceptual approaches presented here have a long and distinguished history. The notions of satisfaction, utility, happiness, value, needs, and capabilities will continue to evolve as long as we strive for improving the quality of our lives with advances in health, medicine, and even broader initiatives of health-care policy, environmental change, and technological advance.

References

Alexander, F. (1950). *Psychosomatic Medicine: Its Principles and Applications*. New York, NY: Norton.

Andrews, F., and Withey, S.B. (1974). Developing measures of perceived life quality: Results from several national surveys. *Soc. Indic. Res.*, 1, 1–26.

Aristotle. (1976). *The Ethics of Aristotle: The Nicomachean Ethics* (J.A.K. Thomson, Trans. Rev. ed./rev. with notes and appendices by Hugh Tredennick ed.). Harmondsworth, UK/ New York, NY: Penguin.

Bandura, A. (1982). Self-efficacy mechanism in human agency. *Am. Psychol.*, 37, 122–147.

Becker, G., Merk, C.S., Meffert, C., and Momm, F. (2014). Measuring individual quality of life in patients receiving radiation therapy: The SEIQoL-Questionnaire. *Qual. Life Res.*, 23, 2025–2030. DOI:10.1007/s11136-014-0661-4

Bentham, J. (1948). *An Introduction to The Principles of Morals and Legislation* (Reprint of 1823 ed.). New York, NY: Hafner Pub. Co.

Bullinger, M. (1999). Cognitive theories and individual quality of life. In: C.R.B. Joyce, H.M. McGee, and C.A.O'. Boyle (eds.), *Individual Quality of Life: Approaches to Conceptualisation and Assessment* (pp. 29–39). Amsterdam: Harwood Academic Publishers.

Diener, E. (1984). Subjective well-being. *Psychol. Bull.*, *95*(3), 542–575.

Diener, E. (1994). Assessing subjective well-being: Progress and opportunities. *Soc. Indic. Res.*, *31*(2), 103–157. DOI:10.2307/27522740

Diener, E., and Biswas-Diener, R. (2008). *Happiness: Unlocking the Mysteries of Psychological Wealth*. Malden, MA: Blackwell Publishers.

Diener, E., and Diener, C. (1996). Most people are happy. *Psychol. Sci.*, *7*(3), 181–185.

Diener, E., Lucas, R.E., and Scollon, C.N. (2006). Beyond the hedonic treadmill: Revising the adaptation theory of well-being. *Am. Psychol.*, *61*(4), 305–314. DOI:10.1037/0003-066x.61.4.305

Diener, E., and Seligman, M.E.P. (2002). Very happy people. *Psychol. Sci.*, *13*(1), 81–84.

Edwards, T.C., Huebner, C.E., Connell, F.A., and Patrick, D L. (2002). Adolescent quality of life, part I: Conceptual and measurement model. *J. Adolesc.*, *25*(3), 275–286.

Farquhar, M., Ewing, G., Higginson, I.J., and Booth, S. (2010). The experience of using the SEIQoL-DW with patients with advanced chronic obstructive pulmonary disease (COPD): Issues of process and outcome. [Randomized controlled trial research support, non-U.S. Gov't validation studies]. *Qual. Life Res.*, *19*(5), 619–629. DOI:10.1007/s11136-010-9631-7

Hunt, S.M., and McKenna, S.P. (1992). The QLDS: A scale for the measurement of quality of life in depression. *Health Policy*, *22*(3), 307–319.

Jahoda, M. (1958). *Current Concepts of Positive Mental Health*. New York, NY: Basic Books.

Kiresuk, T.J., and Sherman, R.E. (1968). Goal attainment scaling: A general method for evaluating comprehensive community mental health programs. *Community Ment. Health J.*, *4*(6), 443–453.

Kobasa, S.C. (1979). Stressful life events, personality, and health: An inquiry into hardiness. *J. Pers. Soc. Psychol.*, *37*(1), 1–11.

Maslow, A.H. (1943). A theory of human motivation. *Psychol. Rev.*, *50*, 370–396.

McGee, H.M., O'Boyle, C.A., Hickey, A., O'Malley, K., and Joyce, C.R. (1991). Assessing the quality of life of the individual: The SEIQoL with a healthy and a gastroenterology unit population. *Psychol. Med.*, *21*(3), 749–759.

Nagel, E. (1961). *The Structure of Science, Problems in the Logic of Scientific Explanation*. London: Routledge.

Nussbaum, M.C., and Sen, A (eds.). (1993). *The Quality of Life*. New York, NY: Oxford University Press.

Patrick, D. (1997). Rethinking prevention for people with disabilities. Part I: A conceptual model for promoting health. *Am. J. Health Promot.*, *11*(4), 257–260.

Patrick, D., Burke, L., Powers, J., Scott, J., Rock, E., Dawisha, S, et al. (2007). Patient-reported outcomes to support medical product labeling claims: FDA perspective. *Value Health*, *10*(Suppl 2), S125–S137. DOI:10.1111/j.1524-4733.2007.00275.x

Patrick, D.L. (2014). Perceived quality of life scale. In: A. Michalos (ed.), *Encyclopedia of Quality of Life and Well-Being Research*. Dordrecht, NL: Springer.

Patrick, D.L., Curtis, J.R., Engelberg, R.A., Nielsen, E., and McCown, E. (2003). Measuring and improving the quality of dying and death. *Ann. Intern. Med.*, *139*(5 Pt 2), 410–415.

Patrick, D.L., Danis, M., Southerland, L.I., and Hong, G. (1988). Quality of life following intensive care. [Research support, non-U.S. Gov't research support, U.S. Gov't, P.H.S.]. *J. Gen. Intern. Med.*, *3*(3), 218–223.

Patrick, D.L., Drossman, D.A., Frederick, I.O., DiCesare, J., and Puder, K.L. (1998). Quality of life in persons with irritable bowel syndrome: Development and validation of a new measure. *Dig. Dis. Sci.*, *43*(2), 400–411.

Patrick, D.L., and Erickson, P. (1993). *Health Status and Health Policy: Quality of Life in Health Care Evaluation and Resource Allocation*. New York, NY: Oxford University Press.

Patrick, D.L., Kinne, S., Engelberg, R.A., and Pearlman, R.A. (2000). Functional status and perceived quality of life in adults with and without chronic conditions. *J. Clin. Epidemiol.*, 53(8), 779–785.

Patrick, D.L., Martin, M.L., Bushnell, D.M., Yalcin, I., Wagner, T.H., and Buesching, D.P. (1999). Quality of life of women with urinary incontinence: Further development of the incontinence quality of life instrument (I-QOL). *Urology*, 53(1), 71–76.

Pyszczynski, T., Greenberg, J., Solomon, S., Arndt, J., and Schimel, J. (2004). Why do people need self-esteem? A theoretical and empirical review. *Psychol. Bull.*, 130(3), 435–468. DOI:10.1037/0033-2909.130.3.435

Rockwood, K., Joyce, B., and Stolee, P. (1997). Use of goal attainment scaling in measuring clinically important change in cognitive rehabilitation patients. *J. Clin. Epidemiol.*, 50(5), 581–588.

Rockwood, K., Stolee, P., and Fox, R.A. (1993). Use of goal attainment scaling in measuring clinically important change in the frail elderly. *J. Clin. Epidemiol.*, 46(10), 1113–1118.

Rosenberg, M. (1979). *Conceiving The Self*. New York, NY: Basic Books.

Sen, A. (1985). Well-being, agency and freedom: The Dewey Lectures 1984. *J. Philos.*, 82(4), 169–221. DOI:10.2307/2026184

Sen, A. (1992). *Inequality Reexamined*. New York, NY: Russell Sage Foundation.

Stewart, A.L., Teno, J., Patrick, D.L., and Lynn, J. (1999). The concept of quality of life of dying persons in the context of health care. *J. Pain Symptom Manage.*, 17(2), 93–108.

Strickland, B. (1984). Levels of health enhancement: Individual attributes. In: J. Matarazzo, S.M. Weiss, J.A. Herd, N.A. Miller, and S.M. Weiss (eds.), *Behavioral Health: A Handbook of Health Enhancement and Disease Prevention* (pp. 101–113). New York, NY: Wiley.

Thurstone, L.L. (1959). *The Measurement of Values*. Chicago, IL: University of Chicago Press.

van Bon-Martens, M.J., van de Goor, L.A., Holsappel, J.C., Kuunders, T.J., Jacobs-van der Bruggen, M.A., Te Brake, J.H, et al. (2014). Concept mapping as a promising method to bring practice into science. *Public Health*, 128(6), 504–514. DOI:10.1016/j.puhe.2014.04.002

von Neumann, J., and Morgenstern, O. (1944). *Theory of Games and Economic Behavior*. Princeton, NJ: Princeton University Press.

Wettergren, L., Lindblad, A.K., Glimelius, B., and Ring, L. (2011). Comparing two versions of the Schedule for Evaluation of Individual Quality of Life in patients with advanced cancer. [Comparative Study Evaluation Studies]. *Acta Oncol.*, 50(5), 648–652. DOI:10.3109/0284186X.2011.557088

WHOQOL Group. (1993). Study protocol for the World Health Organization project to develop a Quality of Life assessment instrument (WHOQOL). *Qual. Life Res.*, 2(2), 153–159.

WHOQOL Group. (1995). The World Health Organization Quality of Life Assessment (WHOQOL): Position paper from the World Health Organization. *Soc. Sci. Med.*, 41(10), 1403–1409.

Wilson, I.B., and Cleary, P.D. (1995). Linking clinical variables with health-related quality of life. A conceptual model of patient outcomes. *JAMA*, 273(1), 59–65.

Windelband, W., and Oakes, G. (1980). History and natural science. *History and Theory*, 19, 165–168.

Zautra, A., and Goodhart, D. (1979). Quality of life indicators: A review of the literature. *Community Ment. Health Rev.*, 4(1), 1 3–10.

4 ICF and other conceptual models: Rethinking the role of context and implications for assessing health

Elizabeth M. Badley

Since its publication in 2001, the World Health Organization (WHO) International Classification of Functioning, Disability, and Health (ICF) has become the most widely used conceptual model of disablement worldwide (WHO, 2001). Although the ICF is ostensibly a revision of the WHO International Classification of Impairments, Disabilities, and Handicaps (ICIDH), its parentage is mixed. The final form of the classification and associated documentation was the result of an international consultative process (WHO, 2001, Appendix 10) with contributions from eight WHO Collaborating Centres, a number of networks and nongovernmental organizations, and consultants. Individual participants in the revision process came from 64 countries with a variety of backgrounds ranging from clinicians of various stripes to researchers, with the notable inclusion of organizations concerned with disability and people with disabilities themselves. This meant that the final version was more than a revision of the ICIDH, but incorporated a variety of perspectives, including those of other disability models and conceptualization of disability processes (Masala and Petretto, 2008).

Earlier models of disability, and the ICIDH in particular, were criticized as reflecting the medical model of disability, an individualistic model that sees disability as caused by disease or trauma and thus residing in the individual (Bickenbach et al., 1999; Pfeiffer, 1998). Social models of disability see disability as socially constructed and the outcome of environmental barriers and attitudes that specifically discriminate against people with impairments and as a matter of basic civil rights (Hurst, 2003; Oliver, 1998; Thomas, 2004; Isaac et al., 2010). The ICF attempts to bring together these two approaches in a biopsychosocial model of disability, where disablement is conceptualized as an interaction between the intrinsic features of the individual and the person's social and physical environment (Bickenbach et al., 1999, Ustun et al., 2003).

The ICF comprises a conceptual model and a classification of all but one of the components of this model, personal factors. The model depicts the relationships between a health condition and its potential impact on body functions and structures, on activities, such as activities of daily living and on participation

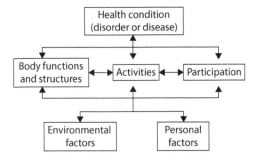

Figure 4.1 The World Health Organization (WHO) International Classification of Functioning, Disability, and Health (ICF) conceptual model.

(Figure 4.1). Participation represents the more social aspects of involvement in life situations. It is important to note that the depiction of the ICF conceptual model is neutral as are the items in the accompanying classification. So, for example, items in the section of the classification on "body functions" include "heart rate," and activity and participation items include "walking short distances," "preparing meals," and "full-time employment." According to the manual of the ICF, functioning is used as an umbrella term to cover all body functions, activities, and participation. The ICF has been mostly used in the context of disability. In this context, the conceptual model is modified to use negative terms. Problems with body functions and structures are called impairments and problems with activity and participation are, respectively, called activity limitations or participation restrictions (WHO, 2001). Disability is the suggested umbrella term for impairments, activity limitations, and participation restrictions. When using the associated classification, any problems or difficulties that arise as a result of a health condition are indicated by the use of qualifiers. So, for example, the qualifiers for activity and participation denote the degree of difficulty.

The conceptual model of the ICF also shows contextual factors. Contextual factors in the ICF are said to represent the complete background of an individual's life and living. The ICF model presents two general categories of contextual factors, environmental factors and personal factors. The ICF includes a classification of environmental factors. Personal factors "are not classified in the ICF because of the large social and cultural variation associated with them" (WHO, 2001).

Contextual factors and conceptual models of disablement

How other conceptual models of disablement contributed to the development of the ICF has been outlined elsewhere (Masala and Petretto, 2008; Whiteneck, 2005), and I will not attempt to review this here. The principal models that influenced the revision were the Nagi model (Nagi, 1965, 1976), the ICIDH (Badley, 1993; WHO, 1980), and the Disability Creation

Process (DCP) (Fougeyrollas, 1995; Fougeyrollas et al., 1998; Fougeyrollas and St Michel, 1991). More generally, the important contribution of people with disability in the revision process is reflected by the influence of theories of disability and movements for the rights of people with disabilities (Masala and Petretto, 2008; Hurst, 2003). The ICF contains elements of these antecedent models, but there are also some major differences. This chapter reviews some of the similarities and differences between these conceptual models with particular attention to how they incorporate contextual factors, and especially personal factors.

To compare conceptual models it is first necessary to establish a terminology. The terminology of conceptual models is complicated because the word "disability" is used in different conceptual models to mean different things. This can cause confusion. Therefore, in this chapter, I use the word disablement for the generic concept, which in the language of the ICF embraces impairment, activity limitation, on participation restrictions.

All the disablement models have common elements. All are tripartite in that they have three components in addition to the health condition, albeit somewhat differently conceptualized (Badley, 2008; Altman, 2001). In a broad overview, the first of these relates to the health condition and its impact on the structure and functioning of the body or body parts. The second usually relates to the performance of activities such as activities of daily living. The third is the more social component, which is called different things in the different models. For convenience here I am going to use the ICF word "societal participation." This is the component that is arguably more closely related to quality of life. I particularly want to focus on this latter component in comparing the way conceptual factors, and particularly on how personal factors are incorporated into disability models.

Although a major claim of the ICF is that it is a biopsychosocial model, the second thing that conceptual models of disablement have in common is that they broadly consider that disablement arises because of an interaction of the features associated with having a health condition and the environment of the individual with the health condition. Although this interaction can result in any one of the three components, in this chapter, I will focus on how the interaction is depicted to give rise to the more social component, the societal participation equivalent. As we will see, a major difference between the models is how this interaction is viewed. I will present the conceptual models in roughly chronological order of development to emphasize their evolution over time, with a focus on the inclusion of the contextual factors.

The first disablement model was a framework published in 1965 by the American sociologist Nagi (Nagi, 1964, 1965). This model was developed in the context of rehabilitation and his work with the US Social Security Administration (SSA). Nagi uses the term disability for what the ICF refers to as societal participation. He wrote, "disability is the expression of a physical or a mental limitation in a social context" (Nagi, 1965). Within this model, the individual is clearly viewed within an environmental context, and it is recognized that the personal component is of two kinds: that related to the person's anatomical, physiological mental, and/or psychological nature, and other characteristics such as age that are culturally important to the nature of social participation and other aspects of functioning (Nagi, 1965). Nagi's approach is conceptual and does not attempt classification of any of the components. The formulation of the model by Nagi was also entirely narrative and did not include a graphic depiction of the conceptual model. This model was largely ignored in the wider literature until it was taken up by others incorporated into the book *Disability in America* in 1991 (Pope and Tarlov, 1991) and in other subsequent publications emanating from the United States (Verbrugge and Jette, 1994; Brandt and Pope, 1997).

The next conceptual model to be published was the WHO ICIDH. It was published in its final form in 1980 (WHO, 1980). This was the first model to include a classification and was developed as an adjunct to the International Classification of Diseases. The depiction of the model as it appeared in the manual for the classification has received considerable criticism because it shows a central pathway starting from a disease or disorder, which may lead to impairment, which may in turn lead to disability and finally to handicap. The depiction shows these concepts linked by arrows, and various authors have interpreted this to mean an inevitable progression from one component of disability to the other (Bickenbach et al., 1999; Pfeiffer, 1998; Colvez and Robine, 1986; Heerkens et al., 1995). The ICIDH was much criticized because the conceptual model did not include an interaction with the environment (Colvez and Robine, 1986; Bury, 1987; Chapireau and Colvez, 1998; Imrie, 1997). However, from the text accompanying the classification and from subsequent publications, it is clear that environmental and other barriers were important, and the experience of disability and handicap is contingent on the environment in which individuals find themselves (Badley, 1993; Bury, 1987; Wood, 1989; WHO, 1993; Wood and Badley, 1981).

Disability in the ICIDH is largely equivalent to activity limitation in the ICF. Handicap is the final socialized outcome and is defined as the disadvantage experience depending on age, sex, and social and cultural factors. Handicap is "characterized by a discordance between the individual's performance or status and the expectation of the particular group of which he [or she] is a member." Handicap is thus contextualized and is relative to what might be expected depending on the circumstances of the individual. In particular, it should be noted here that relevant personal factors, such as those related to age, gender, and culture, are integral to a judgment of what might be expected in terms of social norms and expectations.

The 1990s saw a major evolution in the disablement models. The first was the publication in 1991 of the conceptual model developed in the 1980s by a group in Québec, Canada, led by Fougeyrollas and St Michel (1991). This model was initially called the handicap creation process and later renamed the DCP model as I will refer to it. This is an interactional model where the concept of "handicap" (as it was referred to in the original model) or "life habits" in the neutral form is considered to be the situational result generated by the interaction of two causal (sic) elements; the characteristics of the person (organ systems or impairments and abilities or disabilities) and environmental factors (Fougeyrollas et al., 1998). Like the ICF, this model this has the option for neutral terminology. Although the layout of the conceptual diagram is not linear, the essential elements of the model show the three major components (impairments of organ systems, disability, handicap situations) and an interaction with environmental factors. The model shows impairments of organ systems, which can lead to disability. These can interact with environmental factors to give rise to what are called "handicap situations"—the societal participation equivalent. The documentation implies that the development of this model was influenced by the ICIDH, and this is reflected in the use of similar terminology. One can also see here a clear influence of the thinking reflected in the other North American model, the Nagi model. The DCP model includes both positive and negative aspects: abilities, what a person can do, as well as disabilities. This model was the first to explicitly show environmental factors as part of the conceptual framework. The documentation associated with the DCP model also includes outline classifications of the components of disablement and of environmental factors (Bergeron et al., 1991; Fougeyrollas et al., 2002).

Round about the same time as the publication of the DCP, Nagi further explained his conceptual framework in a chapter of a book, *Disability in America*, which was published in 1991 (Nagi, 1991). According to Nagi, disability is a "limitation in performing socially defined roles and tasks expected of an individual within a socio-cultural and physical environment" and is "the expression of a physical or a mental limitation in a social context disability is a relational concept; its indicators include individuals' capacities and limitations, in relation to role and task expectations, and the environmental conditions within which they are performed." The individual and the individual's performance are thus firmly set at the center of this conceptual model. He further notes that several other factors contribute to shaping the dimensions and severity of disability. These include the individual's definition of the situation and reactions, which at times compound the limitations; the definition of the situation by others, and their reactions and expectations and, finally, the characteristics of the environment and the degree to which it is free from, or encumbered with, physical and sociocultural barriers.

Although Nagi's text made it clear that the environment is important, he did not include a diagram to describe his complex model. This task was undertaken by Verbrugge and Jette in their elaboration of his model (Verbrugge and Jette, 1994). In this model, they show Nagi's main pathway of pathology, which might lead to impairments, which might in turn lead to functional limitations and finally to disability. Pathology is used here to denote the health condition. This model also includes contextual factors, extra- and intraindividual factors, which include those aspects that are relevant to the disability process. In the ICF language, these are factors that might be thought of as being facilitators or barriers in the process that might lead to restriction of societal participation. Extra-individual factors are roughly equivalent to environmental factors in the ICF. This is the first model to explicitly show personal factors as a separate category, labeled intraindividual factors in their paper.

In 1995, Badley published a further elaboration of the ICIDH framework to explicitly show the role of the environment in the genesis of handicap (Badley, 1995). According to this elaboration, handicap is seen to be the result of an interaction of the impairment and/or disability with environmental factors. These include the physical environment, the resources available to an individual including assistive devices, adaptations, and social support, and the social setting. The social setting refers to aspects such as the attitudes of other people and the values of society, which might influence the performance of people with disabilities. These interacting factors come into play in the context of a person's health condition, impairment, or disability and can act as facilitators or barriers in preventing or causing handicap. In this context, they are similar to the extra-individual factors in the Nagi model. Although personal factors are not explicitly shown in this model, key personal factors are included in the definition of handicap: disadvantage depending on age, sex, and social and cultural factors.

An important evolution of the Nagi model is the one published in the book *Enabling America* in 1997 (Brandt and Pope, 1997). The person as a whole is central to this model. This is illustrated by a figure that depicts the person with the health problem in interaction with the environment. It explicitly shows the environment as resembling a safety net supporting the person. An environment that is high in barriers and offers few services fails to support the individual and creates a large displacement of the net, signifying a substantial amount of disablement (difficulties with societal participation). An environment where the resources and support match or exceed what the individual needs shows little deflection, which implies little net disablement.

The DCP model has also undergone further developments over time. Lavasseur slightly reworked the depiction of the conceptual model (Levasseur et al., 2007). According to her depiction, the model risk factors (or cause) lead to what are called personal factors. However, these personal factors are very different from the personal factors in the ICF. They include what are called organic systems and capabilities. The organic systems represent the pathology associated with having a health condition or injury, similar to impairments in the ICF. The capabilities relate to the ability to carry out activities—similar to the activity limitation category in the ICF. These are essentially the same as the categories in the original DCP model. The personal factors box in the model also includes personal characteristics, described as age, gender, sociocultural characteristics that affect the performance of "life habits," the participation equivalent outcome, with the alternative labels social participation or handicap situation. This model is of particular interest in that it explicitly does not separate the fundamental characteristics of the person from the health condition.

Interference with life habits is seen as a result of an interaction of the person with environmental factors, both social and physical. This is very similar to the Institute of Medicine elaboration of the Nagi model with the focus on the person as a whole.

The contextual factors in the ICF and earlier conceptual models

As I have outlined, the different conceptual models of disablement incorporate the person and particularly personal factors in slightly different ways. In the models prior to the ICF, by and large the emphasis on the environment is selective in that it is focused on those features that are relevant to producing disablement, and in particular societal participation restriction. In other words, the models tend to focus on environmental features, which can act as barriers to cause disablement or can act as facilitators to mitigate the impact of the health condition, impairments, and activity limitations on a person. Also, many of the "classic" personal factors such as age, gender, social, and cultural situation are integrated into the model or at the very least in the definition of the societal participation aspect. We see this particularly clearly in the definition of handicap and "handicap situations" in the ICIDH and DCP (Fougeyrollas et al., 1998, 2002; WHO, 1993; Levasseur et al., 2007).

The ICF is somewhat different from earlier models particularly in the way in which personal factors are incorporated. The Nagi model and the DCP refer to the situation of the whole person and the concept equivalent to societal participation restriction is seen to arise from an interaction between the whole person with a health condition (including his or her personal characteristics) and the environment (Fougeyrollas et al., 1998, 2002; Nagi, 1991). In the ICF and ICIHD, the components of disablement related to the health condition, impairment, and activity restriction are seen as distinct from other personal characteristics. This separation is not quite so marked in the ICIDH as in the ICF, because the definition of handicap in the ICIDH includes some personal factors contextualized in terms of what would be expected based on age, sex, and social and cultural factors (WHO, 1993). In the ICF, participation restriction is defined as problems in life situations and the personal characteristics of the individual are explicitly separated from this. This is reinforced by the examples of personal factors given in the manual to the ICF (WHO, 2001). This separation of personal factors from the components of disablement leaves the ICF disablement model in the somewhat awkward situation as being an interaction between a health condition (and associated features: impairment, activity limitation, and participation restriction) and contextual factors, both environmental and personal (Levasseur et al., 2007; Schneidert et al., 2003; Masala and Petretto, 2008). A logical conclusion from this is that all nonhealth condition-related characteristics of the individual can potentially contribute to disablement.

Personal factors in the ICF are personal characteristics that are not included in the structure and functioning of the person's body, their activities, or participation. As listed in the manual to the ICF, these may include gender, race, age, other health conditions, fitness, lifestyle, habits, upbringing, coping styles, social background, education, profession, past and current experience, overall behavioral pattern and character style, individual psychological assets, and other characteristics (WHO, 2001). Although some of these, such as coping style, might be viewed as potentially acting as facilitators or barriers in interaction with a health condition to cause disability, it is also clearly not a reasonable assumption for personal factors, such as age, gender, and race.

The way the role of environmental factors, and by extension personal factors, is described in the ICF manual is somewhat ambiguous. On the one hand, the ICF lists environmental factors that interact with the components to enable the user to "record useful profiles of individuals' functioning, disability and health in various domains" (ICF manual (1) p. 3). This could be interpreted as a listing of factors that are germane to the functioning of an individual without necessarily implying any contributory role to the level of functioning or disability. On the other hand, environmental factors are conceptualized as factors external to the individual that might restrict or enhance the performance of an individual with a health condition (ICF manual (1) p. 16). The suggested qualifiers for environmental factors show their role as facilitators or barriers to functioning, implying that these are factors that are instrumental in the disablement process. If all contextual factors, including personal factors, are viewed in this way, it is hardly surprising that no attempt to classify personal factors was included in the manual of the ICF. Coding personal factors as being facilitators or barriers potentially creates a situation where disablement is an attribute of the individual (Muller and Geyh, 2015). However, ignoring personal factors means taking the person and the person's individual characteristics out of the interaction between the health condition and environment in the process of disablement, which is clearly not the intention behind any of the models of disablement.

Personal factors and the ICF

There have been several attempts to provide a classification of personal factors. The key features of these have been reviewed by Muller and Geyh (2015). The categorizations show considerable diversity. Nevertheless, common to all is the inclusion of sociodemographic factors, and aspects related to behavior/lifestyle, cognitive/psychological factors, and coping. As the authors note, this common core argues against the notion that personal factors are not classified in the ICF because of the large social and cultural variances associated with them. The classifications reviewed illustrate the breath of the range of possible factors, including items not included in the examples in the ICF. They were developed from a number of different perspectives and with different purposes. However, lacking from all is a clear conceptualization of the role of personal factors in the disablement process. A central assumption in most of these categorizations is that personal factors are similar environmental factors, namely potential facilitators or barriers.

I suggest that we may be neglecting important characteristics of the context if we consider contextual factors only as facilitators and barriers. In the ICF contextual factors, both environmental and personal are said to represent the complete background of an individual's life and living (ICF manual (1), p. 16). Surely this background also includes a range of personal and environmental factors, whether or not they are related to the experience of disablement. For all of us, who we are, what we do, and what we aspire to do are influenced by the general background of our lives. In my previous work attempting to develop criteria to differentiate between activity and participation, I suggested that there are two general types of environmental and personal contextual factors (Badley, 2008).

The first category is those that I called scene setters. These are the aspects that in another context were referred to as "givens" (Jahiel and Scherer, 2010). These are the environmental and personal characteristics that determine the repertoire of tasks an individual might undertake, and the manner in which they are carried out, and that which define available options and opportunities for societal participation. Some forms of participation may not be important to the individual or open to them. For instance, not all people can be, or choose to be, parents. Personal factors, which are potentially scene-setting include age, gender, social, and cultural factors, as well as a range of other characteristics such as education, religion, past experience, and so on. The fact that personal factors were not classified in the ICF due to large social and cultural variations associated with them speaks to the need for scene-setting personal contextual factors. The notion of scene-setting contextual factors not unique to the consideration of disablement and is congruent with life course and ecological perspectives on health and human development more generally (Magasi et al., 2015).

One of the characteristics of the ICF is that it is framed neutrally and in principle could be applied to everyone (WHO, 2001; Masala and Petretto, 2008). In this light, one way of thinking of scene-setting contextual factors is to view them as the factors that influence aspects of body, structure and function, and activity and participation in the absence of a health condition. In this way, contextual factors can affect societal participation, in a way unrelated to the activity limitation: as indicated above, this may reflect the social and cultural environment of an individual, including the expectations related to a person's age and gender (Gignac et al., 2008; Herzog and Markus, 1999). Some examples of the role of gender in directly affecting functioning are as follows. There are gender differences in body structure and function (apart from the obvious ones intrinsically related to sexual characteristics): men are usually stronger (and have bigger muscles) than women. In most cultures, the activities people engage in may differ by gender. For example, the tasks involved in dressing may differ related to different types of clothing. Depending on social and cultural factors, opportunities for participation may be available. Even in most Western cultures, the likelihood of participation in various occupations are different. For instance, women are more likely than men to become full-time caregivers especially to young children, and women less likely work as miners, mechanics, or in construction.

The second category of contextual factors are those that can interact with a person's health condition, impairments, or activity limitations to affect the final outcome in terms of participation: these are the contextual factors that can act as facilitators or barriers (Badley, 2008). I further suggest that this type of contextual factor is of two broad types (Badley, 1995). The first I have is called "preexisting." These are those that exist independently of the health condition (and its associated features) but which acquire a different significance (and may be barriers or facilitators) in the face of a potentially disabling health condition. Examples would include barriers in the environment such as steps and stairs, living with others, as well as the wider characteristics of the society in which an individual lives. Personal characteristics would include educational status, personal wealth, as well as some intrinsic personality traits. The second category is those contextual facts that are only mobilized in the presence of potentially disabling health conditions, referred to as responsive factors. Examples include the use of assistive devices, the use of medical or rehabilitation services, and personal factors such as psychological reactions such as hopelessness, anger, frustration, denial, determination, positive self-efficacy, and so forth. An important personal factor in this context is the subjective experience of disability (Lutz and Bowers, 2005; Ueda and Okawa, 2003). Although for both these modes of action, personal factors can theoretically act as barriers or facilitators between activity limitation and the experience of societal participation, in practice viewing them in this way could have the danger of putting the emphasis back on individual behaviors. The bottom line is that extreme care needs to be taken in identifying personal factors to be incorporated in a classification and identifying personal factors as facilitators or barriers (Muller and Geyh, 2015).

There have been various attempts to develop measures to enable environmental factors to be incorporated into research in disablement. These have not been entirely successful (Keysor, 2005; Whiteneck and Dijkers, 2009). As Whiteneck and Dijkers argue in their thoughtful paper, "the environment is so broad, we cannot begin to measure all aspects of it simultaneously. To do this we need a theory of how environments effect functioning" (Whiteneck and Dijkers, 2009). This has yet to be developed. Magasi and colleagues have taken some preliminary steps and reviewed some of the approaches that might contribute to this (Magasi et al., 2015). To date little attention has been given as to how the personal characteristics of an individual might not only affect the disablement process but also determine the nature of the environment in which individuals live. Looking at scene-setting contextual factors, particularly personal factors, raises the question as to the extent to which these factors are truly personal and whether there are personal factors that might be better understood to represent the aspects of environmental factors, especially those related to functioning in society as a whole. Age and gender are quintessential personal factors. However, in the context of activity and participation, they are also socially constructed concepts. Within a given culture, for example, expectations for the range of activities undertaken and the types of societal participation may differ by age and gender, and also evolve over time (Gignac et al., 2008; Herzog and Markus, 1999).

Incorporating the person into the ICF

I suggest that explicitly incorporating contextual scene-setting factors in the ICF conceptual model will provide a background for increased understanding of disability models and processes. This means that we would need to develop a means to do so. At the very simplest, it could be a recording of some of the salient characteristics of an individual, as is done in many, if not all, research studies where data are collected. Explicitly including scene-setting factors will mean that we can include entirely to background to an individual's life and living. It will also serve to remind us that in measuring the impact of health on disability or quality of life, there may be systematic differences independent of the effect of the health condition, including social and cultural differences, depending on the characteristics of the environment and the individual. The types of activities or participation that are important to individuals may vary by level of scene-setting contextual factor, as might any associated difficulty with chosen activities. This has implications for research, particularly for study design and measurement scales. For example, these differences may be important in choosing outcome measures and in understanding how standard measures perform. There may be varying reference points for answering survey or clinical questions. There are also implications for data analysis where we potentially may need to take into account the influence of scene-setting factors. For example, we may need to test for differences between groups (effect modification, also called moderation) by postulated scene-setting variables (Wang et al., 2006).

A more radical approach would be a reconceptualization of the ICF model, more along the lines of the DCP or Nagi models where body structure and function, impairment, and participation are seen to be integral characteristics of the person, taking into account the age gender, culture, and so on. As the ICF evolves it may be that a pragmatic solution will be developed in a more integrated view and simply thinking of contextual factors, without the artificial distinction between environmental and personal. This might require the development of an integrated contextual factors classification. This could be used with qualifiers similar to those suggested for the current environmental factors classification to indicate facilitators or barriers, and with an additional qualifier to indicate the role of a contextual factor as an important scene-setting factor. This would require that the current environmental factors classification be augmented to provide a list of background features, including personal factors that might need to be considered and set the context of the ICF disablement model. Whatever approach is taken, there is a need to further develop our understanding of the role of personal factors, to identify which ones are central to understanding functioning and disablement and come up with an appropriate categorization scheme (Masala and Petretto, 2008; Whiteneck, 2005; Magasi et al., 2015; Alford et al., 2015).

Summary and conclusion

In this chapter, I have traced the development of the ICF and other conceptual models over a time span of almost 50 years, showing how there has been an evolution in the way that environmental and personal contextual factors have been incorporated. The latest conceptual framework, the ICF, was published in 2001, almost a decade and half before the time of writing. The ICF left open a number of aspects for further development. These include the nature and extent of how environmental factors interact with the components of body functions and structures, activities, and participation; the development of a classification for personal factors; and the further elaboration of the conceptual model. In that time, little progress has been made toward the elaborate understanding of the complexity of environmental factors, and in particular making progress toward a classification of personal factors. The development of a classification of personal factors, if this is attempted, will need to start with a better understanding of the role of these factors in the disablement process. It is perhaps time for further development of the ICF conceptual model. One particular such development would be the recognition that environmental and personal contextual factors can be seen scene-setting, as well as acting as facilitators and barriers in the disablement process. Recognizing scene-setting contextual factors has implications for understanding health as these set the background for what people do and aspire to do in the environment and culture in which they live. This recognition also has implications for the way in which we develop and use measures to assess health and health outcomes.

References

Alford, V.M., Ewen, S., Webb, G.R., McGinley J., Brookes A., and Remedios L.J. (2015). The use of the International Classification of Functioning, Disability and Health to understand the health and functioning experiences of people with chronic conditions from the person perspective: A systematic review. *Disabil. Rehabil.*, 37(8), 655–666.
Altman, B.M. (2001). Definitions, models, classification, schemes and applications. In: G.L. Albrect, K. Seelman, and M.R. Bury (eds.), *Handbook of Disability Studies* (pp. 97–123). Thousand Oaks, CA: Sage Publications.
Badley, E.M. (1993). An introduction to the concepts and classifications of the International Classification of Impairments, Disabilities, and Handicaps. *Disabil. Rehabil.*, 15(4), 161–178.
Badley, E.M. (1995). The genesis of handicap: Definition, models of disablement, and role of external factors. *Disabil. Rehabil.*, 17(2), 53–62.
Badley, E.M. (2008). Enhancing the conceptual clarity of the activity and participation components of the International Classification of Functioning, Disability, and Health. *Soc. Sci. Med.* 66(11), 2335–2345.
Bergeron, H., St Michel, G., Cloutier, R., and Fougeyrollas, P. (1991). Impact of the proposed model of impairments: Proposal of a nomenclature of organic systems. *ICIDH Int. Netw.*, 4, 35–37.

Bickenbach, J.E., Chatterji, S., Badley, E.M., and Ustun, T.B. (1999). Models of disablement, universalism and the International Classification of Impairments, Disabilities and Handicaps. *Soc. Sci. Med., 48*(9), 1173–1187.

Brandt, E.N., and Pope, A.M (eds.). (1997). *Enabling America: Asssessing the Role of Rehabilitation Science and Engineering.* Washington, DC: National Academy Press.

Bury, MR. (1987). The ICIDH: A review of research and prospects. *Int. Disabil. Stud., 9*(3), 118–122.

Chapireau, F., and Colvez, A. (1998). Social disadvantage in the International Classification of Impairments, Disabilities, and Handicap. *Soc. Sci. Med., 147*(1), 59–66.

Colvez, A., and Robine, J.M. (1986). Problems encountered in using the concepts of impairment, disability, and handicap in a health assessment survey of the elderly in Upper Normandy. *Int. Rehabil. Med., 8*(1), 18–22.

Fougeyrollas, P. (1995). Documenting environmental factors for preventing the handicap creation process: Quebec contributions relating to ICIDH and social participation of people with functional differences. *Disabil. Rehabil., 17*(3–4), 145–153.

Fougeyrollas, P., Noreau, L., Bergeron, H., Cloutier, R., Dion, S.A., and St Michel, G. (1998). Social consequences of long term impairments and disabilities: Conceptual approach and assessment of handicap. *Int. J. Rehabil. Res., 21*(2), 127–141.

Fougeyrollas, P., Noreau, L., and Boschen, K. (2002). Interaction of environment with individual characteristics and social participation: Theoretical perspectives and applications in persons with spinal cord injury. *Top. Spinal Cord Inj. Rehabil., 7*(3), 1–16.

Fougeyrollas, P., and St Michel, G. (1991). Proposal of a revised nomenclature of life habits. *ICIDH Int. Netw., 4*, 18–20.

Gignac, M.A., Backman, C.L., Davis, A.M., Lacaille, D., Mattison, C.A., Montie, P., Badley, E.M. (2008). Understanding social role participation: what matters to people with arthritis? *J. Rheumatol., 35*, 1655–1663.

Heerkens, Y.F., Van Ravensberg, C.D., and Brandsma, J.W. (1995). The need for revisions of the ICIDH: An example—Problems in gait. *Disabil. Rehabil., 17*(3/4), 184–194.

Herzog, A., and Markus, H. (1999). The self-concept in life span and aging research. In: V. Bengtson, and K. Schaie (eds.), *Handbook of Theories of Aging.* New York, NY: Springer Publishing.

Hurst, R. (2003). The international disability rights movement and the ICF. *Disabil. Rehabil., 25*(11–12), 572–576.

Imrie, R. (1997). Rethinking the relationships between disability, rehabilitation, and society. *Disabil. Rehabil., 19*(7), 263–271.

Isaac, R., Raja, B.W.D., and Ravanan, M.P. (2010). Integrating people with disabilities: Their right—our responsibility. *Disabil. Soc., 25*(5), 627–630.

Jahiel, R.I., and Scherer, M.J. (2010). Initial steps towards a theory and praxis of person-environment interaction in disability. *Disabil. Rehabil., 32*(17), 1467–1474.

Keysor, J.J. (2005). How does the environment influence disability? Examining the evidence. In: Field MJ, Jette AM, and Martin L (eds.), *Workshop on Disability in America: A New Look.* Washington, DC: National Acadamies Press.

Levasseur, M., Desrosiers, J., and St-Cyr, T.D. (2007). Comparing the disability creation process and International Classification of Functioning, Disability and Health models. *Can. J. Occup. Ther., 74*, Spec No: 233–242.

Lutz, B.J., and Bowers, B.J. (2005). Disability in everyday life. *Qual. Health Res., 15*(8), 1037–1054.

Magasi, S., Wong, A., Gray, D.B., Hammel, J., Baum, C., Wang, C.C, et al. (2015). Theoretical foundations for the measurement of environmental factors and their impact on participation among people with disabilities. *Arch. Phys. Med. Rehabil., 96*(4), 569–577.

Masala, C., and Petretto, D.R. (2008). From disablement to enablement: Conceptual models of disability in the 20th century. *Disabil. Rehabil., 30*(17), 1233–1244.

Muller, R., and Geyh, S. (2015). Lessons learned from different approaches towards classifying personal factors. *Disabil. Rehabil.*, *37*(5), 430–438.

Nagi, S. (1965). Some conceptual issues in disability and rehabilitation. In: M. Sussman (ed.), *Sociology and Rehabilitation* (p. 100). Washington, DC: American Sociological Society.

Nagi, S.Z. (1964). A study in the evaluation of disability and rehabilitation potential: Concepts, methods, and procedures. *Am. J. Public Health Nations Health. 54*, 1568–1579.

Nagi, S.Z. (1976). An epidemiology of disability among adults in the United States. *Milbank Mem. Fund. Q. Health Soc.*, *54*(4), 439–467.

Nagi, S.Z. (1991). Disability concepts revisited: Implications for prevention. In: A. Pope and A. Tarlow (eds.), *Disability in America: Toward a National Agenda for Prevention* (pp. 309–327). Washington, DC: National Academy Press.

Oliver, M. (1998). Theories of disability in health practice and research. *BMJ*, *317*(7170), 1446–1449.

Pfeiffer, D. (1998). The ICIDH and the need for its revision. *Disabil. Soc.*, *13*(4), 503–523.

Pope, A.M., and Tarlov, A. (1991). *Disability in America: Toward a National Agenda for Prevention*. Washington, DC: National Academies Press.

Schneidert, M., Hurst, R., Miller, J., and Ustun, B. (2003). The role of environment in the International Classification of Functioning, Disability and Health (ICF). *Disabil. Rehabil.*, *25*(11–12), 588–595.

Thomas, C. (2004). How is disability understood?. An examination of sociological approaches. *Disabil. Soc.*, *19*(6), 569–583.

Ueda, S., and Okawa, Y. (2003). The subjective dimension of functioning and disability: What is it and what is it for?. *Disabil. Rehabil.*, *25*(11–12), 596–601.

Ustun, T.B., Chatterji, S., Bickenbach, J., Kostanjsek, N., and Schneider, M. (2003). The International Classification of Functioning, Disability and Health: A new tool for understanding disability and health. *Disabil. Rehabil.*, *25*(11–12), 565–571.

Verbrugge, L.M., and Jette, A.M. (1994). The disablement process. *Soc Sci Med.*, *38*(1), 1–14.

Wang, P.P., Badley, E.M., and Gignac, M. (2006). Exploring the role of contextual factors in disability models. *Disabil. Rehabil.*, *28*(2), 135–140.

Whiteneck, G. (2005). Conceptual models of disability: Past, present, and future. In: M. Field, A. Jette, and L. Martin (eds.), *Workshop on Disability in America: Summary and Background Papers*. (pp. 50–66). Washington, DC: National Academies Press.

Whiteneck, G., and Dijkers, M.P. (2009). Difficult to measure constructs: Conceptual and methodological issues concerning participation and environmental factors. *Arch. Phys. Med. Rehabil.*, *90*(11 Suppl), S22–S35.

WHO. (1980). *International Classification of Impairments, Disabilities, and Handicaps: A Manual Relating to the Consequences of Disease*. Geneva: World Health Organization.

WHO. (1993). *International Classification of Impairments, Disabilities, and Handicaps—A Manual Relating to the Consequences of Disease (With foreword)*. Geneva: World Health Organization.

WHO. (2001). *International Classification of Functioning, Disability and Health: ICF*. Geneva: World Health Organization.

Wood, P.H.N. (1989). Measuring the consequences of illness. *World Health Stat. Q.*, *42*(3), 115–121.

Wood, P.H.N., and Badley, E.M. (1981). *People with Disabilities: Towards Acquiring Information Which Reflects More Sensitively Their Problems and Needs*. New York, NY: World Rehabilitation Fund.

5 Psychological adjustment to chronic disease

Annette L. Stanton and Michael A. Hoyt

Chronic, noncommunicable diseases affect the majority of adults worldwide and cause 38 million deaths annually (World Health Organization [WHO], 2015). Of the four primary classes of chronic diseases, which account for 82% of chronic disease deaths, cardiovascular diseases are the major causes of mortality (17.5 million), followed by cancers (8.2 million), respiratory diseases (4 million), and diabetes (1.5 million) (WHO, 2015). In the United States, approximately half of the adults have a chronic disease and 25% live with multiple chronic conditions (Ward et al., 2014). In addition to causing profound health threat, chronic diseases confer substantial psychosocial impact. This chapter describes a brief synthesis of the hundreds of studies regarding psychological adjustment to chronic diseases in adults.

Conceptualizations of adjustment to chronic disease

Researchers have proposed several conceptualizations of adjustment to chronic disease. The first involves one's success in negotiating disease-related adaptive tasks. Taylor (1983) offered a model of cognitive adaptation that identifies self-esteem enhancement, maintenance of a sense of mastery, and engagement in a search for meaning as central tasks. Regulating complex emotions, contending with uncertainty, and sustaining close relationships also constitute adaptive tasks. Disease-related tasks, such as pain and symptom management and communication within the medical system, also are prominent (Moos and Schaefer, 1984).

The presence of psychological disorder is also an indicator of adjustment to chronic disease. Elevated prevalence of psychological disorders is documented in samples of individuals with chronic illness (e.g., Golden et al., 2008; Katon, 2011; Mitchell et al., 2011; Müller-Tasch et al., 2008; Van 't Land et al., 2010). For example, in a meta-analysis of 70 studies of more than 10,000 adults treated in oncologic/hematologic settings across 14 countries, the prevalence

Author note: Chapter adapted in part from Hoyt, M.A., and Stanton, A.L. (2012). Adjustment to chronic illness. In: A.S. Baum, T.A. Revenson, and J.E. Singer (eds.), *Handbook of Health Psychology* (2nd Edition, pp. 219–246). New York, NY: Taylor & Francis.

of major depression as indicated by diagnostic interview was 14.9%, anxiety was 10.3%, and adjustment disorder was 19.4% (Mitchell et al., 2011). The experience of symptoms in the subclinical range also is common. In a meta-analysis, 19.3% of adults with heart failure evidenced depression via diagnostic interview versus 33.6% when assessed by self-report questionnaire (Rutledge et al., 2006).

Measures of mood and distress are widely used to indicate adjustment to chronic disease. Assessment includes both general (e.g., anxiety, global distress) and disease-specific (e.g., fear of disease recurrence) measures. Positive mood and other measures of positive functioning are increasingly assessed (see Patrick, 2015 this volume). Reviews demonstrate that chronic disease is associated with both elevated distress and compromised well-being (Steptoe et al., 2015).

Performance in functional roles also signifies adjustment. For example, a meta-analysis revealed that cancer survivors were 1.37 times more likely to be unemployed than the general healthy population (de Boer et al., 2009). Mobility, ability to complete daily activities, and maintenance of social roles are additional examples. Perceptions of quality of life (QoL) in various domains (e.g., social, emotional, physical, spiritual, sexual) also denote adjustment (see Patrick, 2015, this volume). Researchers also typically gather reports of disease- and treatment-related symptoms or related life disruption as markers of adjustment (e.g., Donovan et al., 2007; Gore et al., 2009).

Several general observations emerge from examining the array of conceptualizations of adjustment. First, adjustment to chronic disease is multidimensional, including both intra- and interpersonal domains. Second, adjustment domains are interrelated. For example, depressive symptoms predict functional status (e.g., poor glycemic control) in adults with diabetes (Lustman and Clouse, 2005).

Third, heterogeneity in psychological adjustment is evident across individuals and diseases. Prospective research demonstrates that adults diagnosed with chronic disease are at a heightened risk for distress and dysfunction (e.g., Lazovich et al., 2009; Polsky et al., 2005; Rutledge et al., 2006), although heterogeneity is apparent across and within diseases. Polsky et al. (2005) examined five biennial waves of data for more than 8300 adults and found that individuals diagnosed with cancer had the highest risk of depressive symptoms within 2 years after diagnosis (hazard ratio [HR] = 3.55), followed by chronic lung disease (HR = 2.21) and heart disease (HR = 1.45) versus those with no incident disease. Adults with arthritis did not evidence higher depressive symptoms until 2–4 years after diagnosis (HR = 1.46), and risk for depressive symptoms extended through 8 years after diagnosis for adults with heart disease.

Increasingly, researchers are examining trajectories of adjustment indicators over time to identify heterogeneous patterns of adjustment between subgroups of individuals and over the disease course (e.g., Henselmans et al., 2010; Murphy et al., 2008; Rose et al., 2009). For example, an investigation beginning prior to breast cancer surgery and concluding 6 months after treatment completion indicated four distinct trajectories of psychological distress in 171 women: 36% reported no or minimal distress across the five assessment points, 33% reported distress from the point of diagnosis through medical treatment and then a decline in distress (i.e., recovery), 15% had elevated distress beginning at treatment completion and through the next 6 months (i.e., re-entry phase), and 15% experienced high distress throughout the study period (Henselmans et al., 2010).

A fourth observation is that psychological adjustment involves both negative and positive dimensions. Positive and negative effects are separable constructs with distinct contributors and consequences (Diener, 1984). Even when faced with life-threatening diseases, adults have the capacity to experience joy, discover meaning, and conduct lives of purpose. Comparing positive (e.g., positive affect, social well-being, self-acceptance) and negative (e.g., depressive symptoms, anxiety) markers of adjustment before and after cancer diagnosis to those of a matched healthy control group, Costanzo et al. (2009) found that cancer survivors scored similarly to or better than controls on positive indicators.

Clearly, adjustment to chronic illness is complex and dynamic. It is important that researchers tailor their assessments to the theoretical questions of interest and acknowledge the limitations of any specific approach to conceptualizing adjustment. Both intensive longitudinal and experimental research in the focused adjustment domains and studies tapping multiple dimensions of adjustment are warranted to produce a comprehensive portrait of adaptation to chronic disease.

Theories of contributors to adjustment to chronic disease

General theories of adjustment to stressful experiences, such as that of Lazarus and Folkman (1984), can serve as a foundation for understanding adjustment to chronic disease. Accordingly, characteristics of the situation, personal resources, cognitive appraisals, and individual coping processes all influence adjustment. As depicted in Figure 5.1 (Hoyt and Stanton, 2012), the diverse contexts that influence appraisal and coping processes, ultimately shaping adjustment (e.g., Moos and Schaefer, 1993), include macrolevel factors such as socioeconomic status (SES), gender, and culture, as well as the interpersonal, intrapersonal, and disease-related contexts.

Contextual attributes shape the individual's appraisals of the nature of the threats and benefits arising from the disease experience (i.e., primary appraisal), as well as its controllability (i.e., secondary appraisal; Lazarus and Folkman, 1984). For example, chronic disease can pose threats to one's sense of self and financial standing, as well as destabilize perceived control over bodily integrity, ability to engage in activities, and social and career role fulfillment. Additionally, illness perceptions regarding disease cause, identity, and timeline (e.g., Leventhal et al., 2005) can influence adjustment. For example, adults who view their cancer as chronic (vs. acute or time limited) before chemotherapy report higher distress several months after completing treatment, when

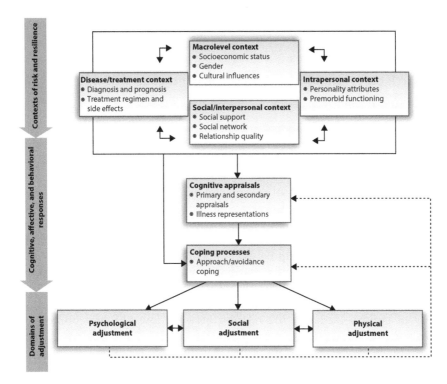

Figure 5.1 Contributors to adjustment to chronic illness. (From Hoyt, M.A., and Stanton, A.L., *Handbook of Health Psychology*, Taylor & Francis, New York, 2012.)

cancer stage is controlled statistically (Rabin et al., 2004). Along with aspects of the intrapersonal, interpersonal, and disease-related contexts, the individual's appraisals and her or his cognitive, emotional, and behavioral efforts to manage the stressor's demands (i.e., coping processes) theoretically determine psychological adjustment to the chronic disease.

Both Lazarus (1991) and other self-regulation theorists (Detweiler-Bedell et al., 2008; Leventhal et al., 2005; Rasmussen et al., 2006; Scheier and Bridges, 1995) also have emphasized the centrality of motivational goal-related processes to adjustment. To the extent that individuals expect to achieve central goals despite chronic illness or are able to identify and pursue alternative goals in the face of goal blockage, engagement in approach-oriented coping strategies and relatively positive adjustment is likely. On the other hand, continued pursuit of unobtainable goals or avoidance of pursuing meaningful alternative goals presages poorer adjustment.

Theories of personal growth following trauma (e.g., Calhoun and Tedeschi, 2006; Janoff-Bulman and Franz, 1997) also are relevant to the well-documented phenomenon of perceiving benefit in the experience of chronic disease (see Park et al., 2009). Adults with chronic disease cite enhanced relationships, life appreciation, personal strength, awareness of priorities, spirituality, and attention to health-promoting behaviors as resulting from chronic disease.

Research on contributors to adjustment to chronic disease

Sociocultural context

SES, as indicated by educational attainment, income, occupational status, geographic location, subjective assessment, or some combination of those variables, affects morbidity and mortality from chronic disease. Environmental and biobehavioral mechanisms, including access to and quality of health care, as well as health-related behaviors (e.g., smoking, substance use, eating patterns, physical activity) account in large part for compromised health outcomes associated with low SES. In a study of more than 11,000 German adults, SES was associated with lower QoL across six chronic diseases (Mielck et al., 2014). Mediators of the relationship between SES and poorer adjustment to chronic diseases require study. Candidate mediators include more consistent exposure to stressful life events and fewer psychosocial resources (Gallo and Matthews, 2003). In a prospective study of older coronary heart disease patients, a lower sense of control mediated the relation between low SES and poorer QoL (Barbareschi et al., 2008).

Although socioeconomic disparities can underlie ethnic/racial and sociocultural differences in psychological adjustment to chronic disease, there is some evidence that SES does not account completely for the obtained differences. With the caveat that relatively few longitudinal studies are available, the research suggests less favorable adjustment among ethnic minorities, particularly among Latino and African American groups in the United States (e.g., Prowe et al., 2006; Yanez et al., 2011). For example, Latinas with breast cancer reported poorer QoL than African American and other women, a relation mediated by mistrust in the medical system (Maly et al., 2008). Research to identify culturally relevant risk and protective processes for adjustment is needed.

As also seen in the general population, women tend to report higher distress than men within groups with chronic disease (Hagedoorn et al., 2008; Polsky et al., 2005; Shanmugasegaram et al., 2012). Gender-linked personality orientations (e.g., agency, communion; Helgeson and Fritz, 1998), role expectations (Hoyt, 2009), and numerous other factors are likely contributors to the gender difference. Beyond the observation of gender differences in adjustment, research is needed to identify the pathways through which gender shapes emotional, behavioral, and biological responses to chronic illness-related stressors.

Disease and treatment context

Prognosis, course (e.g., progressive versus remitting), treatment demands, and pain vary with regard to controllability, predictability, and severity across chronic diseases. However, individual differences can contribute to across- and within-disease variability. Interestingly, studies often demonstrate nonsignificant relationships between objective disease-related factors and psychological adjustment. Bardwell et al. (2006) examined the relative relationships of breast cancer parameters (e.g., stage, treatment, time elapsed since diagnosis), health behaviors, and psychosocial variables (e.g., social support, optimism) with depressive symptoms in more than 2000 women in treatment; disease and treatment factors were not significant predictors. As the authors suggest, subjective appraisals and other psychosocial factors may be more powerful predictors of adjustment than objective variables. For example, women's degree of uncertainty and acceptance regarding the pain of rheumatic disease partially determines the impact of pain on adjustment (Johnson et al., 2006; Kratz et al., 2007).

Interpersonal context

Although findings in the large literature on social support and chronic disease are not entirely consistent, compared with adults reporting less support, chronic disease patients reporting higher levels of social support exhibit more effective coping, higher self-esteem and life satisfaction, and fewer depressive symptoms. Strong social support partially explains trajectories of psychological adjustment to chronic illness (e.g., Helgeson et al., 2004). Both structural (e.g., marital status) and functional (e.g., emotional support provision) aspects of social support can contribute to favorable adjustment on multiple outcomes. For example, prospective studies of rheumatic disease patients demonstrate salutary effects on depressive symptoms (Demange et al., 2004), functional status (Fitzgerald et al., 2004), and disease activity (Holtzman and DeLongis, 2007). Reviewing the literature on coping and social support in chronic disease, Schreurs and de Ridder (1997) reported that prospective studies reveal approach-oriented coping as a consistent mechanism through which social support promotes well-being.

Absent or negative social relationships also are powerful predictors of adjustment to chronic disease. For example, social isolation prior to a breast cancer diagnosis in the Nurses' Health Study cohort predicted poorer QoL 4 years after diagnosis, explaining greater variance than did disease and treatment factors (Michael et al., 2002). Similarly, breast cancer patients without a confiding intimate relationship are more likely to develop depressive symptoms than patients with such a relationship (Burgess et al., 2005). Perceived criticism and avoidant behaviors by family and friends, as well as supportive behaviors, uniquely predicted gynecologic cancer patients' trajectory of depressive symptoms (Manne et al., 2008). Within couples, partners' levels of engagement and satisfaction with the relationship influence adjustment (see Berg and Upchurch, 2007; Revenson and DeLongis, 2011, for reviews). Dismissing emotions to avoid disagreements or protect the patient (i.e., protective buffering) may act to increase distress (e.g., Hinnen et al., 2009; Langer et al., 2009; Manne et al., 2007; Taylor et al., 2008).

Intrapersonal context

Among dispositional and historical factors, a history of depression or psychosocial dysfunction prior to chronic disease predicts vulnerability to unfavorable adjustment (Burgess et al., 2005; Conner et al., 2006; Tennen et al., 2006). Optimism, which is a generalized expectancy for positive outcomes, and pessimism are the most frequently examined dispositional attributes regarding adjustment to chronic disease. Higher optimism predicts reduced risk for depressive symptoms (odds ratio [OR] = 0.82) in the year after acute coronary syndrome (Ronaldson et al., 2015) and faster in-hospital recovery and return to normal life activities 1 year after cardiac surgery (Scheier et al., 2003). Optimism appears to work by enhancing the use of approach-oriented coping strategies, supporting social networks, reducing disease-related threat appraisals and avoidant coping, and prompting health-promoting behaviors (see Carver et al., 2010).

Cognitive appraisals of chronic disease

As postulated in theories of stress and coping, individuals' appraisals and expectancies regarding chronic disease influence adjustment. Prospective studies demonstrate that stronger appraisals of illness as a threat predict increased distress and depressive symptoms (e.g., Hart and Charles, 2013; Park et al., 2006; Lynch et al., 2008). Perceptions of lack of control over aspects of chronic disease in general also predict poorer adaptive outcomes (Bárez et al., 2009; Barry et al., 2006; Hommel et al., 2004).

Consistent with self-regulation theories, perceived disruptions in life goals and diminished ability to navigate them are related to poorer psychological outcomes in cancer patients (Hullman et al., 2015). By contrast, research demonstrates that engagement with alternative goals is associated with lower symptoms of depression and anxiety in cancer samples (Thompson et al., 2013; Zhu et al., 2015).

Evidence for a relation between finding benefit in the chronic disease experience and psychological adjustment is mixed (Algoe and Stanton, 2009). Among the most notable positive findings, perceived positive meaning and benefit finding after a breast cancer diagnosis predicted an increase in positive affect 5 years later (Bower et al., 2005) and lower distress and depressive symptoms 4–7 years later (Carver and Antoni, 2004).

Coping processes and adjustment to chronic disease

The ways in which individuals respond to the demands of illness influence physical and mental health (see Taylor and Stanton, 2007). Broadly, coping efforts are directed toward approaching or avoiding such demands (Suls and Fletcher, 1985). Approach-oriented coping includes active strategies such as problem solving, seeking information or social support, and expressing stressor-related emotions, whereas avoidance-oriented coping involves both cognitive and behavioral attempts at disengagement from the stressor. Avoidant strategies tend to be associated with lower positive affect, higher negative affect, poorer health behaviors, and poorer physical health; approach-oriented coping attempts evidence opposite relations, although they are somewhat less consistent (Carels et al., 2004; Duangdao and Roesch, 2008; Moskowitz et al., 2009; Penley et al., 2002; Roesch et al., 2005; Stanton, 2011).

Directions for research in adjustment to chronic disease

Several opportunities for research are apparent from a synthesis of this large literature. First, it is important to expand outcomes beyond indicators of distress to include functional outcomes and positive markers of adjustment. Second, the examination of interrelations of outcomes also is warranted. For example, depressive symptoms predict nonadherence to medication and completion of medical treatment in patients with chronic disease (Casey et al., 2008; DiMatteo et al., 2000; Mausbach et al., 2015; Rieckmann et al., 2006). Examination of the links between patient-reported psychosocial outcomes and chronic disease morbidities, and mortality is also recommended.

Although cross-sectional studies can hold value for hypothesis generation, longitudinal and experimental research is necessary to approach causal conclusions regarding determinants of psychological adjustment to chronic disease. Progress is evident, in that much of the research cited in this chapter involved longitudinal designs. Such investigations vary significantly in their specific methods, durations, and assessment procedures. Careful attention to methodology will be important to advance the understanding of how variation in adjustment unfolds across the trajectory of a chronic illness and how individuals experience changes in health over time. For example, with changes in physical health, patients might recalibrate their personal concepts of well-being, resulting in a response shift upon reassessment (see Schwartz et al., 2013). Likewise, measurement of personal growth and benefit from the chronic illness experience will need to better distinguish documented growth over time from retrospective reports of growth and preillness beliefs about the self (Taylor and Brown, 1983). Development and utilization of subjective and objective measures of adjustment will be useful.

Relatively few studies have tested comprehensive models of adjustment in longitudinal designs. As an example, support for a stress and coping model emerged in a study of prostate cancer patients and spouses (Kershaw et al., 2008), wherein cognitive appraisals (i.e., uncertainty, hopelessness, negativity) and approach- and avoidance-oriented coping processes mediated the influences of macrolevel (i.e., SES), interpersonal (i.e., social support and communication), intrapersonal (i.e., self-efficacy, current concerns), and disease-related (i.e., physical symptoms, disease phase) contextual factors on psychological and physical QoL. Eight months after study entry, the predictors accounted for 40% and 34% of the variance in QoL in psychological and physical domains, respectively. The use of experimental approaches to allow causal inference and longitudinal methods designed to model the dynamic relationships among risk and resilience contextual factors, cognitive-affective self-regulation and coping efforts, and domains of psychological and physical adjustment will provide the best opportunity to understand patients' diverse experiences and to advance the conceptualization of adjustment to chronic illness.

Identification of psychosocial, biological (e.g., inflammation, neuroendocrine function), and behavioral (e.g., medical regimen adherence) mechanisms of the links between contextual factors and psychosocial, and disease outcomes will pave the way toward efficient and effective interventions to enhance QoL and health in individuals living with chronic disease. As Stanton et al. (2007) suggested, theoretically grounded research on adjustment to chronic illness can refine such interventions by pointing to effective targets of intervention (e.g., Broadbent et al., 2009 on illness perceptions), suggesting potential mechanisms by which interventions may gain their utility (e.g., decreasing avoidant coping and increasing approach-oriented strategies; see Andersen et al., 2007), identifying patient groups to whom interventions might be targeted most productively (e.g., patients low in optimism), and developing intervention components for maximal effectiveness (e.g., increasing specific control appraisals). Greater translation of theory and research on adjustment to chronic disease into evidence-based clinical intervention is a vital goal.

References

Algoe, S.B., and Stanton, A.L. (2009). Is benefit finding good for individuals with chronic disease? In: C.L. Park, S.C. Lechner, M.H. Antoni, and A.L. Stanton (eds.), *Medical Illness and Positive Life Change: Can Crisis Lead to Personal Transformation?* (pp. 173–193). Washington, DC: American Psychological Association.

Andersen, B.L., Shelby, R.A., and Golden-Kreutz, D.M. (2007). RCT of a psychological intervention for patients with cancer: I. Mechanisms of change. *J. Consult. Clin. Psychol.*, *75*, 927–938.

Barbareschi, G., Sandrman, R., Kempen, G.I., and Ranchor, A.V. (2008). The mediating role of perceived control on the relationship between socioeconomic status and functional changes in older patients with coronary heart disease. *J. Gerontol. Psychol. Sci.*, *63B*, 353–361.

Bardwell, W.A., Natarajan, L., Dimsdale, J.E., Rock, C.L., Mortimer, J.E., Hollenbach, K., et al. (2006). Objective cancer-related variables are not associated with depressive symptoms in women treated for early-stage breast cancer. *J. Clin. Oncol.*, *24*(16), 2420–2427.

Bárez, M., Blasco, T., Fernández-Castro, J., and Viladrich, C. (2009). Perceived control and psychological distress in women with breast cancer: A longitudinal study. *J. Behav. Med.*, *32*(2), 187–196.

Barry, L.C., Kasl, S.V., Lictman, J., Vaccarino, V., and Krumholz, H.M. (2006). Perceived control and change in physical functioning after coronary artery bypass grafting: A prospective study. *Int. J. Behav. Med.*, *13*(3), 229–236.

Berg, C.A., and Upchurch, R. (2007). A developmental-contextual model of couples coping with chronic illness across the adult life span. *Psychol. Bull.*, *133*(6), 920–954.

Bower, J.E., Meyerowitz, B.E., Desmond, K.A., Bernaards, C.A., Rowland, J.H., and Ganz, P.A. (2005). Perceptions of positive meaning and vulnerability following breast cancer: Predictors and outcomes among long-term breast cancer survivors. *Ann. Behav. Med.*, *29*(3), 236–245.

Broadbent, E., Ellis, C.J., Thomas, J., Gamble, G., and Petrie, K.J. (2009). Further development of an illness perception intervention for myocardial infarction patients: A randomized controlled trial. *J. Psychosom. Res.*, *67*(1), 17–23.

Burgess, C., Cornelius, V., Love, S., Graham, J., Richards, M., and Ramirez, A. (2005). Depression and anxiety in women with early breast cancer: Five year observational cohort study. *BMJ*, *330*(7493), 702.

Calhoun, L.G., and Tedeschi, R.G. (eds.). (2006). *Handbook of Posttraumatic Growth: Research and Practice*. Mahwah, NJ: Erlbaum.

Carels, R.A., Musher-Eizenman, D., Cacciapaglia, H., Perez-Benitez, C.I., Christie, S., and O'Brien, W. (2004). Psychosocial functioning and physical symptoms in heart failure patients: A within individual approach. *J. Psychosom. Res.*, *56*(1), 95–101.

Carver, C.S., and Antoni, M.H. (2004). Finding benefit in breast cancer during the year after diagnosis predicts better adjustment 5 to 8 years after cancer. *Health Psychol.*, *23*(6), 595–598.

Carver, C.S., Scheier, M.F., and Segerstrom, S.C. (2010). Optimism. *Clin. Psychol. Rev.*, *30*(7), 879–889.

Casey, E., Hughes, J.W., Waechter, D., Josephson, R., and Rosneck, J. (2008). Depression predicts failure to complete phase-II cardiac rehabilitation. *J. Behav. Med.*, *31*(5), 421–431.

Conner, T.S., Tennen, H., Zautra, A.J., Affleck, G., Armeli, S., and Fifield, J. (2006). Coping with rheumatoid arthritis pain in daily life: Within-person analyses reveal hidden vulnerability for the formerly depressed. *Pain.*, *126*(1–3), 198–209.

Costanzo, E.S., Ryff, C.D., and Singer, B.H. (2009). Psychosocial adjustment among cancer survivors: Findings from a national survey of health and well-being. *Health Psychol.*, *28*(2), 147–156.

de Boer, A.G., Taskila, T., Ojajarvi, A., van Dijk, F.J., and Verbeek, J.H. (2009). Cancer survivors and unemployment: A meta-analysis and meta-regression. *JAMA.*, *301*(7), 753–762.

Demange, V., Guillemin, F., Baumann, M., Suurmeiher, B.M., Moum, T., Doelas, D., et al. (2004). Are there more than cross-sectional relationships of social support and social networks with functional limitations and psychological distress in early rheumatoid arthritis? *Arthritis Rheum.*, *51*(5), 782–791.

Detweiler-Bedell, J.B., Friedman, M.A., Leventhal, H., Miller, I.W., and Leventhal, E.A. (2008). Integrating co-morbid depression and chronic physical disease management: Identifying and resolving failures in self-regulation. *Clin. Psychol. Rev.*, *28*(8), 1426–1446.

Diener, E. (1984). Subjective well-being. *Psychol. Bull.*, *95*(3), 542–575.

DiMatteo, M.R., Lepper, H.S., and Croghan, T.W. (2000). Depression is a risk factor for noncompliance with medical treatment: A meta-analysis of the effects of anxiety and depression on patient adherence. *Arch. Intern. Med.*, *160*(14), 2101–2107.

Donovan, K.A., Small, B.J., Andrykowski, M.A., Munster, P., and Jacobsen, P.B. (2007). Utility of a cognitive-behavioral model to predict fatigue following breast cancer treatment. *Health Psychol.*, *26*(4), 464–472.

Duangdao, K.M., and Roesch, S.C. (2008). Coping with diabetes in adulthood: A meta-analysis. *J. Behav. Med.*, *31*(4), 291–300.

Fitzgerald, J.D., Orav, E.J., Lee, T.H., Marcantonio, E.R., Poss, R., Goldman, L., et al. (2004). Patient quality of life during the 12 months following joint replacement surgery. *Arthritis Rheum.*, *51*(1), 100–109.

Gallo, L.C., and Matthews, K.A. (2003). Understanding the association between socioeconomic status and physical health: Do negative emotions play a role? *Psychol. Bull.*, *129*(1), 10–51.

Golden, S.H., Lazo, M., Carnethon, M., Bertoni, A.G., Schreiner, P.J., Diez Roux, A.V., et al. (2008). Examining a bidirectional association between depressive symptoms and diabetes. *JAMA*, *299*(23), 2751–2759.

Gore, J.L., Kwan, L., Lee, S.P., Reiter, R.R., and Litwin, M. (2009). Survivorship beyond convalescence: 48-month quality-of-life outcomes after treatment for localized prostate cancer. *J. Natl. Cancer Inst.*, *101*(12), 888–892.

Hagedoorn, M., Sanderman, R., Bolks, H.N., and Coyne, J.C. (2008). Distress in couples coping with cancer: A meta-analysis and critical review of role and gender effects. *Psychol. Bull.*, *134*(1), 1–30.

Hart, S.L., and Charles, S.T. (2013). Age-related patterns in negative affect and appraisals about colorectal cancer over time. *Health Psychol.*, *32*(3), 302–310.

Helgeson V.S., and Fritz H.L. (1998). A theory of unmitigated communion. *Pers. Soc. Psychol. Rev.*, *2*(3), 173–183.

Helgeson, V.S., Snyder, P., and Seltman, H. (2004). Psychological and physical adjustment to breast cancer over 4 years: Identifying distinct trajectories of change. *Health Psychol.*, *23*(1), 3–15.

Henselmans, I., Helgeson, V.S., Seltman, H., de Vries, J., Sanderman, R., and Ranchor, A.V. (2010). Identification and prediction of distress trajectories in the first year after a breast cancer diagnosis. *Health Psychol.*, *29*(2), 160–168.

Hinnen, C., Ranchor, A.V., Baas, P.C., Sanderman, R., and Hagedoorn, M. (2009). Partner support and distress in women with breast cancer: The role of patients' awareness of support and level of mastery. *Psychol. Health*, *24*(4), 439–455.

Holtzman, S., and DeLongis, A. (2007). One day at a time: The impact of daily satisfaction with spouse responses on pain, negative affect and catastrophizing among individuals with rheumatoid arthritis. *Pain*, *131*(1–2), 202–213.

Hommel, K.A., Wagner, J.L., Chaney, J.M., White, M.M., and Mullins, L.L. (2004). Perceived importance of activities of daily living in rheumatoid arthritis: A prospective investigation. *J. Psychosom. Res.*, *57*(2), 159–164.

Hoyt, M.A. (2009). Gender role conflict and emotional approach coping in men with cancer. *Psychol. Health*, *24*(8), 981–996.

Hoyt, M.A., and Stanton, A.L. (2012). Adjustment to chronic illness. In: A.S. Baum, T.A. Revenson and J.E. Singer (eds.), *Handbook of Health Psychology* (2nd Edition, pp. 219–246). New York, NY: Taylor & Francis.

Hullman, S.E., Robb, S.L., and Rand, K.L. (2015). Life goals in patients with cancer: A systematic review of the literature. *Psycho-Oncology*, *25*(4), 387–399. DOI:10.1002/pon.3852

Janoff-Bulman, R., and Frantz, C.M. (1997). The impact of trauma on meaning: From meaningless world to meaningful life. In: M. Power and C. Brewin (eds.), *The Transformation of Meaning in Psychological Therapies: Integrating Theory and Practice* (pp. 91–106). Sussex, England: Wiley.

Johnson, L.M., Zautra, A.J., and Davis, M.C. (2006). The role of illness uncertainty on coping with fibromyalgia symptoms. *Health Psychol.*, *25*, 696–703.

Katon, W.J. (2011). Epidemiology and treatment of depression in patients with chronic medical illness. *Dialogues Clin. Neurosci.*, *13*, 7–23.

Kershaw, T.S., Mood, D,W., Newth, G., Ronis, D,L., Sanda, M.G., Vaishampayan, U., et al. (2008). Longitudinal analysis of a model to predict quality of life in prostate cancer patients and their spouses. *Ann. Behav. Med.*, *36*, 117–128.

Kratz, A.L., Davis, M.C., and Zautra, A.J. (2007). Pain acceptance moderates the relation between pain and negative affect in female osteoarthritis and fibromyalgia patients. *Ann. Behav. Med.*, *33*, 291–301.

Langer, S.L., Brown, J.D., and Syrjala, K.L. (2009). Intrapersonal and interpersonal consequences of protective buffering among cancer patients and caregivers. *Cancer*, *115*, 4311–4325.

Lazarus, R.S. (1991). *Emotion and Adaptation*. New York, NY: Oxford University Press.

Lazarus, R.S., and Folkman, S. (1984). *Stress, Appraisal, and Coping*. New York, NY: Springer.

Lazovich, D., Robien, K., Cutler, G., Virnig, B., and Sweeney, C. (2009). Quality of life in a prospective cohort of elderly women with and without cancer. *Cancer*, *115*, 4283–4297.

Leventhal, H., Halm, E., Horowitz, C., Leventhal, E.A., and Ozakinci, G. (2005). Living with chronic illness: A contextualized, self-regulation approach. In: S. Sutton, A. Baum and M. Johnston (eds.), *The Sage Handbook of Health Psychology* (pp. 197–240). Thousand Oaks, CA: Sage Publications.

Lustman, P.J., and Clouse, R.E. (2005). Depression in diabetic patients: The relationship between mood and glycemic control. *J. Diabetes Complications*, *19*, 113–122.

Lynch, B.M., Steginga, S.K., Hawkes, A.L., and Pakenham, K.I. (2008). Describing and predicting psychological distress after colorectal cancer. *Cancer*, *112*, 1363–1370.

Maly, R.C., Stein, J.A., Umezawa, Y., Leake, B., and Anglin, M.D. (2008). Racial/ethnic differences in breast cancer outcomes among older patients: Effects of physician communication and patient empowerment. *Health Psychol.*, *27*, 728–736.

Manne, S.L., Norton, T.R., Ostroff, J.S., Winkel, G., Fox, K., and Grana, G. (2007). Protective buffering and psychological distress among couples coping with breast cancer: The moderating role of relationship satisfaction. *J. Fam. Psychol.*, *21*, 380–388.

Manne, S., Rini, C., Rubin, S., Rosenblum, N., Bergman, C., Edelson, M., et al. (2008). Long-term trajectories of psychological adaptation among women diagnosed with gynecological cancers. *Psychosom. Med.*, *70*, 677–687.

Mausbach, B.T., Schwab, R.B., and Irwin, S.A. (2015). Depression as a predictor of adherence to adjuvant endocrine therapy (AET) in women with breast cancer: A systematic review and meta-analysis. *Breast Cancer Res. Treat.*, *152*, 239–246.

Michael, Y.L., Berkman, L.F., Colditz, G.A., Holmes, M.D., and Kawachi, I. (2002). Social networks and health-related quality of life in breast cancer survivors: A prospective study. *J. Psychosom. Res.*, *52*, 285–293.

Mielck, A., Vogelmann, M., and Leidl, R. (2014). Health-related quality of life and socioeconomic status: Inequalities among adults with chronic disease. *Health Qual. Life Outcomes*, *12*, 58.

Mitchell, A.J., Chan, M., Bhatti, H., Halton, M., Grassi, L., Johansen, C., et al. (2011). Prevalence of depression, anxiety, and adjustment disorder in oncological, haematological, and palliative-care settings: A meta-analysis of 94 interview-based studies. *Lancet Oncol.*, *12*, 160–174.

Moos, R.H., and Schaefer, J.A. (1984). The crisis of physical illness. In: R. Moos (ed.), *Coping with Physical Illness* (pp. 3–26). New York, NY: Plenum.

Moos, R.H., and Schaefer, J.A. (1993). Coping resources and processes: Current concepts and measures. In: L. Goldberger and S. Breznitz (eds.), *Handbook of Stress: Theoretical and Clinical Aspects* (2nd Edition, pp. 234–257). New York, NY: The Free Press.

Moskowitz, J.T., Hult, J.R., Bussolari, C., and Acree, M. (2009). What works in coping with HIV? A meta-analysis with implications for coping with serious illness. *Psychol. Bull.*, *135*, 121–141.

Müller-Tasch, T., Frankenstein, L., Holzapfel, N., Schellberg, D., Löwe, B., Nelles, M., et al. (2008). Panic disorder in patients with chronic heart failure. *J. Psychosom. Res.*, *64*, 299–303.

Murphy, B.M., Elliott, P.C., Worcester, M.U.C., Higgins, R.O., Le Grander, M.R., Roberts, S.B., et al. (2008). Trajectories and predictors of anxiety and depression in women during the 12 months following an acute cardiac event. *Br. J. Health Psychol.*, *13*, 135–153.

Park, C.L., Fenster, J.R., Suresh, D.P., and Bliss, D.E. (2006). Social support, appraisals, and coping as predictors of depression in congestive heart failure patients. *Psychol. Health.*, *21*, 773–789.

Park, C.L., Lechner, S.C., Antoni, M.H., and Stanton, A.L. (eds.). (2009). *Medical Illness and Positive Life Change: Can Crisis Lead to Personal Transformation?* Washington, DC: American Psychological Association.

Patrick, D.L. (2017). Conceptual approaches to perceived quality of life. Chapter 3, current volume.

Penley, J.A., Tomaka, J., and Wiebe, J.S. (2002). The association of coping to physical and psychological health outcomes: A meta-analytic review. *J. Behav. Med.*, 25, 551–603.

Polsky, D., Doshi, J.A., Marcus, S., Oslin, D., Rothbard, A., Thomas, N., et al. (2005). Long-term risk for depressive symptoms after a medical diagnosis. *Archiv. Intern. Med.*, 165, 1260–1266.

Prowe, B.D., Hamiliton, J., Hannock, N., Johnson, N., Finnie, R., Ko, J., et al. (2006). Quality of life of African American cancer survivors: A review of the literature. *Cancer*, 109, 435–445.

Rabin, C., Leventhal, H., and Goodin, S. (2004). Conceptualizations of disease timeline predicts posttreatment distress in breast cancer patients. *Health Psychol.*, 23, 407–412.

Rasmussen, H.N., Wrosch, C., Scheier, M.F., and Carver, C.S. (2006). Self-regulation processes and health: The importance of optimism and goal adjustment. *J. Pers.*, 74, 1721–1748.

Revenson, T.A., and DeLongis, A. (2011). Couples coping with chronic illness. In: S. Folkman (ed.), *The Oxford Handbook of Stress, Health, and Coping* (pp. 101–123). New York, NY: Oxford University Press.

Rieckmann, N., Gerin, W., Kronish, I.M., Burg, M.M., Chaplin, W.F., Kong, G., et al. (2006). Course of depressive symptoms and medication adherence after acute coronary syndromes: An electronic medication monitoring study. *J. Am. Coll. Cardiol.*, 48, 2218–2222.

Roesch, S.C., Adams, L., Hines, A., Palmores, A., Vyas, P., Tran, C., et al. (2005). Coping with prostate cancer: A meta-analytic review. *J. Behav. Med.*, 28, 281–293.

Ronaldson, A., Molloy, G.J., Wikman, A., Poole, L., Kaski, J.C., and Steptoe, A. (2015). Optimism and recovery after acute coronary syndrome: A clinical cohort study. *Psychosom. Med.*, 77, 311–318.

Rose, J.H., Kypriotakis, G., Bowman, K.F., Einstadter, D., O'Toole, E.E., Mechekano, R., et al. (2009). Patterns of adaptation in patients living long term with advanced cancer. *Cancer*, 115, 4298–4310.

Rutledge, T., Reis, V.A., Linke, S.E., Greenberg, B.H., and Mills, P.J. (2006). Depression in heart failure a meta-analytic review of prevalence, intervention effects, and associations with clinical outcomes. *J Am Coll Cardiol.*, 48, 1527–1537.

Scheier, M.F., and Bridges, M.W. (1995). Person variables and health: Personality predispositions and acute psychological states as shared determinants of disease. *Psychosom. Med.*, 57, 255–268.

Scheier, M.F., Matthews, K.A., Owens, J.F., Magovern, G.J., Lefebvre, R.C., Abbott, A.R., et al. (2003). Dispositional optimism and recovery from coronary artery bypass surgery: The beneficial effects on physical and psychological well-being. In: P. Salovey and A.J. Rothman (eds.), *Social Psychology of Health: Key Readings in Social Psychology* (pp. 342–361). New York, NY: Psychology Press.

Schreurs, K.M.G., and de Ridder, D.T.D. (1997). Integration of coping and social support perspectives: Implications for the study of adaptation to chronic diseases. *Clin. Psychol. Rev.*, 17, 89–112.

Schwartz, C.E., Ahmed, S., Sawatzky, R., Sajobi, T., Mayo, N., Finkelstein, J., et al. (2013). Guidelines for secondary analysis in search of response shift. *Qual. Life Res.*, 22, 2663–2673.

Shanmugasegaram, S., Russell, K.L., Kovacs, A.H., Stewart, D.E., and Grace, S.L. (2012). Gender and sex differences in prevalence of major depression in coronary artery disease patients: A meta-analysis. *Maturitas*, 73, 305–311.

Stanton, A.L. (2011). Regulating emotions during stressful experiences: The adaptive utility of coping through emotional approach. In: S. Folkman (ed.), *The Oxford Handbook of Stress, Health, and Coping* (pp. 369–386). New York, NY: Oxford University Press.

Stanton, A.L., Revenson, T.A., and Tennen, H. (2007). Health psychology: Psychological adjustment to chronic disease. *Ann. Rev. Psychol., 58,* 565–592.

Steptoe, A., Deaton, A., and Stone, A.A. (2015). Subjective wellbeing, health, and ageing. *Lancet, 385,* 640–648.

Suls, J., and Fletcher, B. (1985). The relative efficacy of avoidant and nonavoidant coping strategies: A meta-analysis. *Health Psychol., 4,* 249–288.

Taylor, C.L.C., Badr, H., Lee, J.H., Fossella, F., Pisters, K., Gritz, E.R., et al. (2008). Lung cancer patients and their spouses: Psychological and relationship functioning within 1 month of treatment initiation. *Ann. Behav. Med., 36,* 129–140.

Taylor, S.E. (1983). Adjustment to threatening events: A theory of cognitive adaptation. *Am. Psychol., 38,* 1161–1173.

Taylor, S.E., and Brown, J.D. (1983). Illusion and well-being: A social psychological perspective on mental health. *Psychol. Bull., 103,* 193–210.

Taylor, S.E., and Stanton, A.L. (2007). Coping resources, coping processes, and mental health. *Annu. Rev. Clin. Psychol., 3,* 377–401.

Tennen, H., Affleck, G., and Zautra, A. (2006). Depression history and coping with chronic pain: A daily process analysis. *Health Psychol., 25,* 370–379.

Thompson, E., Stanton, A.L., and Bower, J.E. (2013). Situational and dispositional goal adjustment in the context of metastatic cancer. *J. Pers., 81,* 441–451.

Van 't Land, H., Verdurmen, J., ten Have, M., van Dorsselaer, S., Beekman, A., and de Graaf, R. (2010). The association between arthritis and psychiatric disorders; results from a longitudinal population-based study. *J. Psychosom. Res., 68,* 187–193.

Ward, B.W., Schiller, J.S., and Goodman, R.A. (2014). Multiple chronic conditions among US adults: A 2012 update. *Prev. Chronic Dis., 11,* 130389.

World Health Organization. (2015). Noncommunicable Diseases. Accessed June, 2015. Available at: http://www.who.int/mediacentre/factsheets/fs355/en/

Yanez, B., Thompson, E.H., and Stanton, A.L. (2011). Quality of life among Latina breast cancer patients: A systematic review of the literature. *J. Cancer Surviv., 5,* 191–207.

Zhu, L., Ranchor, A.V., van der Lee, M., Garssen, B., Sanderman, R., and Schroevers, M.J. (2015). The role of goal adjustment in symptoms of depression, anxiety and fatigue in cancer patient receiving psychosocial care: A longitudinal study. *Psychol. Health., 30,* 268–283.

Section 2

Measurement

6 Contemporary perspectives on the epistemology of measurement in the social sciences

Alain Leplège

The aim of Section 2 is to identify and discuss new perspectives offered by modern psychometric methods for the validation and calibration of measurement and to present two innovative empirical projects that illustrate how these new methods can contribute to the actual development of specific instruments in adequation with concepts and domains of investigation.

To clarify the epistemological context of Section 2, we shall rapidly recall an important issue for the epistemology of measurement in the social sciences. We shall concentrate more particularly on those social sciences in which experimentation and quantification are most developed, for example public health, or the sciences of education, because these disciplines routinely use measurement in experimental designs. In an empirical perspective, every measurement is considered to be the expression of a magnitude (a scalar) by a real number in a reference frame comprising an object to be measured, an agent, and an experimental protocol. The instruments of measurement (the agents) are standardized questionnaires with closed-response choices constructed so as to quantify abstract concepts that cannot be observed directly; these are known as latent variables. The objective is to foster the development of explanatory or even causal hypotheses that can be subjected to empirical testing. We are interested here in the conceptions of measurement that underpin certain measurement models used in the development of standardized questionnaires, in the way the invariance requirement is put into operation, and in the methodological consequences and impact of these conceptions of measurement on the question of demarcation in the social sciences in light of their current applications in research projects.

Many doubts and criticisms have been raised against the scientific pretence of the social sciences. They have been accused of not being mathematical, experimental, and predictive enough. These criticisms take the natural sciences, in particular physics, as a norm for scientificity. Against these criticisms, two lines of defense of the scientificity of the social sciences have been raised:

1   The social sciences are not reducible to any other types of sciences such as biology (e.g., Fodor, 1980), and the specificity of their object implies that the methodological criteria of scientificity that have been identified and developed for the study of the epistemological problems raised by the natural sciences do not apply to the social sciences. This implies that it would be reasonable, in studying the social sciences, to distance oneself from the systematic and depressing reference to physics and other natural sciences (Ogien, 2001). This implies also some kind of methodological eclecticism and to value methodological diversity and triangulation.

2   A different line of defense of the scientificity of the social sciences refuses to call for specific methodological frameworks and for distance from the model of the natural sciences. It may be seen as belonging to a program of naturalization of the social sciences and to the idea that there is some unity among the sciences, at least when it comes to research methodology principles. This can also be called a reductionist perspective because, in principle, the (1) social sciences could be reduced to (2) psychology, which in turn can be reduced to (3) biology, which in turn can be reduced to (4) chemistry, which in turn can finally be reduced to (5) physics. From a methodological point of view, this implies that the nomologico-deductive framework is the framework of choice for the empirical study of human and social facts. For example, Durkheim has held such a position in sociology, Pieron and Watson in psychology, as well as several decision and game theorists. For all these authors, the use of the nomologico-deductive framework is valid, in the social sciences as in the natural sciences, with the aim to enable the identification of invariant relationships (or even universal laws) among variables from which singular facts should be deduced (e.g., Lazarsfeld, 1961).

For this second perspective, which we favor, the epistemological problems of measurement problems are transversal (Leplege, 2003). The validity of the conclusion of the experimental method, which makes it possible to test the consequences of a hypothesis developed inductively by comparing them with empirical observations, is dependent on the validity and precision of the observations and measures being made. This is why Malifaud (2001) has said that measurement in science has two fundamental roles: (1) that of mathematization or quantification of phenomenon and (2) that of empirical touchstone. This is also why the epistemology of measurement questions is as important in the social science as in the natural sciences.

This being said, the specific epistemological question addressed by Section 2 is the following: Should measurement concepts and models in empirical social sciences be different from measurement concepts and models in the natural sciences, or, framed differently, can we conceive of measurement in the social sciences in the same way as measurement in the natural sciences? More specifically, the question is, should measurements developed for the social sciences for the purpose of aggregating or comparing subjects and groups meet the same kind of invariance requirements as those used in the natural sciences? By invariance one means here the absence of item bias (one would not want, for instance, subjects belonging to different groups, e.g., men and women, to understand a given question differently if one wants to use the responses to this question to compare these two groups).

The objective of Chapters 7 and 8 in Section 2 is to present and discuss a class of probabilistic measurement models first published in 1959 by the Danish mathematician Georg Rasch and recently used in the social sciences (Rasch, 1960). This class of measurement models is remarkable by its conception of measurement, which is very similar to the conception of measurement in the natural sciences. After a brief description of the historical circumstances of this discovery, their main common property, named "specific objectivity" by Georg Rasch, will be presented (Rasch, 1977). These two chapters discuss the signification of this discovery for the methodology and epistemology of measurement in the social sciences and its contribution to the debate we alluded to at the beginning of this chapter.

Chapters 9 and 10 aim at illustrating how these epistemological issues and methodological perspectives are operationalized and how they may contribute to the development of outcome measures for contemporary research projects. Chapter 9 by Tamm et al. provides an update on the methodological recommendations regarding the development of contemporary instruments such as the Patient-Reported Outcomes Measurement Information System (PROMIS), which is currently one of the most comprehensive efforts worldwide for the development of tools for assessing a patient's subjective health status (www.nihpromis.org). Chapter 10 by Peter et al. describes a novel method of interacting with the subjects so as to better measure performances in daily life, as opposed to capacities evaluated in laboratory conditions while drawing on modern psychometric methodologies to assess the properties of such an experimental arrangement.

References

Fodor, J. (1980). Methodological solipsism considered as a research strategy in cognitive science. *Behav. Brain Sci.*, *3*, 63–73.

Lazarsfeld, P.F. (1961). Note on the history of quantification in sociology—Trends, sources and problems. In: H. Wolf (ed.), *Quantification, A History of the Meaning of Measurement in the Natural and Social Sciences*. New York, NY: Bobbs-Merril.

Leplege, A. (ed.) (2003). Epistemology of measurement in the social sciences: Historical and contemporary perspectives. *Soc. Sci. Inf.*, *42*(4), 451–462.

Malifaud, P. (2001). "Mesure", *Encyclopaedia Universalis*, CD rom version 6.

Ogien, R. (2001). *Épistémologie des sciences sociales*. In: Jean-Michel Berthelot (dir.) (p. 521 ssq) Paris: Presses Universitaires de France.

Rasch, G. (1960). *Probabilistic Models for Some Intelligence and Attainment Tests*. Danish Institute of Educational Research, 1960; Chicago, IL: University of Chicago Press, 1980; MESA Press, 1993.

Rasch, G. (1977). On specific objectivity: An attempt to formalising the request for generality and validity of scientific statements. *Dan. Yearb. Philos.*, *14*, 58–94.

7 Advances in social measurement: A Rasch measurement theory

David Andrich

Introduction

Although now rendered in a relatively simple form, which makes its principles understandable to elementary school children, measurement is sophisticated, the practice of which has led to the remarkable advancement of the natural sciences. Not surprisingly, therefore, the characteristics of measurement have been of substantial interest to social scientists. This chapter highlights some of these characteristics in making the case that the contributions of the Danish mathematician and statistician Georg Rasch to social measurement can justifiably be called a *measurement theory*, referred to in this chapter as the Rasch measurement theory (RMT). The case is based on three of Rasch's major publications that resulted from a substantial body of empirical and epistemological studies (Rasch, 1960, 1961, 1977). Recently, Stone and Stenner (2014) used the same publications to highlight Rasch's distinctive contribution to epistemology and social measurement—the centrality of invariant comparisons within a frame of reference.

Measurement is concerned with properties considered in terms of more or less, and measured by instruments that operate in some relevant range. In this chapter, the term *property* will be used in general and the term *variable* will be used in the context of measurements. In addition, it is taken for granted that the variable is conceived of as unidimensional and continuous and that, to some specified level of precision, measurements are characterized by real numbers that can be mapped onto a real number line.

In Andrich (2004), it was argued that the controversy that sometimes occurs between proponents of Rasch models and proponents who see the Rasch models as only special cases of general response models can be seen as a clash of paradigms in the sense of Kuhn (1970). That full argument will not be repeated here. Instead, I will draw on features of the Rasch paradigm within a summary of Kuhn's argument to make the case that there is an RMT that has the hallmarks of a scientific theory in general and of a measurement theory in particular. To emphasize the case, brief contrasts are made with classical test theory (CTT) and item response theory (IRT).

An earlier version of this paper was presented at the Scientific Congress meeting on Chronic Diseases, Perceived Health, Stakes and Future, Nancy, France, June 4–6, 2014.

Scientific theory

To set the context for the case for an RMT, some comments on the use of the term theory are required. The term theory has been considered in its many different uses, including, for example, the sense of (1) theory versus practice, (2) a coherent body of problems, (3) a unified conceptual framework, and (4) a scientific theory (O'Connor, 1957). Although these uses can be shown to overlap, the emphasis in this chapter is on the defining elements of a scientific theory.

A scientific theory is seen consistently to summarize a coherent body of knowledge that purports to not only describe but also to *explain* a class of related substantive phenomena. Because they are well developed, examples of scientific theories are readily given in the field of physics. Examples are Newton's theory of gravitation, Einstein's theory of relativity, the theory of thermodynamics, and quantum theory. Other examples in the natural sciences include Wegener's theory of plate tectonics and Darwin's theory of evolution. The well-known examples in psychology are Freud's theory of the subconscious and Piaget's theory of cognitive development.

A scientific theory inevitably has two broad distinctive components. First, it must explain empirical phenomena. A new theory does not have to explain all relevant phenomena immediately, but those it does explain need to be important in the field. The relationship to empirical phenomena concerns the substantive component of the theory. Second, and in addition, it must have its own internal coherence and logic. This internal logic provides the facility for deduction. From these deductions, it is possible to predict or explain new phenomena not immediately evident. If these phenomena are confirmed empirically, it further confirms the substantive theory. Although there is a sense in which each paradigm constrains the evidence that is relevant to a theory within that paradigm, this potential circularity can be broken, and an old paradigm with its own logic and explanations can be overturned. Kuhn (1970) provides an eloquent analysis of episodes when a new theory replaces an existing one. He calls these episodes *scientific revolutions*.

An ultimate form of internal logic, evidenced most clearly in physics, is reached when a theory is expressed in mathematical language. Then mathematical deduction can be used to deduce relationships that otherwise would not have been entertained. It will be seen that mathematical deductions that give new insights are an element of RMT. A very powerful mathematical system that appears in scientific theories involves numbers that arise from measurements.

Definitions of measurement

This section summarizes three related definitions of measurement found in the extensive literature by social scientists on measurement. These are classical, representational, and additive conjoint.

The classical definition of measurement

Measurement is distinguished by a *unit*. The idea of a unit can be illustrated readily with the idea of a beam balance for measuring mass. The two objects constructed or found to have the same mass can be demonstrated readily with a beam balance. The identical mass of the two objects can be declared the unit. Then, if the two objects with the unit mass are placed on one side of the balance, and a new object with a mass balances the beam, the new mass is two times the mass of the unit. The process can, in principle, be continued in establishing a measurement of mass of other objects in a relevant range for the balance. A second feature of measurement that the beam balance exemplifies is that to measure the mass of an object it is necessary to somehow manifest the mass. In the above example, the effect of gravity on the masses is manifested on the instrument, the beam balance, in a controlled way. It is common to suggest that social measurement requires manifestation of variables because, instead of being observable, they are *latent*. The above example indicates that manifesting a variable through some instrument is also necessary in the measurement of mass and is typical in the natural sciences. Therefore, the idea of a latent variable is a feature of all measurement and is not confined to social variables.

The above example of the measurement of mass on a beam balance illustrates the classical definition of measurement (Michell, 2003)—that it is the ratio of the amount of the property of an object relative to an amount declared to be a unit. Historically, the tangible measurement of mass using the beam balance has been very successful without major theoretical conceptualizations. However, because of the pervasive effect of gravity on mass, the separation of the concept of the mass of an object from the effect of gravity on its mass (force of attraction to Earth) was a major conceptual leap that required the geniuses of Galileo and Newton to make. From Newton's laws, the well-known equation $F = ma$ relating the reaction of acceleration when force F impacts on mass m gives

$$a = F/m. \tag{7.1}$$

The beam balance is one way of measuring mass. There are other ways. In general, multiple methods of the measurement of the same property of different objects appear in well-developed sciences (Bock and Jones, 1968). Once the instrument has been well constructed, its application according to established, standardized procedures can be relatively simple.

Representational characterization of measurement

A second definition of measurement is representational—the properties of objects can be assigned numbers in such a way that the relationship among the properties is the same as the relationship among the numbers (Ellis, 1966; Roberts, 1979; Krantz et al., 1971). This relationship permits arithmetical operation on the numbers from which inferences among the properties can be made. Concatenation is an example in which the properties of real numbers can be applied.

The parallel between concatenation and arithmetical operations on measurements is shown in Newton's laws. Thus, if forces F_i and F_j operate on an object n of mass m_n, then

$$a_{ni} = F_i \, / \, m_n, \quad a_{nj} = F_j \, / \, m_n$$
$$a_{ni} + a_{nj} = F_i \, / \, m_n + F_j \, / \, m_n$$
$$a_{ni} + a_{nj} = (F_i + F_j) \, / \, m_n$$
$$a_{n(i+j)} = F_{i+j} \, / \, m_n$$

$$\tag{7.2}$$

which implies that the sum of two forces operating on the same object generates an acceleration, which is the sum of the original accelerations with the form of Equation 7.1 retained. The conceptualization of measurement as representational, with implied concatenation, seems to originate with the work of Campbell (1920).

Additive conjoint measurement

A third definition of measurement, consistently considered in the social sciences, is the idea of *additive* or *simultaneous conjoint measurement* (Luce and Tukey, 1964). Perhaps the reason for its popularity stems from its abstract nature, which liberates it from the literal concatenation exemplified above with masses.

This abstraction implies that, even in the absence of literal concatenation, if the variables in the cells, rows, and columns of a two-way table can be transformed monotonically to produce an additive structure, then a structure analogous to concatenation is preserved. An example of such a two-way table might be one where the rows reflect an assessment of socioeconomic status and the columns reflect an independent test of intelligence, and the cells reflect academic achievement. Then, if there exist transformations of achievement, intelligence, and socioeconomic status that show achievement is the sum of intelligence and socioeconomic status, conjoint additivity is achieved.

All three definitions—classical, representational, and additive conjoint—are compatible with measurement found in the natural sciences, which is sometimes said to characterize *fundamental* measurement. Although there is substantial debate on the relative merits of these definitions, this chapter does not engage in these debates (Schwager, 1991). Instead, it simply notes that these definitions do not lead to incompatible results and suggests that any other definitions or explanations of measurement must be compatible with them. Thus, an RMT would also need to be compatible with them.

It is emphasized that Stevens' (1946) definition that measurement is the assignment of numerals to objects according to rules is not considered because it does not mention *properties* of objects, but simply objects; it does not mention numbers, but simply numerals; and it seems any rule will suffice.

Following the above definitions of measurement and before considering these in relation to Rasch's contribution to a measurement theory, we now summarize the *structure* and *function* of measurements in scientific theories.

Structure among measurements in scientific theories

The *structure* among measurements in any scientific theory (or law) is extremely simple. In a review of Krantz et al. (1971) axiomatization of the representational definition of measurement, Ramsay (1975) notes that

> Also somewhat outside the concerns of the rest of the book, this chapter ... deals with the fact that virtually all the laws of physics can be expressed numerically as multiplications or divisions of measurements. (p. 258)

and

> Although the authors cannot explain this fact to their own satisfaction, the extension to behavioral science is obvious: we may have to await fundamental measurement before we will see any real progress in quantitative laws of behavior. (p. 262)

The multiplicative structure noted by Ramsay is clear, for example, in Newton's law relating force, mass, and acceleration. Thus, a measurement theory should be compatible with a multiplicative structure among measured variables. However, note that Krantz, Luce, Suppes, and Tverskey "cannot explain" this multiplicative structure.

Function of measurement in physical science

The typical perceived *function* of measurement is that it leads to scientific theories; Kuhn's (1961) analysis suggests otherwise:

> In textbooks the numbers that result from measurements usually appear as the archetypes of the "irreducible and stubborn facts" to which the scientist must, by struggle, make his theories conform. But in scientific practice, as seen through the journal literature, the scientist often seems rather to be struggling with facts, trying to force them to conformity with a theory he does not doubt. (Kuhn, 1961, p. 193)

If discovering theories from measurements is not the role of measurement, as portrayed in textbooks, it seems necessary to understand the role it has in the advancement of science. Kuhn gives the answer:

> To the extent that measurement and quantitative technique play an especially significant role in scientific discovery, they do so precisely because, by displaying serious anomaly, they tell scientists when and where to look

for a new phenomenon. To the nature of that phenomenon, they usually provide no clues. (p. 205)

As with the definitions of measurement and the structure of relationships among variables, any measurement theory should be compatible with Kuhn's analysis of the function of measurement in science.

Measurement as a methodological theory—invariance of comparisons

It has been indicated that a scientific theory has the characteristic of explaining substantive, empirical phenomena. This chapter now makes one distinction between such a scientific theory and a measurement theory. The distinction arises because the idea of measurement in the literature, and in this chapter, transcends particular substantive measurements. Thus, although the measurement of mass and the equally familiar measurement of temperature involve substantively different variables with very different instruments, they have features in common. It is these common features that are also common to the measurement of all variables, which suggests that there can be a theory of measurement. Such a theory, relative to substantive theories, might be classed a *methodological* theory (Punch, 2009). The other features of a theory such as explanation, prediction, and so on, are retained. Thus, a measurement theory should apply to measurement in general, both physical and potentially social.

Requirements of a measurement theory

From the above summary of the general properties of a theory, we now summarize the characteristics expected of a measurement theory.

Compatibility with known features of measurement

A measurement theory needs to be compatible with known features of measurement. For this purpose, we take as given (1) the three definitions of measurement: classical, representational, and additive conjoint; (2) that the structure of measured variables in scientific laws is multiplicative; and (3) that the function of measurement is to disclose anomalies. Therefore, any theory of measurement must be compatible with these definitions, structure, and function.

In addition, a measurement theory needs to have two further characteristics, *explanation* and *deduction*.

Explanation beyond description

A measurement theory needs to not only merely *describe* the above properties of measurement, but also go to some length toward *explaining* them. An explanation would contribute to unifying the three definitions, the structure and the function, of measurement and go some way at least to explaining, not merely describing, the multiplicative structure of the laws of physics.

Deduced new insights

Finally, a measurement theory should provide generalizations and deductions that would not be available from a mere description of measurement.

To help make a case that an RMT meets the above criteria, which for the purposes of exposition will not be presented in the same order as above, this section summarizes the historical, ground-breaking work carried out by Rasch. Before doing so, we note the titles of Rasch's publications referenced earlier, which show Rasch working toward a major methodological position regarding not only measurement, but also epistemology. These are

1 Probabilistic models for some intelligence and attainment tests
2 On general laws and the meaning of measurement in psychology
3 On specific objectivity: an attempt at formalizing the request for generality and validity of scientific statements

As shown in this chapter, his position on epistemology is the basis of the case for an RMT.

The multiplicative Poisson model and its elements in an RMT

In the early 1950s, Rasch participated in a study designed to assess an intervention for students who had demonstrated reading difficulties. One of the studies counted the errors students made in reading words in a text. The design required that the texts students read should not be so difficult that they became frustrated but neither should they be so easy that the students were not challenged. The number of errors each student made should be of the order of 5%–10%. Because different students had different initial proficiencies and the improvement over time was studied, it meant that the same text could not be given to all students in the study or to the same student on different occasions. This design is shown in Rasch (1960). For the purpose of this chapter, it is sufficient to focus on the reading of two texts by a single group of persons.

With the probability of an error being relatively small, and the opportunity to make one relatively large, Rasch hypothesized that the Poisson distribution

$$\Pr\{X = x; \lambda\} = [\lambda^x / x!] / \gamma, \tag{7.3}$$

where $\gamma = \exp(\lambda) = \sum_{x=0}^{\infty} \lambda^x / x!$ is the sum of the numerators ensuring that Equation 7.3 is a probability and would characterize the responses. However, rather than characterizing a population of responses among all students that might have been a standard characterization, Rasch resolved the parameter λ

into two components, one for each person, and one for each text: $\lambda_{ni} = \alpha_i/\xi_n$ where $\alpha_i > 0$ is a real number characterizing the difficulty of text I and $\xi_n > 0$ is a real number characterizing the reading proficiency of person n, giving

$$\Pr\{X_{ni} = x; \alpha_i, \xi_n\} = [(\alpha_i/\xi_n)^x/\gamma_{ni}], \tag{7.4}$$

in which

$$E[X_{ni}] = \alpha_i/\xi_n \tag{7.5}$$

is the theoretical mean number of errors. Rasch called Equation 7.4 the multiplicative Poisson model (MPM). It is evident that, as might be expected, the mean number of errors is proportional to the text's difficulty α_i, and inversely proportional to the person's proficiency ξ_n.

Because of his studies with R. A. Fisher where he learned of statistical sufficiency, Rasch obtained the probability of the total score of any person on two texts, and formed the conditional probability of the score on one of the texts given the total score on both texts. The plots resulted in graphs similar to the one shown in Figure 7.1 (Rasch, 1960, p. 25). We do not detail the theory of the graph in Figure 7.1, which follows from Equation 7.4, but note that it includes the line whose slope is given by $\pi_{ij} = \alpha_i/(\alpha_i + \alpha_j)$ and confidence

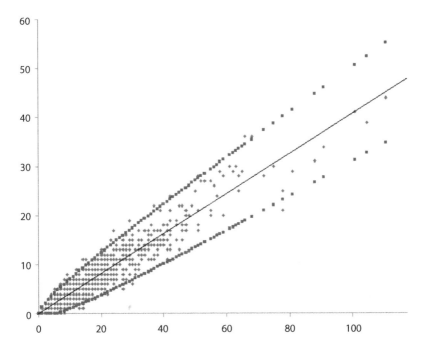

Figure 7.1 Plot of the error count of one text against the total error count on two texts together with binomial 95% confidence limits

limits around this slope. From graphs such as Figure 7.1, Rasch concluded that the data were consistent with the MPM. The estimate of π_{ij} is given by

$$\hat{\pi}_{ij} = x_{+i}/(x_{+i} + x_{+j}) = \hat{\alpha}_i/(\hat{\alpha}_i + \hat{\alpha}_j), \tag{7.6}$$

where the "+" in the subscripts of x_{+j}, x_{+j} indicate summation over the sample of persons.

Compatibility of the MPM with characteristics of measurement

The MPM was the basis of Rasch's insights into measurement. We now consider the degree to which the insights and developments he gained from them can be considered a measurement theory. The required criteria included compatibility with the three definitions of measurement summarized above, with explanation and prediction, and with Ramsay's and Kuhn's respective observations on the structure and function of measurement.

Compatibility with the classical definition of measurement

First, from Equation 7.5, it can be seen readily that an estimate of the relative difficulty of text i to text j is given by

$$\frac{\hat{\alpha}_i}{\hat{\alpha}_j} = \frac{\hat{\pi}_{ij}}{1 - \hat{\pi}_{ij}} = \frac{x_{+i}}{x_{+i}}. \tag{7.7}$$

The example of Figure 7.1 was simulated with 1000 persons and $\alpha_i/\alpha_j = 1.5$. The estimate of this ratio is a very accurate $\hat{\alpha}_i/\hat{\alpha}_j = 9970/6674 = 1.467$.

It is evident that the *relative* difficulties of the two texts can be expressed as a ratio, and that if text i is given the value of 1 unit in reading difficulty, then text j has an estimated difficulty of 1.467 in that unit. Rasch discussed the concept of quantity and formalized the *ability* of a person, referred to in this chapter as *proficiency*, the *difficulty* of a text, and the possibility of choosing one of these to define a unit (Rasch, 1960, p. 16).

In addition, if several texts with different groups of persons are assessed, as in the design in Rasch (1960), and if the responses conform to the MPM, then all texts can be expressed as a ratio of difficulty relative to one text chosen as a unit. Moreover, given an estimate of the difficulty of a text and an error count on just that text, then an estimate of a person's proficiency in the same unit can be obtained from Equation 7.5. This is analogous to obtaining the mass of an object relative to the mass of the other side of a beam balance defined in terms of a unit.

Thus, the MPM example with reading errors is consistent with the classical definition of measurement in that the relative difficulty of two texts is an estimate of the ratio of one quantity to another defined as a unit.

Compatibility with concatenation

Although the full rationale that shows concatenation formally is a little more complex than shown below, it is evident from Equation 7.5 that if person n reads a second text with difficulty α_j, then

$$E[X_{ni}] + E[X_{nj}] = \alpha_i \, / \, \xi_n + \alpha_j / \xi_n,$$
$$E[X_{ni} + X_{nj}] = (\alpha_i + \alpha_j) / \xi_n, \tag{7.8}$$
$$E[X_{n(i+j)}] = \alpha_{i+j} / \xi_n.$$

Equation 7.8 reflects that if two texts of difficulties α_i, α_j were concatenated and a person reads both texts, the expected value for the total number of errors is the sum of the errors on each of the texts and the difficulty of the combined text α_{i+j} is simply the sum of the difficulties of the individual texts $\alpha_i + \alpha_j$ with Equation 7.8 retaining the same structure as Equation 7.5. This concatenation is entirely consistent with the concatenation in classical physics.

Compatibility with a multiplicative structure

Third, the relationship between the person and text parameters in the MPM is multiplicative, again consistent with Ramsay's observation.

We consider compatibility with additive conjoint measurement and the function of measurement in science following a consideration of Rasch's generalization from the above example that meets the criterion of *explaining* measurement.

Explaining measurement

It was indicated above that a theory should *explain*, rather than merely describe, its domain of relevance. It is suggested that the three definitions of measurement, though sophisticated, are essentially descriptive summaries of measurement rather than explanations. In addition, Ramsay stresses that the multiplicative structure of measured variables is not explained in general, nor in particular, by Krantz et al. (1971) axiomatization of the representational measurement. In this section, the case is made that Rasch's abstraction from the MPM contributes to *explaining* aspects of measurement.

First we note that the MPM is not only compatible with all three definitions of measurement and the multiplicative structure of theories in classical physics, but also Rasch recognized these compatibilities in the publications cited above. However, rather than focusing on any of these, he made a different generalization from the MPM that leads to a measurement theory that explains measurement. The significance of the MPM in making this generalization was not immediately obvious even to Rasch, but depended on a conversation with Frisch, a Norwegian economist with whom Rasch was acquainted (Rasch, 1960, 1977; Andrich, 2004). Once Rasch made the abstraction, he proceeded to make a case for what effectively is an explanation of measurement.

A key feature of Equation 7.6, from which an estimate of the ratio of the difficulties of two texts can be calculated, is that it has *no person param-eter*. This results because the total score of a person, $r_n = x_{+i} + x_{+j}$, on the two texts is a *sufficient* statistic for the person parameter ξ_n; that is, all the information that the data can provide about the parameter ξ_n is contained in r_n (Rasch, 1960). Thus, r_n can be used directly to estimate ξ_n. However, for Rasch, even this result was not the main feature. Instead, he focused on a second feature: He recognized that if, given the fit of the data to the model, the relative difficulties of the texts could be estimated *independently* of the proficiencies of the persons, then the check that responses fitted the model involved checking if the ratio was consistent across different proficiencies. This check was done using the plot of the kind shown in Figure 7.1 and the related statistics.

Instead of simply observing the two features of the MPM in the above para-graph, Rasch specified them as a requirement—that is, if there is to be a single ratio of the relative difficulties of the two texts that is general, then this ratio must hold for persons with different proficiencies. Complementary-wise, if the ratio was different for persons with different proficiencies, there would be no single, general, summary ratio.

Invariant comparisons within a frame of reference

Rasch generalized the *ratio* of the difficulties of two texts to the concept of a *comparison*, and the requirement that the comparison be constant across pro-ficiencies, *to a requirement of the invariance of comparisons within a specified frame of reference.*

Beginning with a two-way frame of reference:

> The comparison between two stimuli should be independent of which par-ticular individuals were instrumental for the comparison; and it should also be independent of which other stimuli within the considered class were or might also have been compared.

> Symmetrically, a comparison between two individuals should be independ-ent of which particular stimuli within the class considered were instru-mental for comparison; and it should also be independent of which other individuals were also compared, on the same or on some other occasion. (Rasch, 1961 p. 332)

The two-way frame of reference is captured in Table 7.1, in which Rasch (1977) generalizes *individuals* to be any *objects* of measurement and *stimuli* to be *agents* of measurement. The frame of reference defines the class of objects, the class of agents, and all features that are concerned with the administration of the engagement between the objects and agents that might be relevant for comparisons. For example, if objects are persons and agents are texts, and age

Table 7.1 Two-way frame of reference

		Agents (items)					
Response x	X_{ni}	A_1	A_2	·	$A_i(\delta_i)$	·	A_I
	O_1	x_{11}	x_{12}	–	–	–	x_{1I}
	O_2	–	–	–	–	–	
	–	–	–	–	–	–	
Objects (persons)	$O_n(\beta_n)$.	x_{n1}	–	–	x_{ni}	–	x_{nI}
	–	–	–	–	–	–	–
	O_N	x_{N1}	–	–	x_{Ni}	–	x_{NI}

grouping is relevant in making comparisons, then age grouping would also be included in the specification of the frame of reference. Furthermore, it would be required that the relative difficulties of the texts are invariant with respect to age groupings. And if gender were relevant for making comparisons, then it would be required that the relative difficulties are also invariant with respect to gender.

The nature of the engagement between objects and agents in the frame of reference is part of the empirical design. For example, the beam balance in the example of measurement of mass defines the nature of the engagement between the two masses—it is through the balance of the beam, which, in its design, must not bias to one side or the other. Then the response depends on the relevant property of the object and the agents that engage each other, both characterized by their respective parameters. Indeed, it is the relevant property of the agent that is engaged to provoke the relevant property of the object. Thus, under controlled conditions, a reading text provokes the manifestation of reading proficiency, just as under controlled conditions, a beam balance provokes the manifestation of mass. Rasch's generalization does not require these parameters to be quantitative, that is, to be characterized by real numbers. However, if they are characterized by real numbers, as he postulated with the parameters of his class of models, then the comparisons have the key properties of measurement. This understanding arises from two generalizations, which Rasch derives from the requirement of invariant comparisons within a specified frame of reference.

Rasch's generalization of models that provide invariant comparisons

First, Rasch asked the question: "Which class of probability models has the property in common with the MPM, that one set of parameters can be eliminated by means of conditional probabilities while attention is concentrated on the other set, and vice versa?" (Rasch, 1977, p. 65). To answer this question he wrote the general expression in the form of Equation 7.9 and then proceeded to derive the class of probabilistic models that satisfy it in which the right side does not involve the object parameter β_n:

$$\Pr\{(x_{ni}, x_{nj}); \beta_n, \delta_i, \delta_j \mid f(x_{ni}, x_{nj})\} = \vartheta(x_{ni} x_{nj}, \delta_i, \delta_j). \tag{7.9}$$

Derivations in Rasch (1961), demonstrated constraints on the properties of the model to show sufficient in Andersen (1977), interpretation of the parameters in terms of thresholds and discriminations at the thresholds in Andrich (1978), and an algebraic generalization to structures where not all items have the same number of categories in Wright and Masters (1982) led to the model for discrete ordered categories where $x_{ni,} = 0,1,2,...m_i$ is an ordered count of the successive categories and where m_i is the maximum score of agent i, taking the form

$$\Pr\{X_{ni,} = x; \beta_n, (\delta_{ik})\} = \left[\exp\left(x\beta_n - \sum_{k=0}^{x} \delta_{ik} \right) \right] / \gamma_{ni}, \tag{7.10}$$

where the vector (δ_{ik}), $k = 1,2,3,..., m_i$ is a set of thresholds at which the probability of a response in adjacent categories is identical. Equation 7.9 will be referred to as the polytomous Rasch model (PRM). In the case of dichotomous responses, there is only the one threshold, $\delta_i = \delta_{i1}$, and the equation specializes to

$$\Pr\{X_{ni,} = x; \beta_n, (\delta_i)\} = [\exp(x(\varsigma_{ni})]/\gamma_{ni} = [\exp(x(\beta_n - \delta_i))]/\gamma_{ni}. \tag{7.11}$$

Relative to the MPM, two notational modifications result—the parameters are expressed in natural logarithms, thus $\exp(\beta_n) = \xi_n$, and the greater the score on an agent (item), the greater the proficiency. Thus, in Equation 7.10, the parameter β_n appears in the numerator and because the greater the difficulty and the smaller the response score, the thresholds (δ_{ik}), $k = 1,2,3, ...,m_i$ take the opposite role to the single text parameter α_i in Equation 7.4. The relative locations of the items, δ_i, in the dichotomous case help define what it means to have more or less of the property measured, and in addition, the relative locations δ_{ik} in the PRM help characterize how the successive categories reflect more or less of the property being measured.

The now familiar parameterizations of this model are the rating scale, in which threshold mean deviates $\tau_{ik} = \delta_{ik} - \bar{\delta}_i$, $k = 1, 2, 3,..., m_i$ are the same for each item, and partial credit is shown in Equation 7.9. In the case of the MPM, $m_i \to \infty$. Masters and Wright (1984) summarize these specific parameterizations, which satisfy the necessary and sufficient conditions in providing the kind of invariance of comparisons required by Rasch. We return to this general model later in this chapter.

The requirement of invariance as a property of measurement was not unique to Rasch. Both Thurstone (1928) and Guttman (1950) articulated its centrality to measurement. They saw it as a requirement of data. Significantly for the development of a measurement theory, in addition to a property of data, Rasch formalized invariance as a property of a model, and as a result, was able to carry out mathematical derivations that led to further insights not otherwise available. In particular, the class of probabilistic models is constrained not only by the structure of the parameters that must be multiplicative (or equivalently based on a monotonic transformation, additive), but also by the probabilistic element of the model that must have sufficient statistics for all parameters. The mathematical rendition of the requirement of invariance in a probabilistic framework, with accompanying new insights obtained from further mathematical derivations, is the major contribution to Rasch's work having the characteristics of a theory.

Additive conjoiwnt measurement

In addition to deriving a class of probabilistic models that permit the separation of parameters, Rasch considered frames of reference in which the responses were deterministic. That is, taking the parameters of objects and agents in Table 7.1 to again be characterized by positive real numbers, but replacing the response x_{ni} by a scalar reaction χ_{ni} giving $\chi_{ni} = \rho(\beta_n, \delta_i)$, Rasch (1977) states that the necessary and sufficient condition for invariant comparisons is that there exist strictly monotonic functions $\beta_n' = \phi(\beta_n)$, $\delta_i' = \psi(\delta_i)$, and $\chi_{ni}' = P(\chi_{ni})$, which transform the parameters into the additive form

$$\chi_{ni}' = \beta_n' + \delta_i'. \tag{7.12}$$

In the above form, the characterization of the objects, agents, and the reaction function and the transformations, in a sense, assumes and defines measurement simultaneously. Thus, if transformations that give Equation 7.12 cannot be found, then the numerical characterizations of the parameters β_n, δ_i are not measurements. There is not enough space in this chapter to further consider these deterministic formulations except to emphasize that they are entirely consistent with Luce and Tukey's (1964) condition of additive conjoint measurement (Wright, 1985, 1997).

However, not only is the deterministic case of invariance compatible with additive conjoint measurement, but also the deeper point is that because of their parametric structure (multiplicative or equivalently additive in the logarithmic scale), the Rasch class of probabilistic models is also entirely compatible with deterministic, additive conjoint measurement (Wright, 1985, 1997; Karabatsos, 2004). This synthesis between probabilistic and deterministic response structures is a major theoretical contribution to explaining measurement in terms of invariant comparisons.

Invariant comparisons and scientific inquiry beyond measurement

Rasch goes on further to consider the significance of a comparison, and then argues that for comparisons to be general, rather than merely local, they need to be invariant within a specified frame of reference. Rasch considers that although they are a requirement for measurement, such comparisons go beyond measurement and are the basis of scientific enquiry. Stone and Stenner (2014) summarize the key passages of Rasch's publications in which he develops these claims. These claims for the centrality of invariance in scientific discovery are consistent with those of Nozick (2001).

If the objects, agents, and reactions are characterized by real numbers, the result is a class of models that Rasch called *models for measurement*. Thus, measurement is explained as having a scalar characterization of invariant comparisons within a specified, empirical frame of reference. For example, the typical instrument that shows the magnitude of a property in terms of units (a ruler, thermometer) implies many simultaneous comparisons with a unit. In a well constructed and calibrated set of instruments, the comparisons are invariant across measuring instruments.

Therefore, unlike derivation where concatenation and conjoint additivity follow from a set of *axioms*, for Rasch these properties, and others, follow mathematically from an a priori requirement of invariant comparisons within an empirical, specified frame of reference, and where the characterizations of reactions are with real numbers. And invariant comparisons are justified as a requirement because of their centrality to scientific enquiry and scientific generalization, not just to measurement.

Rasch studied the deterministic case within the framework of the probabilistic models that had the properties of invariance described above. It seems most unlikely that if he, or anyone else, set out to unify probabilistic and deterministic structures for measurement, then he would have come up with a solution. The solution came before the problem was recognized, a characteristic of a Kuhnian revolution (Kuhn, 1970, Andrich, 2004). The significance of Rasch's synthesis of probabilistic and deterministic responses in the realization of measurement cannot be overstated. Apart from its conceptual leap, one reason for its significance is that most data in the social sciences are stochastic in nature. Thus, Guttman's (1950) formulation for dichotomous responses, which is the deterministic counterpart of Rasch's formulation (Andrich, 1985), has had little practical impact except that it is invoked as an idealization of a required structure for measurement. On the other hand, from the MPM, which has as its maximum score a nonfinite integer count and which therefore has very tractable properties, the abstraction of sufficiency generalizes to the PRM for any finite maximum score, beginning with a maximum score of 1. This makes the application of the PRM practical with common assessment instruments where the agents in the frame of reference of Table 7.1 are items and the objects are persons.

Implications for data analysis: An example with dichotomous responses

To make the generality of the PRM concrete, and to illustrate not only its profundity but its practical implications, we now consider briefly the case of just two dichotomous items.

Let (x_{ni}, x_{nj}) be an ordered set of responses of person n to items i, j, respectively, where $x_{ni} = 0.1$; $x_{nj} = 0.1$. The estimation equation for the relative difficulties of the items is given simply by

$$\frac{Pr\{(1;0) \mid (1,0)\ OR\ (0,1)\}}{Pr\{(0;1) \mid (1,0)\ OR\ (0,1)\}} = \frac{\exp(\delta_2)}{\exp(\delta_1)} = \exp(\delta_2 - \delta_1), \tag{7.13}$$

which is independent of the person parameter β_n. Recognizing that the sample space $\{(1,0)\ OR\ (0,1)\}$ can be summarized as a person's total score of $r_n = x_{ni} + x_{nj} = 1$, the estimate of the difference on the right side of Equation 7.13 is given by the ratio

$$\frac{F\{(1;0) \mid r = 1\}}{F\{(0;1) \mid r = 1\}} = \exp(\hat{\delta}_2 - \hat{\delta}_1), \tag{7.14}$$

where $F\{(1;0) \mid r = 1\}$, $F\{(0;1) \mid r = 1\}$ denotes the respective frequencies of the probabilities in Equation 7.13, and from which

$$\ln\left(\frac{F\{(1;0) \mid r = 1\}}{F\{(0;1) \mid r = 1\}}\right) = \hat{\delta}_2 - \hat{\delta}_1. \tag{7.15}$$

Equations 7.14 and 7.15 are remarkable. Despite each response from a person engaging with an item being governed by a different parameter $\zeta_{ni} = \beta_n - \delta_i$, and the response being dichotomous and therefore discrete and finite, the data can be recast to give replications with respect to the same comparison parameter $\delta_2 - \delta_1$, independently of any person parameter β_n, and from which the comparison can be estimated in terms of a real number. That is, by selecting a subset of all data, an estimate of the ratio (or difference in the logarithmic scale) is available independently of all person parameters. Rasch established that Equation 7.11 is necessary and sufficient for an invariant comparison of item parameters, and symmetrically, if persons are to be compared. Although the invariance is a property of the model, in any real measurement, the invariance needs to be a property of the responses. The function of the PRM has as a measurement model helped to establish evidence that the invariance holds in responses. For example, without the derivations that lead to Equations 7.10, 7.11, and 7.13, it is not immediately obvious how the comparison of the difficulty of two items could be made independently of the proficiencies of the persons and neither is it obvious which sample space should be used. These mathematical derivations, and their implications, are part of the case that Rasch's contribution constitutes a measurement theory.

Clearly, the features of Equation 7.13 are generalized for the joint comparison of multiple dichotomous items that are explicated in references made earlier. Again, how this generalization would be made without a mathematic model in which the condition of invariant comparisons and sufficient statistics is built into as an integral property is not clear.

Mathematical derivations and further insights into measurement and data analysis

One of the requirements of a measurement theory rendered mathematically is that it provides new insights that follow from further mathematical deductions. One example, the choice of a model and a sample space for data that provides evidence of invariant comparisons of item difficulties, was illustrated above with a pair of dichotomous items. That there is such a restricted model for ordered categorical data, the PRM, is in itself significant. This model has become popular and is one of two classes of models routinely applied to responses in ordered categories. Ordered categorical data are common in the social and behavioral sciences. Dawes (1972) estimated that approximately 60% of variables were of this kind. This percentage is likely to have increased since Dawes' estimate.

However, the PRM, itself arising from the theory of invariant comparisons, permits deductions through mathematical derivations. This section gives two examples of such deductions that lead to new, and initially even counterintuitive, insights. These are the nonarbitrary combination of adjacent categories and the interpretation of the threshold parameters.

Combining adjacent categories in ordered, categorical response data

The PRM has the distinctive property that if the probabilities of responses in two adjacent categories are summed, then the new model is no longer a Rasch model (Rasch, 1966). This result implies that if the responses fit the PRM, then if frequencies in adjacent categories are amalgamated into a smaller number of categories, the data will not fit as well and the invariance of parameter estimates will be distorted, and that amalgamating categories before responses are made are not the same as amalgamating them after they are made. Jansen and Roskam (1986) considered this result so counterintuitive that they argued that the PRM should not be used for ordered categorical data. Andrich (1995) explained this property in terms of how the PRM accounted for the precision of measurement, where more categories implied greater precision. However, the result that categories cannot be amalgamated arbitrarily gives further insights. It indicates that the structure and format of the categories of an item are an integral part of the responses, and that it is *because amalgamating categories is not arbitrary* that the model can provide evidence regarding the empirical operation of the categories and hypotheses as to how many might be optimal in any particular context. In contrast, if the categories can be combined arbitrarily in the model, then the model could not provide evidence about whether or not the categories are working as intended, for example, if there might be too many or if they are unstable because they are ill-defined, and so on. Anderson (1984) expresses similar sentiments. "For example, it is well known in questionnaire design that a change in the form of words of a question can lead to an unpredictable change in the pattern of observed responses. Hence, it is not obvious that the change in the form of a question corresponding to the amalgamation of two categories would simply result in the amalgamation of responses in the two categories" (Anderson, 1984, p. 2).

Empirical evidence of order in ordered, categorical response data

Following from the result of the nonarbitrary combining of adjacent categories, a more specific insight follows from the interpretation of the threshold parameters of the PRM of Equation 7.10. These thresholds are points on the continuum where the probabilities of responses in adjacent categories are identical. If ostensibly ordered categorical data are operating as required, then the *estimates* of the thresholds, which are the only item parameters in the model and therefore must have something to do with the ordering of the categories, need to be ordered (Andrich, 2011). It is possible for the model to provide this evidence because the ordering of the thresholds is a required property of the responses and not of the model itself—estimates, therefore, can take any value as a reflection of the property of the responses. Similar to the implications that categories cannot be amalgamated arbitrarily, which some considered counterintuitive, so the implications that the PRM can provide evidence of the empirical ordering of categories has been rejected by Adams et al. (2012). Their misunderstandings between requiring the ordering of estimates to be a property of the model, irrespective of the data, and a property of the data as revealed by the model, have been explained by Andrich (2013). Because the successive categories are intended to define what it means to have successively more of the property being measured, it seems critical that the empirical ordering is consistent with the intended ordering; otherwise, misleading interpretations can follow readily. It seems that only Fisher (1958) had ever considered the relevance of empirical ordering of categories rather than merely taking the ordering for granted, and the contribution of the PRM in this regard is a novel contribution in analyzing such data.

Thus, the requirement that to be justified as a measurement theory, there should be derivations that generate genuinely new insights, is met: the ones shown above are derivations of the model and sample space that gives evidence of invariant comparisons in dichotomous items and the nonarbitrary combining of adjacent categories and the empirical evidence of the ordering of categories in polytomous items. Although initially nonstandard in the body of knowledge on social measurement, because these insights follow, not merely from attempting to model data, but from the a priori property of invariant comparisons within a frame of reference that is independent of any data, their implications need to be understood and exploited and not dismissed. Whether or not any data set fits with the relevant Rasch model is irrelevant to the case for the model (Duncan, 1984).

To reinforce the earlier criterion of a theory—that it provides new insights—it is suggested that the three insights described above could have arisen only from a series of mathematical derivations and not because anyone set out to produce the insights. It is noted that the key successive derivations in Rasch (1961), Andersen (1977), and Andrich (1978), all resting on the criterion of invariance and its complement of sufficiency with probabilistic models, had no empirical examples.

The function of measurement in science—disclosing anomalies

The final feature listed that is necessary for Rasch's work to be considered a theory of measurement is that it was consistent with Kuhn's analysis that the function of measurement in science is to disclose anomalies. The defining reason that RMT is consistent with disclosing anomalies is that the case for any model that arises from it for any particular context is independent of the data that are collected. Then, in principle, if there is incompatibility between the data and the model, where the model is chosen because it is considered relevant to the checking the degree to which the data achieve measurement, it is not a problem with the model, but an anomaly in the data. This contrasts with the standard statistical paradigm to which IRT belongs, where if there is incompatibility between the model and the data, it is seen as a problem with the model, and another model that accounts for the data better is sought (Andrich, 2004, 2011). Rasch was very aware of this apparently novel relationship between a model and data:

> It is tempting, therefore, in the case with deviations of one sort or other to ask *whether it is the model or the test that has gone wrong.* (Rasch, 1960, p. 51. Emphasis in the original.)

To appreciate why the model discloses what are justifiably called anomalies, it may be useful to recount the justification that data from an instrument might be subjected to a Rasch model analysis. The kind of instrument considered is one in which multiple items are used to assess a property of persons. Multiple items are used to increase both validity and precision of measurement. Then following the construction of the items based on the understanding of the property, the class of persons for whom it is deemed relevant, and the full frame of reference, it is expected that the responses to the items will conform with each other; that is, the items will all contribute to an estimate of a single location parameter β for each person. If the data fit the PRM, the total score of the responses on the items contains all the information about β and its estimate can be located on a real number line. From a perspective of the RMT, the application of the PRM to responses is a test of the hypothesis that the responses to the items will conform to the model and in turn that the single value is invariant with respect to different subsets of items. Because the model is a mathematical rendition of the requirement of invariant comparisons for ordered, discrete responses, the degree to which responses violate the model with respect to different aspects of invariance (e.g., across gender, age, proficiency levels) indicates the degree to which they do not provide invariant comparisons with respect to a single estimate for each person.

It is stressed again that the application of the Rasch model, and evidence of fit, is not sufficient to claim that useful measurement is possible with an instrument. Thus, simply applying a Rasch model to data, even if the data fit the model, is not sufficient to establish that measurement has been achieved. The fact that measurement has been achieved needs to be established with triangulated empirical evidence, where the Rasch model provides a necessary, although not a sufficient, condition to demonstrate the degree to which valid and reliable measurements have been achieved. The point that the application of the Rasch model "... does not revoke the criteria scientists normally cite in deciding whether the right variables have been measured" must be taken seriously (Duncan, 1984, pp. 398, 399). Thus, a great deal of explication of the experimental and empirical context, the specified empirical frame of reference, together with a nonmechanical application of statistical inference, is required to claim that fit of data to the Rasch model has resulted in measurement.

Contrasts with CTT and IRT

To emphasize its distinctive features, this section highlights briefly some contrasts between RMT and both CTT and IRT. The contrasts highlighted, though necessarily brief, are considered defining and help justify RMT as a theory of measurement. A publication from which the contrasting perspectives of CTT, IRT, and RMT can be obtained is Engelhard (1997) in which Traub (1997), Bock (1997), and Wright (1997) provide comprehensive respective histories of the fields.

Classical test theory

First, a feature of CTT, explicated in many books (e.g., Lord and Novick, 1968; Gulliksen, 1950; Magnusson, 1966), is that it *presumes* that each response is already a measurement. It does this even though the responses are generally discrete with a small finite number of ordered categories, including often just two ordered categories. The basic CTT equation is

$$y_n = \tau_n + e_n, \tag{7.16}$$

where $y_n = \sum_{i=1}^{I} x_{ni}$ is the total score of person n on a test composed of I items where each response is $x_{ni} \in \{0,1, ...m_i\}$, τ_n is the person's true score, and e_n is the error around the true score. The core of the development of CTT from this definition rests on the idea of taking means of measurements, where the mean of measurements provides a better estimate of a person's true score than each of the measurements. (For the purpose of increasing the precision of the estimate of the true score, taking the sum of responses to all items is equivalent to taking the mean of the responses to all items.) The history of CTT that high-lights the principle of taking the mean of measurements as providing a more precise estimate than any one measurement (which itself has an interesting history; Eisenhart, 1983) is described in excellent detail in Traub (1997). By assuming that the responses are measurements, the theory has little to contribute to explain the measurement.

Second, unlike the PRM, Equation 7.16 has no item parameter, where items are taken as simply random replications of each other and therefore do not contribute to the operational and empirical rendition of a variable. In addition, although features of items are inevitably used in assembling a test, because it has no item parameter, there are no variables in the theory to conjoin in the sense that it is articulated in Luce and Tukey, and in RMT. Not having item parameters in the CTT creates major problems for constructing tests for longitudinal and cross-sectional studies. Generally, properties of CTT such as test reliability are anchored to a particular population.

CTT can be considered a theory in the sense of a body of problems and knowledge regarding those problems (O'Connor, 1957) concerned with assessment and tests, and therefore it is justifiably referred to, as it is currently in the literature, as a *test* theory (rather than a *measurement* theory).

Item response theory

IRT has also been explicated in many books (Lord, 1980; van der Linden and Hambleton, 1997; Embretson and Reise, 2000; Raykov and Marcoulides, 2011; Hambleton et al., 1991) and many papers. One paradigmatic distinction between IRT and RMT is that in the former there is *no* a priori criterion for a choice of the model, and the choice of the model from a very general class of models is primarily a function of whether or not the model accounts for a particular set of responses. If the model does not account for these particular responses, a different model is sought. For example, in the case of dichotomous responses to items, if they do not show adequate fit to the model of Equation 7.11, then the model

$$\Pr\{X_{ni,} = x; \beta_n, (\delta_i)\} = [\exp(a_i x(\beta_n - \delta_i))] / \gamma_{ni}, \tag{7.17}$$

where a_i is a discrimination parameter that is applied. Wright (1997) analyzes the problems these additional parameters cause with respect to the condition of invariance of comparisons.

An equation of the form of Equation 7.13, in which the estimates of the item parameters can be obtained independently of the person parameters, is of no concern in IRT. As a result, there is little discussion in IRT regarding the foundations and principles of measurement. In particular, the invariance and sufficiency of models on which RMT is based are not properties of general IRT models. This distinction between the criterion of fit to responses as the choice of a model in IRT on the one hand and an a priori choice of the model governing valid empirical research that generates responses to fit the model in RMT on the other has been elaborated in Andrich (2004, 2011) and is not repeated here.

Like CTT, IRT can be considered a theory in the sense of a body of problems and a body of knowledge regarding those problems (O'Connor, 1957) concerned with responses to assessment instruments, and therefore it is justifiably referred to, as it is currently in the literature, as a *response* theory (rather than a *measurement* theory).

Current status of RMT applications

Two summary points are made regarding the current status of applications of the RMT and not merely a Rasch model. First, although the concept of sufficiency was first understood and formalized by Fisher (1934), the way Rasch exploited sufficiency for the purpose of separating parameters in a frame of reference led to his measurement theory based on the requirement of invariant comparisons. With the development of the models with sufficient statistics that provide the separation, the conditional estimation of parameters and a range of tests of fit are now available and are a distinct body of knowledge. Andersen's (1980) publication, together with publications of many others, has contributed to this knowledge. Thus, this knowledge is not only consistent with features of a theory that there is a coherent body of knowledge that flows from it, but it has also been made available for application through software and has been applied in many settings.

One important conceptual elaboration arises from RMT: that between a *reflective* and a *formative* relationship between the variable and the items used to assess it (Stenner et al., 2008). In the reflective relationship, responses to items are taken as manifestations of the same variable that provides a nonunique, operationalization of the variable; in the formative relationship the specific collection of items, characterized as indexes, defines the variable. Traditionally measured variables in the natural sciences are reflective. In contrast, in general, in the social sciences, variables can have elements of reflective and formative relationships (Tesio, 2014). Having these elements does not preclude the power of demonstrated invariant, relevant, comparisons.

An advanced and exceptional application of RMT carried out at *Meta-Metrics* (http://www.metametricsinc.com), the basis of which is described in Stenner et al. (1983), has resulted in the assessment of the variable of reading proficiency in a well-defined unit called a *lexile*. In this assessment, the substantive theory is used to generate nonunique items while a person is reading a text.

Whether RMT can be fully exploited in other fields will depend on the ingenuity of substantive, empirical research, not simply psychometric research. RMT invites, and requires, such empirical research. A compelling precedent for such work, details of which have been comprehensively described in Olsen (2003), is provided in Rasch (1960), which reports integrated theoretical developments and empirical studies. At the same time, however, if the measurement is not achieved even when applying a relevant Rasch model and RMT, there is no evidence against Rasch's epistemological case for invariant comparisons and his rendition of this case in the form of a class of applicable probabilistic models as a theory of measurement.

Summary

Within the practice and literature concerned with attempts at social measurement, there is now a vast literature on Rasch models and their applications, including books (Andrich, 1988; Smith and Smith, 2004; Olsen, 2003; Salzberger, 2009; Fischer and Molenaar, 1995; Christensen et al., 2013), which indicates that the application and justification of Rasch models is not the same as the application and justification of CTT and IRT. However, there is no distinct, separate nomenclature for an RMT. Instead reference is made to *Rasch models* and *Rasch analyses*, rather than RMT. This chapter sets out to make a case that the contributions of Rasch in articulating a case for invariant comparisons as fundamental to generalizable knowledge, and rendering these in the form of probabilistic models that can be used for a range of derivations of new insights and applications, constitute a measurement theory and therefore justifies being referred to as *RMT*. Because of the empirical implications of RMT, rather than *modeling* as in IRT and *description* as in CTT, it might help develop strong empirical studies designed to construct measuring instruments in the social sciences. However, irrespective of whether or not, or the degree to which, these empirical endeavors succeed, they will not detract from Rasch's articulation of the requirements of invariant comparison within an empirical, specified frame of reference, and the rendering of these in a probabilistic mathematical framework, being a very general and powerful *theory of measurement* relevant to both the natural and the social sciences.

Acknowledgment

The author would like to thank Barry Sheridan, Irene Styles, Pender Pedler, and an unknown reviewer for providing valuable comments for this chapter.

References

Adams, R.J., Wu, M.L., and Wilson, M. (2012). The Rasch rating model and the disordered threshold controversy. *Educ. Psychol. Meas.*, 72, 547–573.
Andersen, E.B. (1977). Sufficient statistics and latent trait models. *Psychometrika*, 42, 69–81.
Andersen, E.B. (1980). *Discrete Statistical Models with Social Science Applications*. Amsterdam, the Netherlands: North Holland.
Anderson, J.A. (1984). Regression and ordered categorical variables. *J. R. Stat. Soc. Ser. B.*, 46, 1–30.
Andrich, D. (1978). A rating formulation for ordered response categories. *Psychometrika*, 43, 561–574.
Andrich, D. (1985). An elaboration of Guttman scaling with Rasch models for measurement. In: N. Brandon-Tuma (ed.), *Sociological Methodology* (Chapter 2, pp. 33–80). San Francisco, CA: Jossey-Bass.

Andrich, D. (1988). *Rasch Models for Measurement*, Newbury Park, CA: Sage Publications.

Andrich, D. (1995). Models for measurement, precision and the non-dichotomization of graded responses. *Psychometrika, 60*(1), 7–26.

Andrich, D. (2004). Controversy and the Rasch model: A characteristic of incompatible paradigms? *Med Care, 42*, 7–16. Reprinted In: E.V. Smith and R.M. Smith. *Introduction to Rasch Measurement: Theory, Models and Application* (Chapter 7, pp. 143–166). Minnesota, MN: JAM Press.

Andrich, D. (2011). Rating scales and Rasch measurement. *Expert. Rev. Pharmacoecon. Outcomes Res., 11*(5), 571–585.

Andrich, D. (2013). An expanded derivation of the threshold structure of the polytomous Rasch rating model which dispels any "threshold disorder controversy." *Educ. Psychol. Meas., 73*(1), 78–24.

Bock, R.D. (1997). A brief history of item response theory. *Educ. Meas. Issues Pract., 16*(4), 21–33.

Bock, R.D., and Jones, L.V. (1968). *The Measurement and Prediction of Judgement and Choice*. San Francisco, CA: Holden Day.

Campbell, N.R. (1920). *Physics: The Elements*. London, UK: Cambridge University Press.

Christensen, K.B., Kreiner, S., and Mesbah, M. (2013). *Rasch Models in Health*. London, UK: Wiley.

Dawes, R.M. (1972). *Fundamentals of Attitude Measurement*. New York, NY: John Wiley.Ellis, B. (1966). *Basic Concepts in Measurement*. Cambridge: Cambridge University Press.

Duncan, O.D. (1984). Rasch measurement further examples and discussion. In: C.F. Turner and E. Martin (eds.), *Surveying Subjective Phenomena* (Vol. 2). New York, NY: Russell Sage Foundation.

Eisenhart, C. (1983). Law of error I: Development of the concept. In: S. Kotz and N.L. Johnson, (eds.), *Encyclopedia of Statistical Sciences* (Vol. 4, pp. 530–547). Toronto, ON: Wiley.

Ellis, B. (1966). *Basic Concepts in Measurement*. Cambridge: Cambridge University Press.

Embretson, S.E., and Reise, S.P. (2000). *Item Response Theory for Psychologists*. London: Erlbaum.

Engelhard, G. (1997) (ed.). Special issue: Theory of modern psychometrics. *Educ. Meas. Issues Pract., 16*(4), 4–58.

Fisher, R.A. (1934). Two new properties of mathematical likelihood. *Proc. R. Soc. A., 144*: 285–307.

Fisher, R.A. (1958). *Statistical Methods for Research Workers* (13th Edition). Edinburgh: Oliver and Boyd.

Fischer, G.H., and Molenaar, I.W. (eds.) (1995) *Rasch Models: Foundations, Recent Developments, and Applications*. New York, NY: Springer.

Gulliksen, H. (1950). *Theory of Mental Tests*. New York, NY: Wiley.

Guttman, L. (1950). The basis for scalogram analysis. In: S.A. Stouffer, L. Guttman, E.A. Suchman, P.F. Lazarsfeld, S.A. Star, and J.A. Clausen (eds.), *Measurement and Prediction* (pp. 60–90). New York, NY: Wiley.

Hambleton, R.K., Swaminathan, H., and Rogers, J. (1991). *Fundamentals of Item Response Theory*. Newbury Park, CA: Sage.

Jansen, P.G.W., and Roskam, E.E. (1986). Latent trait models and dichotomization of graded responses. *Psychometrika, 51*(1), 69–91.

Karabatsos, G. (2004). The Rasch model, additive conjoint measurement, and new models of probabilistic measurement theory. In: E.V. Jr. Smith and R.M. Smith (eds.), *Introduction to Rasch Measurement* (pp. 630–664). Minnesota, MN: JAM Press.

Krantz, D.H., Luce, R.D., Suppes, P., and Tversky, A. (1971). *Foundations of Measurement* (Vol. 1). New York, NY: Academic Press.

Kuhn, T.S. (1961). The function of measurement in modern physical science. *Isis.*, *52*, 161–190.

Kuhn, T.S. (1970). *The Structure of Scientific Revolutions* (2nd Edition enlarged). Chicago, IL: University of Chicago Press.

Lord, F.M. (1980). *Applications of Item Response Theory to Practical Testing Problems.* Hillsdale, NJ: Lawrence Erbaum Associates.

Lord, F.M., and Novick, M.R. (1968). *Statistical Theories of Mental Test Scores.* Reading, MA: Addison-Wesley.

Luce, R.D., and Tukey, J.W. (1964). Simultaneous conjoint measurement: A new type of fundamental measurement. *J. Math. Psychol.*, *1*, 1–27.

Magnusson, D. (1966). *Test Theory.* Reading, MA: Addison-Wesley.

Masters, G.N., and Wright, B.D. (1984). The essential process in a family of measurement models. *Psychometrika*, *49*, 529–544.

Michell, J. (2003). Measurement: A beginner's guide. *J. Appl. Meas.*, *4*, 298–308.

Nozick, R. (2001). *Invariances: The Structure of the Objective World.* Cambridge, MA: Bellknap Press of the Harvard University Press.

O'Connor, D.J. (1957). *An Introduction to the Philosophy of Education.* London: Routledge & Kegan Paul.

Olsen, L.W. (2003). *Essays on Georg Rasch and His Contributions to Statistics.* Copenhagen: University of Copenhagen, Institute of Economics.

Punch, K.F. (2009). *Introduction to Research Methods in Education.* Los Angeles, CA: Sage.

Ramsay, J.O. (1975). Review of foundations of measurement. Vol. I, by Krantz D.H., R.D. Luce, P. Suppes, A. Tverskey. (1971). *Psychometrika.*, *40*, 257–62.

Rasch, G. (1960). *Probabilistic Models For Some Intelligence and Attainment Tests.* (Copenhagen, Danish Institute for Educational Research). Expanded edition (1980) with foreword and afterword by B. D. Wright. Chicago, IL: University of Chicago Press. Available from www.rasch.org/books.htm.

Rasch, G. (1961). On general laws and the meaning of measurement in psychology. In: J. Neyman (ed.), Proceedings of the Fourth Berkeley Symposium on Mathematical Statistics and Probability. IV (pp. 321–334). Berkeley, CA: University of California Press. Reprinted In: Bartholomew D.J. (2006) (ed.). Measurement Volume I, 319–334. Sage Benchmarks in Social Research Methods, London: Sage.

Rasch, G. (1966). An individualistic approach to item analysis. In: P.F. Lazarsfeld and N.W. Henry (eds.), *Readings in Mathematical Social Science* (pp. 89–108). Chicago, IL: Science Research Associates.

Rasch, G. (1977). On specific objectivity: An attempt at formalising the request for generality and validity of scientific statements. *Dan. Yearb. Philos.*, *14*, 58–94.

Raykov, T., and Marcoulides, G.A. (2011). *Introduction to Psychometric Theory.* New York, NY: Routledge.

Roberts, F.S. (1979). *Measurement Theory.* Reading, MA: Addison-Wesley.

Salzberger, T. (2009). *Measurement in Marketing Research: An Alternative Framework.* Cheltenhavem: Edward Elgar.

Schwager, K.W. (1991). The representational theory of measurement: An assessment. *Psychol. Bull.*, *110*, 618–626.

Smith, E.V. Jr., and Smith, R.M. (2004) (eds.). *Introduction to Rasch Measurement.* Minnesota, MN: JAM Press.

Stenner, A.J., Burdick, D., and Stone, M.H. (2008). Formative and reflective models: Can a Rasch analysis tell the difference? *RMT*, *22*, 1059–1060.

Stenner, A. J., Smith, M., and Burdick, D.S. (1983). Toward a theory of construct definition. *J. Educ. Meas.*, *20*(4), 305–316.

Stevens, S.S. (1946). On the theory of scales of measurement. *Science*, *103* (June), 677–680. Reprint. In: A. Haber, R.P. Runyon and P. Badia. (1970) (eds.), *Readings in Statistics.* Reading, MA: Addison-Wesley.

Stone, M.H., and Stenner, A.J. (2014). Comparison is key. *J. Appl. Meas.*, *15*(1), 26–39.

Tesio, L. (2014). Causing and being caused: Items in a questionnaire may play a different role, depending on the complexity of the variable. *RMT*, 28(1), 1454–1456.

Thurstone, L.L. (1928). Attitudes can be measured. *Am. J. Sociol., 33,* 529–554.

Traub, R.E. (1997). Classical test theory in historical perspective. *Educ. Meas. Issues Pract., 16*(4), 8–14.

van der Linden, W.J., and Hambleton R.K. (eds.). (1997). *Handbook of Item Response Theory.* New York, NY: Springer.

Wright, B.D. (1985). Additivity in psychological measurement. In: E.E. Roskam (ed.), *Measurement and Personality Assessment.* Selected papers, XXIII International Congress of Psychology (Vol 8, pp. 101–111). Amsterdam, NL: North Holland.

Wright, B.D. (1997). A history of social science measurement. *Educ. Meas. Issues Pract., 16*(4), 33–45.

Wright, B.D., and Masters, G.N. (1982). *Rating Scale Analysis: Rasch Measurement.* Chicago, IL: MESA Press.

8 A matter of convergence: Classical and modern approaches to scale development

Alan Tennant

Introduction

How we measure the efficacy of a particular intervention to improve (or recover) our health is a matter of concern to all of us. While some interventions can use directly ascertained measures such as blood pressure or grip strength, most health outcomes, particularly in the context of long-term conditions such as arthritis or multiple sclerosis, use patient completed questionnaires to ascertain the magnitude of some relevant construct, for example, fatigue (Mills, 2010). A cursory examination of PubMed or Scopus for new Patient Reported Outcomes Measures (PROMs) in any of the common diagnostic groups will elicit a constant flow of such PROMs, covering a wide range of constructs (theoretical perspective) consistent with the biopsychosocial model, as defined within the International Classification of Functioning, Disability and Health (ICF), ranging from fatigue (Impairment of Function), through work limitations or restrictions (Activity and Participation), to the availability of services (Environmental) (WHO [World Health Organization], 2001). For the purpose of this chapter, a PROM is here defined as any self (or proxy, e.g., carer) completed summative scale, resulting in a total score, or one or more "domain" scores. Thus, it will exclude the single item (e.g., a Visual Analog Scale [VAS] for pain), and any assessment whereby a patient is "rated" by a health professional on a set of items (which may subsequently be summed to give a total score). In the literature, PROMs may be referred to as an "instrument," a "scale," a "self-completed questionnaire," a "test," or an "assessment."

There are a vast number of PROMs, some of which are deemed "generic" and apply to any health condition and others that are designed for use with a specific condition, often referred to as a "disease-specific" scale. All such instruments, be they generic or disease-specific, share a common set of indicators with regard to their quality. These indicators are defined by psychometrics. Psychometrics is "the science of measuring mental capacities and processes," reflecting its early origins in measuring intelligence (Thurstone, 1919). It is the field of study concerned with the theory and technique of (psychological) measurement and is concerned with the construction of instruments and the procedures for measurement, as well as the development and refinement of theoretical approaches to the latter. Many of the basic concepts were elaborated by Thurstone in the 1920s and 1930s. For example, he stated that the measurement of any object or entity describes only one attribute of the object measured (Thurstone, 1931). This, he argued, was a universal characteristic of all measurement and thus emphasized the concept of unidimensionality for the measurement of psychological attributes. He also anticipated a key epistemological requirement of measurement that relative scale locations must "transcend" the group measured; that is, scale locations must be invariant to (or independent of) the particular group of persons instrumental to comparisons between the stimuli (Thurstone, 1928). This property of invariance is seen as the cornerstone of "fundamental measurement" in the health and social sciences (Engelhard, 2013). Thus, the relative distance (difficulty/impact) between any two items must remain invariant, irrespective of how much of the construct a person possesses, or to which group (e.g., sample or gender) they belong. Today psychometrics is applied to any attribute that cannot be directly observed, or only with considerable, time, effort, and cost! Thus, the ubiquitous questionnaire applied in health outcomes can have a wide range of concepts, not just psychological attributes such as self-esteem, but all aspects of functioning as defined by the ICF, as well as quality of life (QoL). Items from such scales are summated to ascertain the level of magnitude of a hypothesized latent (underlying) construct.

The most famous recent exposition of psychometrics is that by Nunnally in the book Psychometric Theory (Nunnally, 1978), and many readers will be familiar with the quality indicators relevant to PROMs, which are to be found in this book, including reliability and validity. Somewhat later, aspects such as responsiveness were included in the set of quality indicators (Kirshner and Guyatt, 1985). Various statistical techniques have been utilized to ascertain the quality of these attributes, such as test–retest reliability and factorial validity (unidimensionality), the latter introduced by the English statistician and psychologist Charles Spearman in an article in the *American Journal of Psychology* in 1904.

More recently, the various quality indicators have been cataloged within the COSMIN checklist (Mokkink et al., 2010). Based upon the three domains of Reliability, Validity, and Responsiveness, along with interpretability, the checklist delineates each domain in great detail. For example, the validity can be seen to encompass Content (Face), Structural, Criterion, Cross Cultural, and hypothesis testing, which incorporates other types of validity such as Known Groups (expected difference in means between groups, part of hypothesis testing in COSMIN), and convergent validity. All these different aspects essentially measure the same thing from a different perspective, that is, does the scale measure what is intended? Thus, we can ask health professionals if the item set is consistent with what they expect for the construct under consideration; we can test the score against some "gold standard," for example, the summed score from a scale for depression against some clinical structured test for depression. However, to test these aspects, the summed score itself must be a valid and sufficient statistic to represent the construct under consideration. It is structural validity, which effectively indicates whether or not the items can be summated to form a total score, a form of "internal" construct validity, focusing on the assumptions of unidimensionality and invariance. It precedes all other indicators as this is a requirement to be able to test any indicator based upon the total score (as in classical test theory [CTT]), as well as being an assumption of modern test theory approaches. However, although it does indicate if the item set is measuring a single construct, and is free of group bias in doing so, it does not confirm which construct is being measured, which is the province of the other types of validity. Neither does it indicate if the item set is reliable, rather offering the basis of testing reliability.

Thus, it is important to understand that there is a hierarchical ordering of these indicators. Structural validity is a necessary but not sufficient condition for the testing of reliability and "external" construct validity. Nunnally, for example, also states that validity is never more than the square root of reliability (Nunnally, 1978). This suggests that no matter how valid the scale, it will be of little value if the reliability is low. Unfortunately, there are many different types of reliability, as the COSMIN checklist shows, and there are also circumstances where it is possible to obtain a low reliability from a perfectly good test, such as where subjects have very similar scores in a test (i.e., a homogeneous sample) and as a consequence there is little dispersion in the test scores. Consequently, it is usual practice to obtain as many indicators as possible to make judgments about the quality of the scale.

Collectively, these indicators, the ways of assessing them, and the theory behind the approach have been given the label "CTT." For the latter, the observed score (i.e., the sum of the items in a questionnaires) added to the error associated with that score provides the "True" score of the individual. One assumption of this approach is that each item of the questionnaire is deemed to have equal "difficulty" or "impact," unless they have been explicitly weighted to be otherwise.

More recently, another set of indicators has appeared within the framework of item response theory (IRT). IRT is a general statistical theory about item (question) and scale performance, and how that performance relates to the abilities that are measured by the items in the scale (Hambelton and Jones, 1993). IRT includes a "family" of different models with different attributes, although many share the same underlying assumptions such as unidimensionality. Recent IRT literature is replete with concepts such as "differential item functioning" (DIF), which assesses group invariance; that is, given the same level of the construct being measured, the response to an item differs by group membership, for example, gender (Teresi et al., 2000). "Targeting" is where the people and scale items are congruent, such that it can be said that the scale items are "well-targeted" to the sample of people.

Overall there is an emphasis upon the individual item and its behavior with respect to the construct being measured, and how persons interact with those items. Collectively, these IRT-based approaches can be considered as "modern test theory" (although in practice they go back to the 1950s). In this approach, items are given a differential "weight" according to their difficulty level (e.g., the task of dressing oneself) and persons are given an ability estimate derived from their response to items. The probability that a person can (in the above example) dress themselves is therefore the difference between their ability and the difficulty of the task, expressed initially in a log-odds (Logit) framework (Rasch, 1960).

It is important to note that within IRT in general there are two distinct, and for some incompatible, approaches, that is, the approach belonging to the Rasch family of models and those belonging to all other IRT models (Rasch, 1960; Andrich, 2011). The former, it is argued, is consistent with the principals of fundamental invariant measurement, whereas the latter is concerned with finding the model that best explains the data (Mislevy, 1987; Hobart and Cano, 2009). Notwithstanding these potentially incompatible approaches within the modern test theory framework, the approaches share many attributes. However, do classical and modern test theories manifest different approaches to scale construction and validation, or are they simply much the same but from a different perspective, or are they different but complementary?

Comparative approaches

To best illustrate the different approaches, a comparison will be made between CTT and the Rasch model, with occasional reference to IRT in general. The principal reason for making this particular comparison is that there are fundamental differences between the application of the Rasch model and CTT that are not shared by other IRT models. For example, when data satisfy the Rasch model expectations, the item and person estimates are sample independent (Hambelton, 1993), whereas CTT and IRT are sample dependent. Furthermore, IRT models have distributional assumptions that are absent from the Rasch model. This latter aspect is important for clinical populations, as they rarely have the same distributional properties as, for example, the population at large. Finally, for the Rasch model, due to the parameter separation applied through a conditional maximum likelihood algorithm, person estimates are independent of the item parameters, and vice versa, so providing the ability to satisfy (in a probabilistic manner) the axioms of additive conjoint measurement such that estimates are provided on an interval scale, whereas for CTT and IRT these estimates remain ordinal (Luce and Tukey 1964; Lord, 1975; Mislevy, 1987; Reise and Waller, 2009; Van Newby et al., 2009; Hobart and Cano, 2009).

Acknowledging these fundamental differences, consider the process involved with developing and testing a new instrument to be applied as a self-reported outcome measure in a health-care setting, a typical PROM:

1   A theoretical and/or clinical framework to define the construct(s) to be measured.
2   Derivation of potential items from qualitative work with patients, focus groups, or other sources.

3 Decisions about the appropriate response format.
4 Cognitive debriefing of a draft questionnaire.
5 Consideration of what other scales are required to support construct (concurrent) validity.
6 Design of study to include baseline data and test–retest reliability. Consideration of group invariance to be tested (DIF).
7 Data collection and associated quality control.
8 Analytical strategy to test the new scale:
   a Unidimensionality (including separate domains if relevant)
   b Local independence assumption
   c Response option analysis (for polytomous items—is it working as intended?)
   d Group invariance
   e Internal consistency reliability
   f Test–retest reliability
   g Targeting
   h Conversion of ordinal to interval scale
   i Validity testing (e.g., known groups; concurrent)
   j Responsiveness

Most of what is generally understood to belong to the application of both classical and modern test theory can be found in point 8 of the above list, testing both the assumptions and quality indicators for a scale. Modern Test Theory also has additional assumptions relating to the stochastic ordering of items; that is, there is a probabilistic relationship between the items in any domain or scale (Gustafsson, 1980). This requirement generally forms the "tests of fit" of data to the model in the case of the Rasch model (Van der Linden, 1998). Format decisions and study design will set out some of the parameters to be analyzed in point 8 of the above list. It is also unusual for responsiveness (J) to be tested in the original scale development, as this requires a reliable and valid scale to measure change over time. Table 8.1 provides the main classical and modern test theory approaches to the quality indicators a–i in point 8 in the above list.

For illustrative purposes, a simulated data set of 300 cases and 20 items, scored 0–4 has been prepared. The data have some multidimensionality (two equally sized domains with latent correlation 0.9), DIF by gender on two items, and a pair of locally dependent items embedded within each domain. A total score is proposed, ranging from 0 to 80. The item set can also be analyzed per domain (i.e., 10 items) for illustrative purposes.

A–B. Unidimensionality and local independence assumptions

Both classical and IRT approaches would undertake a confirmatory factor analysis (CFA) on an existing scale prior to further analysis (Hahn et al., 2010; Brown, 2015). Marais and Andrich pointed out that the local independence

Table 8.1 Classical and modern test theory approaches to scale development

| Point 8 | Assumption/ indicator | Classical | Modern | |
			IRT	Rasch
a	Unidimensionality assumption	Factor analysis	Prior factor analysis	Post-hoc PCA of residuals
b	Local independence assumption	Factor analysis showing required correlations of errors	Magnitude of residual correlation	Magnitude of residual correlation
c	Category response working	None	Generally cumulative threshold estimates cannot be disordered	Threshold estimates which can be disordered
d	Group invariance	Logistic (multinomial) regression Group invariance within SEM	DIF	DIF
e, f	Reliability	Various, including alpha, test–retest	Alpha	Person separation, alpha
g	Targeting	Floor and ceiling effects	Person–item distribution maps	Person–item distribution maps
h	Ordinal to interval	No	No, proofs of such not published	Yes, proofs published
i	Validity	Various, including "external" validity	Structural validity	Structural validity
j	Responsiveness	MID/MCID	MID/MCID	On the metric

IRT, item response theory; DIF, differential item functioning; MID/MCID, minimally (clinical) important difference; PCA, principal component analysis; SEM: structural equation modeling.

assumption is an "umbrella" term including "trait" dependence (unidimensionality) and "response" dependence, which is the clustering of items such as "climbing a single flight of stairs" with "climbing several flights of stairs." In this instance, if the latter item is affirmed, so must the former, and thus the items are not truly independent (Marais and Andrich, 2008). A CFA would ascertain both these aspects.

In the case of our example, using a polychoric correlation-based analysis in MPlus, the initial CFA gives a χ^2 670.379 [df 170] p = <.001; root mean square error of approximation (RMSEA) 0.103 (90% confidence interval [CI]: 0.095–0.112); comparative fit indices (CFI) 0.959, Tucker Lewis Index (TLI) 0.954 (Muthén and Muthén, 1998–2010). Kline is very clear that the true fit is the χ^2, which should be nonsignificant, and that other fit statistics are just ancillary, except perhaps where sample sizes are very large (Kline, 2010). There is also some debate over the acceptable levels of the RMSEA, but 0.6 will usually be accepted by reviewers in the context of CFA. For a more detailed discussion see the paper by Chen et al. (2008). Other fit indices such as the TLI, and the CFI, usually carry a threshold of 0.95 but are not without their detractors. What is clear from the above analysis is that this data set has failed the CFA. However, in health outcomes it is quite common for items to reflect nuances of a particular attribute, which may have clinical relevance. For example, in a rehabilitation outcome assessment, items such as "dressing the upper body" and "dressing the lower body" may appear as separate items, albeit locally dependent upon one another. In the simulated data two pairs of such items appeared, 4 dependent upon 3 (strong), and 14 dependent upon 13 (weak). What did the CFA recover? The modification indices (MIs) showed that A4 with A3 has the highest MI value or 65.884 (it would reduce the χ^2 by this value), and so it has recovered this simulated dependency. In contrast, A14 with A13, although present, is not that high. There can be a very close relationship between clusters of locally dependent items and multidimensionality, with the former leading to what psychologists refer to as "bloated specific" factors (Cattell, 1978). Nevertheless, allowing for correlated errors with these two pairs did not resolve the dimensionality problem; the item set remains multidimensional.

What happens if the data are fitted to the Rasch model? Using the RUM2030 software package the same information is provided (Andrich et al., 2009). There is some misfit to the model expectations indicated by a summary χ^2 value of 134.5 (df 80) (p = .0001) when good-fit would show a nonsignificant χ^2. The item set indicates multidimensionality in that the post hoc test of unidimensionality shows that 10% of estimates (95% CI: 7.5–12.5) based upon independent sets of items are significantly different (Smith, 2002), whereas 5% or less (for the lower confidence interval of the test of proportions) would be indicative of unidimensionality. Items A3 and A4 are identified as having a residual correlation of 0.345; however, A13 and A14 at 0.170 are not really distinguishable from other low-level dependencies, which may themselves have been caused by the multidimensionality. Creating testlets (adding the pair of items together to make a super item) to absorb the local dependency (equivalent to correlating the errors in the CFA) does not resolve the dimensionality issue, neither does it improve fit (Wainer and Kiely, 1987).

C. *Response option analysis*

This indicator is unique to modern test theory and can differ considerably between IRT and Rasch. Generally, within IRT the transition between categories (threshold) is estimated as a cumulative probability. This means that the point on the underlying latent trait (of whatever is being measured) always increases as the response option chosen increases. Figure 8.1 shows how this would look. The items are scored 0–4, and the probability of response in a particular category increases in a manner consistent with the increase in the underlying trait. This is what is expected when the polytomous items are designed. Some IRT and Rasch applications report the average latent estimate within each category, which is very similar, but not identical, to a cumulative probability of response at the threshold. The threshold is the transition point between adjacent categories. It is more common within the Rasch framework to test if the response options are working correctly by a close examination of the threshold pattern. Figure 8.2 shows an item where the thresholds have become "disordered" (Andrich, 2013). Note that the transition between categories 2 and 3 is higher on the latent trait than that between categories 3 and 4, which should not be the case.

There are many reasons for this, in that the words attached to each category may be confusing; there may be too many categories representing small differences, but also multidimensionality may cause disordering. Often overlooked, the reading age and level of literacy may also affect responses (Chachamovicha et al., 2009). In these simulated data, the 10 items belonging to domain 1 show five disordered thresholds when analyzed in the context of all 20 items, but none are disordered when analyzed as a subset of 10 items. Thus, the analyst must consider all relevant aspects before deciding what action (if any) to take about disordering. The principal difference within modern test theory with regard to the response structure is whether disordering of thresholds is considered or not. It is rarely if ever considered within IRT (e.g., the graded response model has Thurstone cumulative thresholds) and some applications within the Rasch framework do not report on this aspect (e.g., see Luo, 2005 for further discussion).

D. Group invariance

DIF occurs when construct-irrelevant covariates interfere with the relationship between construct levels and item response (Mukherjee et al., 2013). Originally

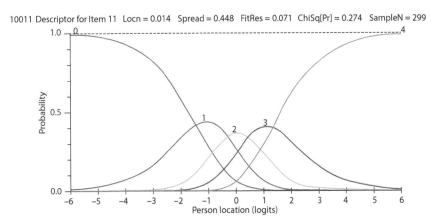

10011 Descriptor for Item 11 Locn = 0.014 Spread = 0.448 FitRes = 0.071 ChiSq[Pr] = 0.274 SampleN = 299

Figure 8.1 Response option profile.

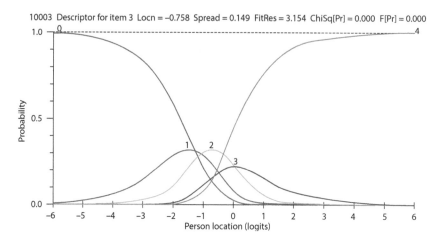

Figure 8.2 Disordered thresholds.

referred to as "item bias," in an educational setting and early health settings, it was used to ascertain bias in testing by race or gender (Teresi et al., 1995). For example, *at the same level of ability*, the response to a test item should be the same for both males and females. Thus, the response to an item by group membership is conditioned on the total score, most preferably a subset of that score that is free from DIF (Lange et al., 2000). In health sciences, the approach is widely used to test for DIF by age and gender and other aspects, such as diagnostic group (in generic instruments) or cross-cultural validity (Tennant et al., 2004).

Classical approaches to DIF include tests such as Mantel–Haenszel or (ordinal) logistic regression (Mantel and Haenszel, 1959; Swaminathan and Rogers, 1990). More recently, there is a potential elegant approach within structural equation modeling (SEM), but this has yet to be refined. It has the potential to provide, within the Classical Test Theory Framework, an integrated approach similar to that found within modern test theory, that is, testing the structural validity, including trait and response independence, and group invariance all within its measurement model perspective. Thus, a CFA can be established within an SEM framework and group invariance can be tested and items whose loadings are statistically different across groups can be identified.

Unfortunately, there are problems when some variables display considerable DIF. In domain 2, the first of 10 items (item 3 in the total set) shows considerable DIF (Figure 8.3). The Rasch analysis on the 10 items of domain 2 (to avoid confounding by dimensionality issues) shows that at any level of the construct being measured, males will report a much higher score than females. Note that this is an example of uniform DIF, where there is a consistent difference between males and females across the whole trait. Should the trace lines for males and females cross, then this would be nonuniform DIF (e.g., see Teresi et al., 2000).

Unfortunately, the third item also displays DIF in the opposite direction, which was not simulated to be so, and illustrates the problem of "artificial" or compensatory DIF, where the item is forced to be biased in the opposite

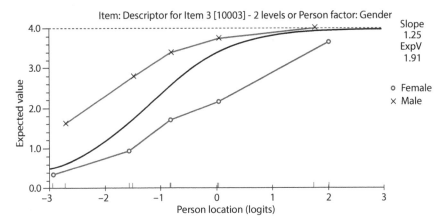

Figure 8.3 Differential item functioning.

direction because of strong DIF in another item (Andrich and Hagquist, 2012). This can be addressed within the Rasch framework by allowing the item with the most DIF to be split such that (in this case) males and females have a different item difficulty estimate for the first item and then this resolves the artificial DIF, which disappears. The SEM group invariance post hoc test for significant differences when the coefficients are constrained to be equal between groups, clearly identifies the first variable to be biased, by a significant order of magnitude greater than all other variables (i.e., it clearly stands out as lacking invariance—Wald test p <.0001; score test p <.001). Males have a much higher loading on this item than do females. So the SEM analysis identifies the simulated DIF, in the context of all the other items in domain 2. Just as with the Rasch analysis, a second variable shows marginal DIF, in this case with females loading higher than males. The MIs in the SEM point to the need for separating males and females on the first item. As the latest strategy within the Rasch framework would be to resolve the variable showing the highest DIF first, and then see what happens, this would seem to be a useful solution within the SEM framework, constraining the coefficients for the DIF variable to be different by group (in this example by gender), after which the remaining DIF can be reviewed. Although this may be a strategy for DIF within the classical test framework, it does not indicate whether the item has uniform or nonuniform DIF, the latter, for example, expressed as an interaction between the item and the trait within an ordinal logistic regression (e.g., see Cameron et al., 2014).

E–F. Reliability

Cronbach's alpha (α) is the most recognizable form of reliability in CTT. It indicates the lower bound of the reliability of a test. It *assumes* unidimensionality and cannot indicate such an attribute; rather it expresses the interconnectedness of items (Green et al., 1977). It is linked to the discriminative ability of a test, whereby an α of 0.7 can distinguish two groups of respondents, 0.8 three groups,

0.9 four groups, 0.92 five groups, and so on (Fisher, 1992). In this respect, it can be interpreted as an indicator of the degree of precision of a test, which is why common practice would suggest a minimum of 0.7 for group comparisons, but much higher (e.g., 0.9) for individual or "high stakes testing" (Bland and Altman, 1997). The α of the 20-item simulated set is 0.957, despite the multidimensionality.

It is just one of many forms of reliability in CTT with, perhaps, "test–retest" reliability being the next most familiar. Here the new scale would be tested to see if it was stable over a short period where no change would be expected. Originally, this would be a simple (Spearman) correlation, often accompanied by the median score for the two time points. The latter was necessary as a correlation would not be able to uncover a systematic bias across time. More recent approaches to test–retest reliability have emerged, notably the intraclass correlation coefficient (Weir, 2005). What is apparent about this approach is that it ignores the ordinal nature of test scores, and applies parametric procedures (e.g., analysis of variance [ANOVA]) in its calculations. Such misuse of ordinal data could lead to incorrect inference (Khan et al., 2015).

Modern test theory equivalents center upon "Person Separation" Indices (PSIs) (Andrich, 1982). These have traditionally had a close link to α, although recently the RUMM2030 has changed the calculation of PSI such that it still remains equivalent to α when the data are normally distributed but deviates when the data are skewed and, particularly when there are substantial floor or ceiling effects. Indeed, substantial floor or ceiling effects may inflate α, given the responses to random sets of items (split-half reliability) as they will give perfect correlations under these circumstances. The PSI of the 20-item set is 0.960 (also reporting α as 0.957). Quite often within the modern test theory framework, α is still reported (Kirisci et al., 1996).

G. Targeting

The presence of minimum (floor) and maximum (ceiling) scores has always been understood to be problematic and is often reported (Alonso et al., 1998). It can constrain the ability of a scale to both show the full range of the construct relevant to a particular sample, as well as to show change (for example, it is unknown how far above the ceiling an individual may be, and thus despite showing a decline in the construct being measured, they may nevertheless still be above or at the ceiling). In educational testing this would be equivalent to giving students a test that was too easy (ceiling effect) or too hard (floor effect). It would be seen as a poor test, but in health this may not be so uncommon. For example, screening a population for depression may give a left-skewed effect (low scores) with a sizeable floor effect. In the simulated 20-item scale, only one person out of 300 was at the extreme. The Rasch analysis has the ability to graphically show the relationship between the distribution of persons and items on the same interval scaled metric (Figure 8.4). Thus, the average person ability (–0.030 logits, upper level of graph) matches almost exactly the average difficulty of the item set (centered on zero logits), and consequently the scale is deemed to be perfectly targeted at the people (it was simulated to be so). Logits, or log odds ratio is the unit of measurement

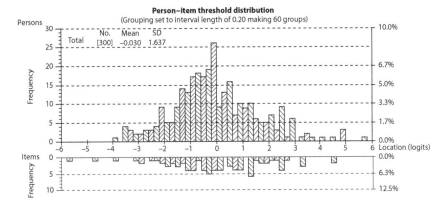

Figure 8.4 Persons and item distributions on the same metric scale.

derived from modern test theory, but the invariance requirement is only available within the Rasch model, so giving interval scaling (Fischer and Molenaar, 1995).

H. *Ordinal to interval*

All PROMs in their "raw" state provide an estimate of the trait at the ordinal level. In other words, the magnitude of the attribute is being assessed. Many articles have, over the years, given a warning about the misuse of such data, such as the calculations of means and standard deviations, or change scores, including such aspects as minimally important differences (MID) (Forrest and Andersen, 1986; Merbitz et al., 1989; Doganay Erdogan et al., 2015). Where data are shown to satisfy the assumptions of the Rasch model then a transformation is available to provide an interval scale latent estimate. This should avoid the possible pitfalls of misusing ordinal data and drawing the wrong inference from the results of a study (Merbitz et al., 1989; Khan et al., 2015). The Rasch transformation shows clearly the non-linear nature of the ordinal raw score (Figure 8.5). The data from domain 1 (10 items) satisfied all the Rasch model assumptions (χ^2 35.2 [df 40] p = 0.684; PSI and α 0.94; no residual item correlation >0.1; lower CI: *t*-test for unidimensionality 3.5%).

I. *Validity (external)*

Validity is asking the question: Does the scale measure what is intended? Excluding structural validity, at the present time it appears to remain in the domain of CTT. Thus, all the various types of validity indexed in the COSMIN checklist can be found in the literature. Of note, the most ascertainment of validity uses the ordinal raw score but not all use appropriate nonparametric based statistics for this purpose. The reporting of concurrent validity and, for example, known groups validity can all be accomplished by nonparametric approaches, for example, a Kruskal–Wallis one-way ANOVA.

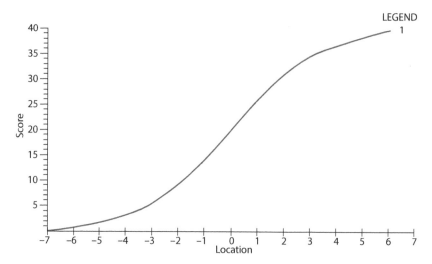

Figure 8.5 Raw score to interval scale (location) transformation for domain 1.

It is possible that modern test theory approaches may emerge, for example, by the cocalibration of scales to show that they measure the same construct (Fisher et al., 1995). Thus, for example, in the development of a new fatigue scale, with an existing comparator fatigue scale, rather than (or as well as) reporting the correlation between the two scales, reporting the result of considering the item sets of both scales to belong to one item set. There may have to be some adjustment for local response dependency, in that some items may be very similar, but it would be an interesting adjunct to the classical way of reporting validity.

J. Responsiveness

The ability to detect change is an important characteristic of most health outcome scales, and comparisons of responsiveness are often made between different scales (Guyatt et al., 1992; de Yébenes Prous et al. (2008); Hsieh et.al., 2009). There are various indicators for responsiveness such as the effect size (Kaziz et al., 1989), the standardized response mean (Liang et al., 1990), and the responsiveness statistic (Guyatt et al., 1987). They all have something in common, mathematical calculations (e.g., change score) on mostly ordinal scales. As such, little confidence can be placed in the various reported levels. It can be seen from Figure 8.5 that a raw score change at the margins of a PROM is likely to represent a substantial larger change (on the metric) than such a change in the middle of the scale. Calculations such as minimally (clinical) important difference (MCID/MID) are similarly affected (Doganay Erdogan et. al., 2015). Over 25 years ago, Merbitz et al. made it very clear that such calculations are not valid on ordinal scales and, despite continuing evidence that this is the case, this practice of misusing ordinal scales remains widespread (Merbitz et al., 1989; Grimby et al., 2012).

Summary

Both classical and modern test theory share some common aspects in the ascertainment of indicators of psychometric quality. This is particularly the case for structural validity, the very basis of the validity for PROMs, where evidence is presented that a set of items can be summated to provide a total score. All other indicators of psychometric quality are based upon this foundation. Using simulated data as an example, it has been shown that much the same results can emerge from either approach. The more recent analytical strategies such as structural equation modeling also offer a more integrated approach, similar to that found in Rasch analysis and IRT in general, such that several indicators—local response dependence, unidimensionality, group invariance—can all be ascertained at the same time. Modern test theory has some additional benefits, notably the ability to check if polytomous items are working as intended, and the Rasch model provides an interval scale transformation when data satisfy its assumptions. This may be one way of improving the confidence in the various responsiveness indices, although carrying out such calculations on the metric. On the other hand, modern test theory has little to add to the tests of external validity, other than providing a confirmation that the item set can be summated and, again for the Rasch model, confirmation that this raw score is a sufficient statistic (all you need for the estimate of the persons level of the construct) (Fisher, 1934). Without needing the transformation to the interval scale, the nonparametric Mokken scale model will also confirm sufficiency (Mokken, 1971).

For the debate between Rasch and the remainder of IRT, Mislevy argues that the link to additive conjoint measurement theory "is a central issue in the unresolved (and possibly unresolvable) debate between those who advocate the exclusive use of Rasch models and those who forgo its satisfaction by using other models in order to fit data better." The desirable inferential properties of the restricted family of Rasch models are played off against their ability to capture the patterns present in real data" (Mislevy, 1987). Thus, as Andrich points out, this may well be a case of incompatible paradigms (Andrich and Hagquist, 2012). Fortunately, CTT and modern test theory as applied in the Rasch model do appear to complement one another and together can provide strong evidence of the structural validity of a PROM, as well as, in the latter case, additional indicators such as sufficiency and interval scaling.

References

Alonso, J., Prieto, L., Ferrer, M., Vilagut, G., Broquetas, J.M., Roca, J., et al. (1998). Testing the measurement properties of the Spanish version of the SF-36 Health Survey among male patients with chronic obstructive pulmonary disease. Quality of Life in COPD Study Group. *J. Clin. Epidemiol.*, 51(11), 1087–1094.

Andrich, D. (1982). An Index of person separation in latent trait theory, the Traditional KR-20 Index, and the Guttman Scale Response Pattern. *Educ. Res. Perspect.*, 9, 95–104.

Andrich, D. (2011). Rating scales and Rasch measurement. *Expert Rev. Pharmacoecon. Outcomes Res.*, *11*, 571–585.

Andrich, D. (2013). An expanded derivation of the threshold structure of the polytomous rasch model that dispels any "Threshold disorder controversy". *Educ. Psychol. Meas.*, *73*(1), 78–124.

Andrich, D., and Hagquist, C. (2012). Real and artificial differential item functioning. *J. Educ. Behav. Stat.*, *37*, 387–416

Andrich, D., Sheridan, B.E.D., and Luo, G. (2009). *RUMM2030: Rasch Unidimensional Models for Measurement.* Perth, Western Australia: RUMM Laboratory.

Bland, M.J., and Altman, D.G. (1997). Crombach's alpha. *BMJ.*, *314*, 572.

Brown, T.A. (2015). *Confirmatory Factor Analysis for Applied Research, (Methodology in the Social Sciences)* (2nd Edition). New York, NY: Guilford Press.

Cameron, I.M., Scott, N.W., Adler, M., and Reid, I.C. (2014). A comparison of three methods of assessing differential item functioning (DIF) in the Hospital Anxiety Depression Scale: Ordinal logistic regression, Rasch analysis and the Mantel chi-square procedure. *Qual. Life Res.*, *23*(10), 2883–2888.

Cattell, R.B. (1978). *The Scientific Use of Factor Analysis in Behavioral and Life Sciences.* New York, NY: Plenum.

Chachamovicha, E., Flecka, M.P., and Power, M. (2009). Literacy affected ability to adequately discriminate among categories in multipoint Likert Scales. *J. Clin. Epidemiol.*, *62*(1), 37–46.

Chen, F., Curren, P.J., Bollen, K.A., Kirby, J., and Paxton, P. (2008). An empirical evaluation of the use of cut points in RMSEA test statistic in structural equation models. *Social Methods Res.*, *36*, 462–494.

de Yébenes Prous, M.J.G., Salvanés, F.R., and Ortellsa, L.V. (2008). Responsiveness of outcome measures. *Rheumatol. Clin.*, *4*(6), 240–247.

Doganay Erdogan, B., Leung, Y.Y., Pohl, C., Tennant, A., and Conaghan, P.G. Minimal clinically important difference as applied in rheumatology: An OMERACT Rasch Working Group Systematic Review and Critique. *J. Rheumatol.*, *43*, 194–202. 2015 Jun 1. pii: jrheum.141150. [Epub ahead of print]

Engelhard, G., Jr. (2013). *Invariant Measurement: Using Rasch Models in the Social, Behavioural and Health Sciences.* New York, NY: Routledge.

Fischer, G.H., and Molenaar, I.W (eds.). (1995). *Rasch Models: Foundations, Recent Developments, and Applications.* New York, NY: Springer.

Fisher, R.A. (1934). Two new properties of mathematical likelihood. *Proc. Royal Soc. A*, *144*, 285–307.

Fisher, W.P. Jr. (1992). Reliability statistics. *Rasch Measure Trans.*, *6*, 238.

Fisher, W.P., Jr., Harvey, R.F., Taylor, P., Kilgore, K.M., and Kelly, C.K. (1995 Feb). Rehabits: A common language of functional assessment. *Arch. Phys. Med. Rehabil.*, *76*(2), 113–122.

Forrest, M., and Andersen, B. (1986). Ordinal scales and statistics in medical research. *BMJ*, *29.*, 537–538.

Green, S.B., Lissitz, R.W., and Mulaik, S.A. (1977). Limitations of coefficient alpha as an index of test unidimensionality. *Educ. Psychol. Meas.*, *37*, 827–838.

Grimby, G., Tennant, A., and Tesio, L. (2012 Feb). The use of raw scores from ordinal scales: Time to end malpractice? *J. Rehabil. Med.*, *44*(2), 97–98.

Gustafsson, J.E. (1980). Testing and obtaining fit of data to the Rasch model. *Br. J. Math. Stat. Psychol.*, *33*, 205–233.

Guyatt, G.H., Kirshner, B., and Jaeschke, R. (1992). Measuring health status: What are the necessary measurement properties? *J. Clin. Epidemiol.*, *45*, 1341–1345.

Guyatt, G., Walter, S., and Norman, G. (1987). Measuring change over time: Assessing the usefulness of evaluative instruments. *J. Chronic Dis.*, *40*, 171–178.

Hahn, E.A., Devellis, R.F., Bode, R.K., Garcia, S.F., Castel, L.D., Eisen, S.V, et al. (2010). PROMIS Cooperative Group Measuring social health in the patient-reported outcomes measurement information system (PROMIS): Item bank development and testing. *Qual. Life Res.*, *19*, 1035–1044.

Hambleton, R.K., Jones, R.W., and Rogers, H.J. (1993). Influence of item parameter estimation errors in test development. *J. Educat. Measurem.*, 30, 143–155.

Hobart, J., and Cano, S. (2009). Improving the evaluation of therapeutic interventions in multiple sclerosis: The role of new psychometric methods. *Health Technol. Assess.*, *13*(12), 1–177.

Hsieh, Y.W., Wu, C.Y., Lin, K.C., Chang, Y.F., Chen, C.L., and Liu, J.S. (2009). Responsiveness and validity of three outcome measures of motor function after stroke rehabilitation. *Stroke.*, *40*, 1386–1391.

Kaziz, L., Anderson, J.J., and Meenan, R.F. (1989). Effect sizes for interpreting changes in health status. *Med. Care.*, *27*, S178–S189.

Khan, A., Chien, -W., and Bagraith, K.S. (2015). Parametric analyses of summative scores may lead to conflicting inferences when comparing groups: A simulation study. *J. Rehabil. Med.*, *47*, 300–304.

Kirisci, L., Moss, H.B., and Tarter, R.E. (1996 May–Jun). Psychometric evaluation of the Situational Confidence Questionnaire in adolescents: Fitting a graded item response model. *Addict. Behav.*, *21*(3), 303–317.

Kirshner, B., and Guyatt, G. (1985). A methodological framework for assessing health indices. *J. Chronic Dis.*, *38*, 27–36.

Kline, R.B. (2010). *Principles and Practice of Structural Equation Modelling* (3rd Edition). New York, NY: Guilford Press.

Lange, R., Irwin, H.J., and Houran, J. (2000). Top-down purification of Tobacyk's revised paranormal belief scale. *Pers. Individ. Dif.*, *29*, 131–156.

Liang, M.J., Fossel, A.H., and Larson, M.G. (1990). Comparisons of five health status instruments for orthopedic evaluation. *Med. Care*, *28*, 632–642.

Lord, F.M. (1975). The "ability" scale in item characteristic curve theory. *Psychometrika*, *40*, 205–217.

Luce, R.D., and Tukey, J.W. (1964). Simultaneous conjoint measurement: A new type of fundamental measurement. *J. Math. Psychol.*, *1*(1), 1–27.

Luo, G. (2005). The relationship between the Rating Scale and Partial Credit Models and the implication of disordered thresholds of the Rasch models for polytomous responses. *J. Appl. Meas.*, *6*(4), 443–455.

Mantel, N., and Haenszel, W. (1959). Statistical aspects of the analysis of data from retrospective studies of disease. *J. Natl. Cancer Inst.*, *22*, 719–748.

Marais, I., and Andrich, D. (2008). Formalising dimension and response violations of local independence in the unidimensional Rasch model. *J. Appl. Meas.*, *9*, 200–215.

Merbitz, C., Morris, J., and Grip, J.C. (1989). Ordinal scales and foundations of misinference. *Arch. Phys. Med. Rehabil.*, *70*, 308–312.

Mills, R.J., Young, C.A., Pallant, J.F., and Tennant, A. (2010). Development of a patient reported outcome scale for fatigue in multiple sclerosis: The Neurological Fatigue Index (NFI-MS). *Health Qual. Life Outcomes.*, *8*, 22.

Mislevy, R.J. (1987). Recent developments in item response theory. *Rev. Res. Educ.*, *15*, 239–275.

Mokken, R.J. (1971). *A Theory and Procedure of Scale Analysis with Applications in Political Research*. New York-Berlin, NY: de Gruyter (Mouton).

Mokkink, L.B., Terwee, C.B., Patrick, D.L., Alonso, J., Stratford, P.W., Knol, D.L, et al. (2010 Jul). The COSMIN study reached international consensus on taxonomy, terminology, and definitions of measurement properties for health-related patient-reported outcomes. *J. Clin. Epidemiol.*, *63*(7), 737–745.

Mukherjee, S., Gibbons, L.E., Kristjansson, E., and Crane, P.K. (2013). Extension of an iterative hybrid ordinal logistic regression/item response theory approach to detect and account for differential item functioning in longitudinal data. *Psychol. Test Assess. Model.*, *55*, 127–147.

Muthén, L.K., and Muthén, B.O. (1998–2010). *Mplus User's Guide* (6th Edition). Los Angeles, CA: Muthén & Muthén.

Nunnally, J.C. (1978). *Psychometric Theory*. New York, NY: McGraw-Hill Book Company.

Rasch, G. (1960/1980). *Probabilistic Models for Some Intelligence and Attainment Tests*. Copenhagen, Danish Institute for Educational Research), expanded edition (1980) with foreword and afterword by B.D. Wright. Chicago, IL: The University of Chicago Press.

Reise, S.P., and Waller, N.G. (2009). Item response theory and clinical measurement. *Annu. Rev. Clin. Psychol.*, *5*, 27–48.

Smith, E.V. (2002). Detecting and evaluation the impact of multidimensionality using item fit statistics and principal component analysis of residuals. *J. Appl. Meas.*, *3*, 205–231.

Swaminathan, H., and Rogers, H.J. (1990). Detecting differential item functioning using logistic regression procedures. *J. Educ. Meas.*, *27*, 361–370.

Tennant, A., Penta, M., Tesio, L., Grimby, G., Thonnard, J-L., Slade, A, et al. (2004). Assessing and adjusting for cross cultural validity of impairment and activity limitation scales through differential item functioning within the framework of the Rasch model: The Pro-ESOR project. *Med. Care.*, *42*(Suppl. 1), 37–48.

Teresi, J.A., Kleinman, M., and Ocepek-Welikson, K. (2000). Modern psychometric methods for detection of differential item functioning: Application to cognitive assessment measures. *Stat. Med.*, *19*, 1651–1683.

Teresi, J.A., Golden, R.R., Cross, P., Gurland, B., Kleinman, M., and Wilder, D. (1995). Item bias in cognitive screening measures: Comparisons of elderly white, Afro-American, Hispanic and high and low education subgroups. *J. Clin. Epidemiol.*, *48*, 473–483.

Thurstone, L.L. (1919). A scoring method for mental tests. *Psychol. Bull.*, *16*, 235–240.

Thurstone, L.L. (1931). Measurement of social attitudes. *J. Abnorm. Soc. Psychol.*, *26*, 249–269.

Thurstone, L.L. (1928). The measurement of opinion. *J. Abnorm. Soc. Psychol.*, *22*, 415–430.

Van der Linden, W.J. (1998). Stochastic order in dichotomous item response models for fixed, adaptive, and multidimensional tests. *Psychometrika*, *63*, 211–226.

Van Newby, A., Conner, G.R., and Bunderson, C.V. (2009). The Rasch model and additive conjoint measurement. *J. Appl. Meas.*, *10*, 348–354.

Wainer, H., and Kiely, G. (1987). Item clusters and computer adaptive testing: A case for testlets. *J. Educ. Meas.*, *24*, 185–202.

Weir, JP. (2005). Quantifying the test-retest reliability using the intra-class correlations coefficient and the SEM. *J. Strength Conditioning Res.*, *19*, 231–240

World Health Organization. (2001). *International Classification of Functioning, Disability and Health: ICF*. World Health Organization.

9 Item generation and construction of questionnaires

Nina Tamm, Janine Devine, and Matthias Rose

Abbreviations

A-CAT	anxiety-CAT
CAT	computerized adaptive test
CTT	classical test theory
D-CAT	depression-CAT
DIMDI	German Institute for Medical Documentation and Information
DRM	day reconstruction method
DSM-IV	diagnostic statistical manual of mental disorders IV
EMA	ecological momentary assessments
EMR	electronic medical records
FDA	Food and Drug Administration
GAD-7	generalized anxiety disorder scale
ICD-10	*International Classification of Diseases 10*
IRT	item response theory
PHQ-9	patient health questionnaire-depression scale
PRO	patient-reported outcomes
PROMIS	patient-reported outcomes measurement information system

Background

Historically, medicine was focused on the treatment of acute diseases, and today's paradigms are still profoundly influenced by the treatment of infectious diseases with "cure" being the natural treatment target. However, as most diseases today are chronic disorders (Vos et al., 2012) complete recovery or "cure" is much less likely to be achieved (see Chapter 1). Instead the goals of most medical interventions today are to prevent further morbidity and to improve the functionality of the patients as well as their perceived health status.

Thus, within the framework of an evidence-based medicine a precise, reliable, and valid, that is, "objective," empirical assessment of the patient's reported "subjective" health status is warranted. Patient self-reported health measures are used (1) to monitor treatment success, (2) to predict other health outcomes,

(3) to screen for health disorders, or (4) to allocated resources. There is a plethora of instruments available today, which can assess a wide range of health constructs with excellent psychometric properties. For practical, economic, and scientific reasons, it is generally recommended to use one of the instruments available.

However, new research questions evolve and new tools will need to be developed. Several federal institutions, including the U.S. Food and Drug Administration (FDA, 2009) or the German Institute for Medical Documentation and Information (DIMIDI) (Brettschneider et al., 2011), have issued guidance documents for the development of self-assessment instruments. Within the next paragraphs we will focus on those steps, which are generally recommended and also used for the development of the Patient-Reported Outcomes Measurement Information System (PROMIS). The PROMIS initiative, which we are part of, is the most comprehensive and well-funded effort worldwide for the development of tools for the assessment of the patient's subjective health status (www.nihpromis.org).

Construct definition—"The work before the work"

The adequacy of new instruments depends most of all on the theoretical concepts of the construct aimed to be measured. For some it may seem rather obvious, for example, like pain. However, even for a straightforward construct that may be assessed by a single question (e.g., "Do you have pain?"), in most cases different theoretical aspects need to be considered before a measurement tool can be built. For our example, the developer needs to decide if pain existence, severity, duration, or frequency is of main interest; if different pain qualities should be weighted; or different locations considered. From a measurement perspective, the first step of selecting an appropriate measurement approach is to decide whether the assessment shall focus on generic symptoms of pain relevant for many conditions, or specific symptoms of one particular disorder.

One standard way is to screen the literature very carefully (using keywords and medical/psychological literature databases) to define the construct theoretically, as well as gather expert input on the construct at hand, for example, using standardized interviews. Also, in structured interviews, ask the patients and caregivers involved about the construct/chronic condition and its impact as it helps to fully understand all aspects of the construct and inform the next steps of item development. Furthermore, it may help to identify tools that already measure the construct in the specific field, and carefully inspect their content (validity), psychometric properties, practical advantages, as well as their limitations.

Conceptional framework

For many higher order constructs such as physical functioning (see Chapter 4 about the International classification of functioning [ICF]), those theoretical considerations are even more complex. Researchers need to define which

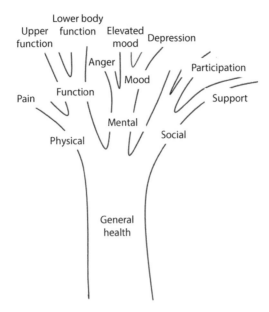

Figure 9.1 Example of a health domain hierarchy, including subdomains and facets.

subdomains (e.g., function of the upper, or lower extremity, back, and neck) should be included in one comprehensive score. In general, higher order domains (e.g., physical health or mental health) need to include a larger number of subdomains and facets for a comprehensive assessment (Figure 9.1). To make claims on a particular hierarchy level (e.g., "drug X improves your physical health"), the FDA requires a complete assessment of all subdomains' contribution to the higher order construct (FDA, 2009).

In addition, different underlying conditions may influence different subdomains of a higher order constructs differently. Thus, weighting of subdomains within one comprehensive score may influence the responsiveness of the tool (e.g., a physical function questionnaire including more items asking about musculoskeletal functions may be most responsive for patients with rheumatoid arthritis, whereas a physical function instruments primarily including items asking about cardiopulmonary functioning may be most responsive for patients with heart failure).

Polarity of the construct

From a measurement perspective, a dimensional construct with lower or higher quantities needs to be assumed. For many health constructs, it has been extensively discussed whether the assumption of the construct being "unipolar" is appropriate (e.g., from "no depression" to "high depression"). This model is usually favored by clinicians by using a pathology model where "depression" is a symptom of a disease and no symptom of the disease would be health. Another model, more often favored by epidemiologists, is to assume "bipolar"

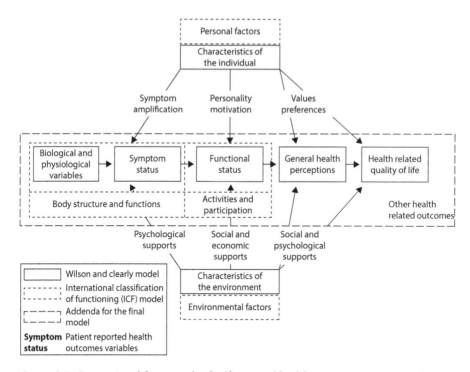

Figure 9.2 Conceptional framework of self-reported health status measurements. (From Valderas, J.M., and Alonso, J., *Qual. Life Res.*, 17, 1125–1135, 2008.)

health states, that is, a continuum from positive health to negative health states. This model has a larger measurement range and allows the assessment of different health levels in the normal population as well (e.g., from elevated to depressed mood states).

Relation to other health constructs

Once the construct is determined, its position within a framework of health outcome tools should be determined. Probably the most well-known framework is from Wilson and Cleary (1995). A more comprehensive model is provided by Valderas and Alonso (2008) (Figure 9.2; see also Chapter 12). Essentially, self-assessment tools can be distinguished into the following four categories: assessment of (1) symptoms, (2) functions, (3) their specific impact on the patient's perceived heath status, and (4) a generic assessment of health-related quality of_life_(QoL).

Item generation—"The art work"

The item generation includes a number of practical steps, which should be followed to ensure acceptance of the tool being developed. If the instrument is intended to be used to support labeling claims for product development, an item-tracking matrix (FDA, 2009) is usually recommended, which includes all steps mentioned below. In general, the development of the tool is an iterative process where first several items are written by the author—based on knowledge gained from literature reviews, initial focus groups, interviews with patients and family members, or other sources—presented to patients or experts to evaluate content validity and item comprehension by cognitive testing (Collins, 2003; Drennan, 2003; Irwin et al., 2009; Napoles-Springer, 2006; Willis, 1999, 2005a, 2005b), and refined and reconsidered until the first instrument is compiled for field testing.

Literature review

The first step in the creation of a content valid item pool usually includes a systematic literature review, among other approaches. To identify all existing instruments that measure the concept of interest or some subconcepts, a systematic literature review should be performed, for example, using an approach developed by Klem et al. (2009). According to this approach, controlled vocabularies are developed that operationalize, for example, (1) the concept of interest, (2) measurement, and (3) mode of administration. These vocabularies are applied to scientific databases, for example, PubMed or PsycINFO. To select relevant articles, inclusion and exclusion criteria are specified. Abstracts of identified articles are reviewed. Subsequently articles that conform to the inclusion criteria are retrieved. Authors of the instruments of interest are then contacted to obtain approval to review items. When an item pool of existing instruments is successfully retrieved and permission to review items is obtained, relevant concepts can be extracted by experts.

Expert involvement

Qualitative input from clinical experts is crucial to determine the current knowledge base regarding the concept of interest, to propose a definition of the concept of interest, to specify the relation to subconcepts, and to generate ideas for possible draft items. Research questions are specified before semistructured interviews or open interviews with clinical experts are conducted. Additionally, experts could be asked to prepare for interviews by reviewing definitions and specifications of the concept of interest. Following each interview, concept specification is iteratively revised (Ravens-Sieberer et al., 2014).

Focus group sessions with health professionals discussing the specification of the concept are often used in item generation. Concept mapping (e.g., using an approach by Novak and Canas, 2008) is a useful tool in guiding the generation of ideas during focus group sessions. Concept maps are graphical tools for organizing and representing knowledge. They include concepts and relations between concepts. Relations are indicated by a connecting line, and are labeled by a term, which specifies the relationship. The concepts are represented in a hierarchical fashion: Broader concepts are arranged at the top of the map, while more specific are arranged hierarchically below. Cross-lines link concepts of different (sub-)domains. Often a focus question like "What Is Health-Related Quality of Life for You?" is used to initiate the design of a concept map.

Patient involvement

It is recommended that input from the target patient population is included in the item generation. Qualitative interviewing is essential to support content validity of the instrument. The aim is the identification of item concepts comprehensively covering the full spectrum of the concept of interest and the contribution to its evaluation. It is quite important to understand the patient's perspective of the concept of interest to generate content valid items. During patient interviews, interviewees are asked to describe how they understand the concept of interest. Additionally, they respond to more specific questions regarding thoughts, feelings, and behavior toward the concept of interest. In the course of this process, audio tapes and/or transcripts are registered. These transcripts are subjected to thematic analysis to summarize key findings. Specific expressions used by patients could be retained for item generation. If a new relevant concept emerges during patient interviewing, the conceptualization is iteratively revised (Ravens-Sieberer et al., 2014).

The involvement of patients in the early stages of item generation allows the development of items that are closer to the "real world." The patient population studied in the instrument development process should represent the target population enrolled in subsequent clinical trials. It is vital to gain input from a variety of patients within the population of interest to represent variations in health condition severity and in characteristics such as age, sex, and ethnicity. This will ensure that the instrument is applicable for the specific population (FDA, 2009). The development and testing of items in student populations are important disadvantages of many existing instruments, since the representation of the target population is not given.

The sample size cannot be determined in advance. It should depend on the completeness of information gained. Saturation is reached when no new relevant information is generated by the patients and further interviews are not likely to add to the understanding of the patient's perspective of the concept of interest. The quality of the interviews performed with patients and the diversity of patients included are key factors for a comprehensive understanding of the patients' view of the concept of interest. Qualitative interviews can also be held with other information sources such as family members.

Item construction

Literature review and expert and patient or other source input lead to the specification of themes and domains within the concept or even to a concept map. These concepts and subconcept specifications or the resulting concept map are used to create item expressions (item context, item stem, and response set). These draft items are discussed in several focus group sessions with the following aims: identification of gaps in concept specification and item wording and the establishment of face and content validity. The concept specification and the draft items are modified iteratively after each focus group session. Initial big item pools can be systematically grouped by using "binning" (i.e., classification of items into domains according to their content) and "win-nowing" (elimination of items that lack face validity or are similar to better worded items) during focus group sessions.

Instruction and recall period

Instructions allow patients to understand to which recall period they should refer and how they should use the response options. As many respondents just briefly run over instructions, important information such as the recall period is recommended to be printed in bold (see Irwin et al., 2009). The instruction should be as clear and brief as possible. Sometimes it is necessary to provide a general instruction at the beginning and then give specific instructions for sub-scales or separate instructions for specific items or item sets, in case different recall periods or response options are used in subsets of items (Rauchfleisch, 2009). New instructions for each item should be avoided to keep the respond-ent burden as low as possible.

The choice of recall period depends on the instrument's purpose, intended use, the variability, duration, frequency, intensity of the concept of interest, the disease or condition's characteristics, and the tested treatment (FDA, 2009). If we are interested in changes in the concept of interest (state assessment), short recall periods (e.g., integrated effect over a short period of 2 weeks) have to be estab-lished. Patients can be requested to respond on current state, so, for example, the effect at regular time intervals (e.g., every 2 weeks) can be collected. Short recall periods or current state reporting are preferable to avoid respondent bias. However, sometimes long recall periods are necessary (e.g., if a trait variable is measured). If outcomes are expected to be stable over time (trait assessment), a long recall period (e.g., patients shall refer to "the last 3 months" or patients are requested to describe themselves "in general") is assigned.

When integrated effects over a long time period are surveyed, some prob-lems may occur. Patients may be influenced by their state (current mood). As a consequence, their responses may be biased and patients are likely to add noise and mask treatment effects (FDA, 2009). If detailed recall of experience over a long period is necessary, appropriate methods should be used to increase the validity and reliability of retrospectively reported data (e.g., ask patients to respond on the basis of their worst or best experience over the recall period or to make use of a diary as reported below). When using a method of unsuper-vised data entry, it is important to train patients to make entries according to the clinical trial design. Thereby, respondent bias can be limited.

The FDA (2009) shows increasing interest in the use of Ecological Momentary Assessments (EMAs) or Day Reconstruction Methods (DRMs) (Dockray et al., 2010; Kahneman et al., 2004; Stone etv al., 2010). These methods address the problem of recall bias. It has been frequently questioned what the tool meas-ures, when a patient is asked to report on his or her health state over a time span of 1 or 4 weeks, that is, to what extent does the current health state distort the evaluation of the recall assessment. This may be particularly important for the assessment of emotional distress (Edmondson et al., 2013; Kashdan and

Collins, 2010; Pfaltz et al., 2010). DRM and EMA typically use some kind of electronic data capturing device (e.g., a smart phone) to assess the patient's health status under daily life conditions. The patient is being asked in different planned or randomly selected intervals to report their current health status frequently. All collected time points are later integrated for a comprehensive picture of the health status over a given time span. Although the use of EMA or DRM is rare until now, this may become a relevant upcoming technology for patient-reported outcome assessments outside clinical environments.

Item stem and item content

Instrument design involves the development of item wording that permits respondents successfully to answer the question that is asked. It is important to ensure that not only all patients understand the item in the same way, but also that patients understand the item in the way it is intended by the researcher and that response is not biased by the way the item is worded. Generally, an item stem, for example, "Are you able to" or "Does your health now limit you to" can be distinguished from the item content, for example, "walk a mile" or "turn the faucets."

Items are recommended to be as simply worded and clear as possible to guarantee that all patients understand the item regardless of their academic background or cognitive skills. Ambiguous wording has to be avoided, as well as the use of colloquial or technical terms, and academic expressions. In developing items assessing chronic diseases and their impact on QoL, dependency, or medical care it is crucial to consider the health literacy of respondents. Health literacy is "the degree to which individuals have the capacity to obtain, process, and understand basic health information and services to make appropriate health decisions" (Selden et al., 2000). Furthermore, it is recommended to ask for concrete behavioral criteria rather than asking hypothetical questions. When asked hypothetically, patients may be tempted to respond on the basis of their desired condition rather than on their actual condition (FDA, 2009). When statements are created, the use of "I" rather than "You" is assumed to support the identification of the respondent. The sentence structure should not be too complex to avoid that respondents experience the instrument as exertive. When pediatric instruments are constructed, the age-related differences in respect to development processes should be taken into consideration. As the development of abstract reasoning and metacognitions starts at the age of 8 and progresses across adolescence, younger children could experience difficulties with more abstract evaluations or comparisons with inner experience points (Ravens-Sieberer et al., 2014). Quantifications in both item text and response options should be avoided as they may confuse patients. Double negations should be eliminated. They occur when the item is negated and the patient negates the negation, for example, by choosing the response option "do not agree." Such complicated thinking processes have to be prevented to minimize confusion of patients and to facilitate completion of the instrument. All items should be relevant for most of the patients in the clinical trial, as the use of not applicable response options creates problems with scoring. Skip patterns may create difficulties in administration and patients may fail to understand the instructions to skip questions. It is important to create sensitive items, which detect changes when there is a known change in the concept of interest. Items should be included that discriminate between patients either at the upper or the lower end of the normal distribution. Items for which no variation in answers is elicited (all patients respond in marking the same response option, e.g., all patients affirm the item) should be avoided as they carry no information. Further considerations affect the respondent burden, which should be as low as possible. The font size should be easy to read (in special consideration of the target group, e.g., visually impaired people and children).

Response options

Response options for each item should be consistent with its purpose and intended use. There are different types of item response options, which can be used. They are described in detail in this section.

Response format can be unstructured, that is, open entry fields for qualitative input or structured with given response options. Structured single option formats are generally used as they are easier to analyze. Visual analog scales (VAS) are lines of fixed length (usually 100 mm) with words that anchor the scale at the endpoints and no words anchoring the intermediate positions. Patients respond to the item by marking the location on the line corresponding to their perceived state. VASs are frequently used in pain assessment. Anchored or categorized VASs are VASs with one or more additional intermediate marks anchored by reference terms to facilitate the identification of the locations between the two endpoints of the scale (e.g., halfway). Likert scales are ordered sets of discrete terms or statements. Patients are instructed to choose the response option that best describes their state or experience. Often a statement is followed by different levels of agreement, for example, strongly agree, rather agree, rather disagree, and strongly disagree. Rating scales are sets of numerical categories with the endpoints of the rating scales being anchored with words and the categories between being numbered rather than labeled with words. Patients are instructed to choose the category that best describes their state or experience. Recordings of events as they occur refer to event logs that can be included in a patient diary or other reporting systems. The patient is instructed to record specific events as they occur. Pictorial scales are sets of pictures applied to any of the other response option types (e.g., Self-Assessment Manikins scales, Bradley and Lang (1994), for ratings of subjectively experienced affect). They are often used in pediatric questionnaires, questionnaires for cognitive impaired patients, or patients who are otherwise unable to speak or write. Checklists comprise a limited set of options, such as "Yes," "No," and "Don't know." The patient is instructed to place a mark in the option that applies to him or her or in some checklists that comprise statements to place a mark in a space if the item is true. Checklists should be complete and not redundant.

There are some recommendations to ensure appropriateness of item response options, which are described in the following. Wording used in response options should be clear and appropriate (e.g., anchoring a scale using the term "normal" assumes that patients understand what is normal for the general population). Item response option type should be suitable for the intended population (e.g., no use of VAS for visual impaired patients). There should be a clear distinction between response options (e.g., the distinction between "intense" and "severe" could be difficult for patients who are asked to describe their pain). The number of response options should be empirically justified based on existing literature, qualitative research, or initial instrument testing. The following questions have been discussed extensively: Is it better to use a 4-, 5- or 7-point scale? Is there a bias toward the middle? Are decisions being forced when the middle option is omitted? There are no simple answers to those questions. However, we recommend using a 4-point scale in items, which ask for the level of agreement with a statement. Using an even number of response choices forces the respondent to mark the direction of their attitudinal tendency. A neutral middle point risks to be attempting for respondents who did not understand the item or who do not want to reflect about the item. In our experience, four response options show the best distributions for this type of question.

For items that ask for frequency or intensity we recommend a 5-point scale, as patients are often overstrained when choosing between more than five response options, and fewer response options provide less information when using item response theory methods (see below).

Response options should be appropriately ordered and represent similar intervals. Potential ceiling or floor effects should be avoided. It may be necessary to add more response options or modify the item wording to allow better differentiation at the higher or lower end of the response scale. Thereby, it is avoided that almost all patients respond at the maximum or minimum endpoint of the scale and a better discrimination between respondents at the higher or lower end is reached. Response options should not bias the direction of responses. It is crucial to provide an equal number of options toward the two ends of the scale (e.g., possible response options for a severity spectrum should be weighted equally at the mild and the severe end).

Patients may want to conform to notions of social desirability and self-presentation, even when the impact of social desirability factors is often limited to questions perceived as being sensitive and potentially threatening. The problem of social desirability bias is more present in face-to-face or telephone interviews but has to be taken into account in deciding on the mode of data collection and the privacy of the setting in which the instrument is completed.

Cognitive testing

Traditional piloting of an instrument can detect overt problems that disrupt the response elicitation process. To detect covert problems and to understand why problems arise in answering the questions, cognitive interviewing has to be performed. Cognitive interviewing is necessary to evaluate whether or not respondents can understand the item, or if respondents understand the item in a consistent way and in the way the researcher intended. It can be used to better understand the potential sources of measurement error, to identify reasons why certain items cannot be answered by some patients, and to provide concrete ideas how to modify wording to reach a better understanding.

Cognitive interviewing is crucial for the evaluation of comprehensibility and the identification of problematic items that may create response error and decrease questionnaire response rates. It allows direct input from respondents on item content, format, and comprehensibility. Cognitive interviewing helps to understand the mental steps that patients go through when they respond to a specific item. The theoretical underpinning of cognitive methods is the four-stage cognitive model introduced by Tourengeau (1984). In its simplest form, the model suggests that there are four components of the response process: comprehension, retrieval, judgment, and response (Tourangeau et al., 2004).

The two main cognitive techniques are think aloud interviewing and probing. The think-aloud technique is a method in which patients are instructed to tell all their thoughts in answering the items. The think-aloud method is usually used concurrently, that is, information about thoughts of the patient is collected during the completion of the instrument. The probing method is an approach in which the interviewer asks specific questions or *probes,*which helps to identify the cognitive processes of the patient. Probing can be either retrospective or concurrent (e.g., "What does the term X mean to you?").

Standardized probing questions focus on different aspects of the instrument. They can be included into the think-aloud technique. Questions concerning the instruction (e.g., "What does 'in the past 7 days' mean to you?"), items (e.g., patients can be asked to rephrase the items in their own words), domains (e.g., "How do you think these items are related?"), response choices (e.g., "What do you think about the response choices?"), and overall assessment (e.g., "Would you change anything in the questionnaire?") can be asked (Irwin et al., 2009).

To reduce respondent burden, a sampling scheme is applied. It allows each respondent to be tested on a limited set of items rather than all items of the instrument. Some authors suggest that every single item should be tested in 10–15 cognitive interviews (Willis, 2005).

There are some limitations of cognitive interviewing (Collins, 2003). Cognitive interviews are qualitative in nature and, therefore, they can neither provide quantitative information on the extent of comprehension problems nor quantitative evidence on whether or not the revised version of the instrument is better than the original. The researcher has to evaluate the importance of an item problem and the necessity to revise the item on the basis of qualitative feedback. Furthermore, respondents can experience difficulties in "thinking aloud," because not all cognitive processes can be verbalized as they occur very fast. Respondents who have difficulties in verbalizing their thoughts are less prone to participate in cognitive testing. Therefore, the sample on which cognitive interviewing is performed could be not representative for the target population. Besides, the cognitive interview process can affect the way respondents answer questions and as a result bias the responses. Despite these limitations, cognitive interviewing allows a better understanding of sources of measurement error and enables researchers to integrate input from the target population in the early development stages of the instrument. As mentioned before, the involvement of patients into the development and revision of an instrument helps to create items that are higher in content validity and better in comprehensibility.

Literacy level evaluations should be performed to judge if instruction and item text are understandable for children of a certain grade-school level. Common analyzing methods are the Flesch–Kincaid method in Microsoft Word and the Lexile Analyzer (2013; MetaMetrics, Durham, NC). The Flesch–Kincaid method analyzes and rates text on a U.S. grade-school level based on the average number of syllables per word and words per sentence to calculate a readability score that indicates the school reading level required to understand the text (Klare, 1976).

When item banks are translated in different languages to establish the instrument internationally, translation experts and content experts review each item concerning translatability and cultural adaptability following international and PROMIS standards (Adler and Fagley, 2005; Kim et al., 2005; Wild et al., 2005). If items are not generated in all language groups included in subsequent clinical trials, the appropriateness of the content should be evaluated in cognitive interviewing within each language group of the target population (FDA, 2009).

To ensure comprehension of the revised items, cognitive interviews should be performed again after deletion and modification of items. Items that continue to create problems in understanding should either be modified or deleted. It is pivotal to evaluate iteratively if deletion and modifications of items affect content coverage of the respective subconcepts to which each item is assigned (Collins, 2003; Drennan, 2003; Irwin et al., 2009; Napoles-Springer, 2006; Willis, 1999, 2005).

Comprehensive documentation

A detailed documentation of all steps in the development process of the instrument is recommended, including documentation of the complete list of items generated, the modifications, and deletions made and the reasons for those changes (item-tracking matrix). Documentation should include all item generation techniques used, the populations studied, source of items, selection, editing and reduction of items, cognitive interview summaries or transcripts, pilot testing, importance ratings, and quantitative techniques for item evaluation. Documentation of patient input in item generation as well as cognitive interviewing transcripts is crucial to support content validity. This documentation contributes to prove the instrument adequacy in measuring the concept of interest. The FDA published a list of recommended documents that should be generated and evaluated in detail to ensure the quality of the new developed or revised instrument (FDA, 2009).

Scale development—"The hard work"

The main goal of any instrument development is to provide a valid and precise tool. As the validity of the tool is largely determined by the qualitative work described above, choosing the right items for a scale largely determines the measurement precision and measurement range. There are excellent textbooks describing the construction of scales (Allen and Yen, 2001; Moosrugger and Kelava, 2012), and a comprehensive description of all methods for scale development is beyond the scope of this chapter. Within the next paragraphs, we will highlight a few examples to demonstrate the potential advantages of more recently established methods.

Scoring algorithms

The majority of tools used today are constructed based on the assumption of the classical test theory (CTT). The CTT was developed at the start of the nineteenth century (Spearman, 1907) and put into axiomatic measurement formulas by Gulliksen (1950) and Novick (1966). The main axiom is that any test score is a result of a "true score" and a "measurement error." CTT methods have been used to develop highly informative instruments (like the SF-36, McHorney et al., 1993, 1994; Ware and Sherbourne, 1992), which are widely accepted in the medical field. Most instruments assessing perceived health states sample items from different domains (e.g., mood, cognition, behavior, somatic symptoms) to capture a comprehensive set of manifest indicators of the underlying latent construct. CTT tools usually use sum scores to aggregate the responses to the items of the scale to one combined total score. Summing up equally weighted responses to each item is appropriate when responses to items are independent and items have the same item difficulty. However, if two items are dependent (which is often the case), their summed information is less than two independent items and they are overweighted when they are treated as two equally weighted items. This overweighting is especially problematic if the number of response categories varies by item and if (sub)scale scores are aggregated into a single test score.

The probabilistic test theory, or often also called Item Response Theory (IRT), provides a solution to many of the limitations of the CTT, including the issue of overweighting. IRT methods were developed more than four decades ago (Lord and Norvick, 1968; Rasch, 1960), and numerous attempts have been made to exploit their potential (Bech et al., 1978; Fisher, 1993). Today, IRT-based tests are well established in the educational field (Wainer et al., 2000; Cohen et al., 1989), but have just been introduced into health care during the past decade (Ware et al., 2003, 2000; Cella and Chang, 2000; Bjorner et al., 2003).

Like factor analysis, IRT models assume that the measured construct is a latent variable, referred to as the IRT score, theta, or θ that cannot be observed directly but can be estimated based on responses to different items measuring the construct. An IRT item bank consists of items measuring the same construct and a mathematical description of the items' measurement properties (Bjorner et al., 2004). The IRT model (van der Linden and Hambleton, 1997; Fischer and Molenaar, 1995) describes the probability of choosing each response on a questionnaire item as a function of theta (Embretson, 1996, 2000). There are several different models being used for health-care applications with unique psychometric properties (Wainer et al., 2000; van der Linden and Hambleton, 1997; Embretson and Reise, 2000; van der Linden and Glas, 2000). One important distinction of all IRT methods from classical test theory methods is that theta can be estimated from the responses to *any* subset of items in the bank (Bjorner et al., 2004). Accordingly, researchers or clinicians can select items that are most relevant for a given group or an individual patient and score the responses on one common metric that is independent of the choice of items. In addition, if the item bank contains items from established questionnaires, scores on these questionnaires can be predicted from estimates of theta even if the questionnaires themselves have not been administered. Thus, comparisons of results from different questionnaires are expected to be facilitated with the introduction of comprehensive IRT item banks (Bjorner et al., 2003; Rose et al., 2008; Wahl et al., 2014).

Today, the most recently developed comprehensive tests are using IRT methods (Alonso et al.,. 2013; Cella et al., 2007). Chapter 7 discusses the differences between CTT and IRT methods in great detail, thus we can focus on some practical implications for scale development here.

Item information

For any scale construction a decision needs to be made on which items should be included. IRT methods provide several methods to make a rational choice about the use of the best items in a particular questionnaire. The item information curve (IIC) visualizes the information of each item in relation to the measurement range (Figure 9.3). The item information of all items determines the measurement precision of the IRT score. CTT methods only allow the evaluation of the measurement range and precision on a scale (not item) level.

For example, Figure 9.3 shows the IICs of three established physical functioning items asking about similar content (Rose et al., 2008). The figures show that the LSU7 item provides the most information over the largest measurement range. Thus, when constructing a scale one would probably prefer this item over the SF-36 item (PF7). The figure also shows that the item with three response options provides the least overall information. To explore this further we have deliberately included a number of permutations of items measuring the same content in the PROMIS data collection (Fries et al., 2014). Figure 9.4 shows an example that IRT curves allow to make a rational choice about response options as well as the use of the item stem. To construct a scale, those IIC curves can be easily used to inform the developer which items cover which range of measurement with high precision.

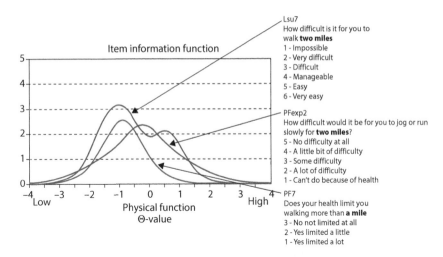

Figure 9.3 Item information functions of three items from different existing instruments. (Data from Rose, M. et al., *J. Clin. Epidemiol.*, 61, 17–33, 2008.)

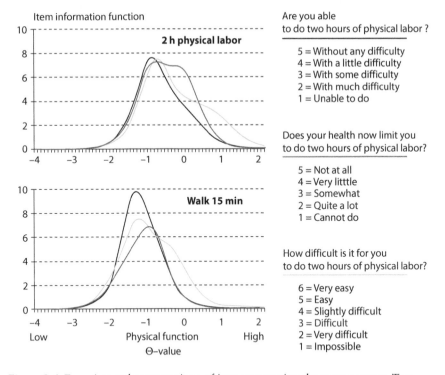

Figure 9.4 Experimental permutations of items measuring the same content. Two items with different content are displayed: "Do two hours of physical functioning" and "Walk for 15 minutes on even ground." Item stems and response options are the same for both items and shown for the first item on the right side of the figure. (Data from Rose, M. et al., *J. Clin. Epidemiol.*, 67, 516–526, 2014.)

Reliable range

The main goal of any instrument is to provide maximum precision with a minimal number of items. Usually, the "precision" of an instrument is described using a measure of internal consistency, like the Cronbach α coefficient. However, Cronbach α does not reflect a sample independent measurement and does not provide information about the precision of the tool in relation to its measurement range. In fact, all static tools do have floor and ceiling effects, that is, low precision at the low and top end of their measurement range, which cannot be captured by Cronbach α values. (For detailed information on reliability assessment, please see Garson, 2013.)

IRT methods offer more informative methods to evaluate the measurement precision in relation to the measurement range on the item and scale level. In our opinion, the term "reliable range" is a useful term to describe this relation. The reliable range can be determined when inspecting the test information function, which is a combined function of all information of the items of a scale. As an example, Figure 9.5 shows that the measurement precision and range of different established depression measures differ substantially (Wahl et al., 2014). The graphs show that some tools are more reliable in the general population, whereas others are more suited for clinical samples. We believe that those methods are intuitively informative to improve scale construction by adding more precise items and choosing the scales most suited for the purpose of the study.

Norming

One aspect of scale development is becoming more relevant in recent years. Scales covering more generic aspects of health, like physical function, depression, etc., are becoming more often centered based on representative population data. The idea behind this is to facilitate an intuitive interpretability of scale scores. It has been discussed if a Z-scale, that is, a zero representing the population mean, or a T-metric should be favored, that is, with 50 representing the population mean. Others have suggested a score of 100 like for the assessment in intelligence. In our view, today mostly a score of 50 is recommended, with a standard deviation of 10. Thus, a score of 60, for example, on a depression scale would indicate that the respondent is one standard deviation above the general population mean.

Respondent burden

The most precise and comprehensive health assessment questionnaires are usually rather lengthy and complex, leading to a level of respondent burden that hampers their use in routine care and leads to substantial problems of missing data. Therefore, tools that are popular are relatively short questionnaires (Snaith, 2003; Spitzer et al., 2006; Zigmon and Snaith 1983). They represent a compromise in measurement precision, range, and other desirable attributes

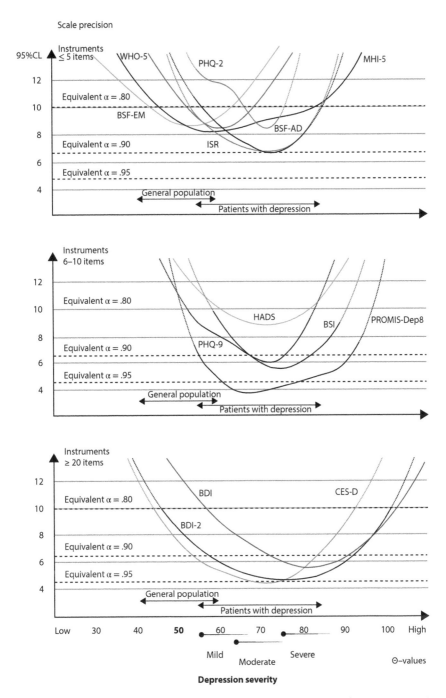

Figure 9.5 Reliable range of different static instruments measuring depression severity. (From Wahl, I. et al., *J. Clin. Epidemiol.*, 67, 73–86, 2014.)

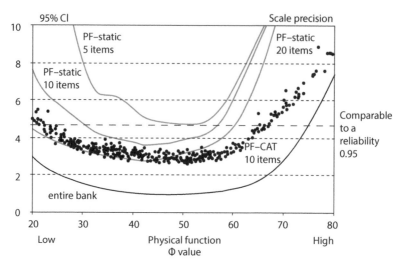

Figure 9.6 Reliable range of static and dynamic instruments measuring physical function. (From Rose, M. et al. *J. Clin. Epidemiol.*, 67, 516–526, 2014.)

in favor of practicality (Lowe et al., 2010). These short forms are useful for measuring/screening the health status of large samples, but in a small sample, or, when test scores of individual patients are monitored over (treatment) time their reduced precision causes concerns (McHorney and Tarlov, 1995).

Individually tailored, dynamic tools (computer adaptive tests, CATs) can provide shorter and more precise measures (Becker et al., 2008; Fliege et al., 2005; Walter et al., 2007). There is an extensive explanation of CATs in other chapters of this book. Figure 9.6 compares the reliability range of static instruments to a CAT. It illustrates that a 10-item CAT can provide as much information like a 20-item instrument over a much larger measurement range.

Modes of assessment

There are several different modes of assessment as described in the following chapters. The most established forms are paper–pencil assessments. However, mainly for economic reasons electronic modes of assessment are becoming more popular. All modes of assessment have their unique advantages, and the study design is likely to decide which mode of assessment will be favored. In general, paper–pencil assessments, interactive voice recognition, or computer assisted assessments provide comparable results (Bjorner et al., 2014).

Instrument validation—"The true work"

After an instrument is carefully developed, its validity needs to be demonstrated. There are several approaches to assess the validity of a scale: evaluating the *content validity*, that is, whether the instrument truly measures the intended content of the target construct; the *criterion validity* investigating the relationship of the target construct to external criteria (like Diagnostic Statistical Manual of Mental Disorders IV [DSM-IV] diagnoses); and the *construct validity*, which can be tested by hypotheses of associations of the target construct to *similar* constructs (assessed by similar measures, like other depression scales) also called the *convergent* validity, or to different constructs (measured by different scales) also called the *discriminant* validity. *Responsiveness to change* needs to be demonstrated for outcome assessments, as well as *minimal clinical important differences* to assess meaningful differences between or within group comparisons. Other chapters in this book describe these issues in detail (Campbell and Fiske, 1959).

Outlook

The empirical assessment of health symptoms from the patient's perspective is essential for an evidence-based medicine in general and in particular to monitor treatment success for chronic diseases. Modern methods allow developing instruments, which can provide valid and reliable assessments of most health constructs. This chapter describes most of the issues that need to be considered to build and chose new items for instruments with excellent psychometric properties.

However, despite the immense methodological progress being made over the last decades, the measurement of the self-reported health status is not as established as the measurement of biomarkers in medical routines. One reason for this may be that all current instruments provide different scores making an intuitive interpretation and communication more difficult. In addition, if the same construct is being measured with different tools, scores cannot be easily compared. The situation is as if body temperatures assessed in different settings were not comparable with one another but were dependent on the particular thermometer used (Ware, 1993, 2008).

Thus, we encourage all readers to consider carefully if an existing instrument may be available before constructing a new instrument as not to contribute to a situation that already reminds us of the Tower of Babel.

To make the measurement of self-reported health constructs more similar to biomedical ones, we strongly believe that a standardized, efficient approach for a variety of applications including ambulatory monitoring, clinical trials research, and population monitoring needs to be developed, so that results can be compared across conditions, therapies, trials, and patients. IRT methods allow building large item banks, which have the potential to provide those common metrics and first studies have been published in this direction (Wahl et al., 2014; Choi et al., 2014; Schalet et al., 2014). Future developments will show if these efforts will be adopted by the scientific community.

Acknowledgment

We like to acknowledge the valuable, thoughtful comments and careful edits from our colleague and coworker Melanie Conrad from the Department for

Psychosomatic Medicine, Center for Internal Medicine and Dermatology, Charité, Universitätsmedizin Berlin.

References

Adler, M.G., and Fagley, NS. (2005). Appreciation: Individual differences in finding value and meaning as a unique predictor of subjective well-being. *J. Pers.*, 73, 79–114.

Allen, M.J., and Yen, W.M. (2001). *Introduction ot Measurement Theory*. Long Grove, IL: Waveland Press.

Alonso, J., Bartlett, S.J., Rose, M., Aaronson, N.K., Chaplin, J.E., Efficace, F., Leplège, A., Lu, A., Tulsky, D.S., Raat, H., Ravens-Sieberer, U., Revicki, D., Terwee, C.B., Valderas, J.M., Cella, D., Forrest, C.B.; PROMIS International Group. (2013). The case for an international patient-reported outcomes measurement information system (PROMIS(R)) initiative. *Health Qual. Life Outcomes*, 11, 210.

Bradley, M.M., and Lang, P.J. (1994). Measuring emotion: The self-assessment manikin and the semantic differential. *J. Behav. Ther. Exp. Psy.*, 25, 49–59.

Brettschneider, C., Luehmann, D., and Raspe, H. (2011). *The Value fo the Patient-Reported Outcome (PRO) for Health Technology Assessments (HTA) (German)*. Cologn., Germany: DIMDI - German Institute for Medical Documentation and Information.

Bech, P., Allerup, P., and Rosenberg, R. (1978). The Marke-Nyman temperament scale. Evaluation of transferability using the Rasch item analysis. *Acta. Psychiatr. Scand. Suppl.*, 57, 49–58.

Bjorner, J.B., Kosinski, M., and Ware, J.E., Jr. (2003a). Calibration of an item pool for assessing the burden of headaches: An application of item response theory to the headache impact test (HIT™). *Qual. Life Res.*, 12, 913–933.

Bjorner, J.B., Kosinski, M., and Ware, J.E., Jr. (2003b). Using item response theory to calibrate the Headache Impact Test (HIT) to the metric of traditional headache scales. *Qual. Life Res.*, 12, 981–1002.

Bjorner, J.B., Kosinski, M., and Ware, J.E., Jr. (2004). Computerized adaptive testing and Item banking. In: P.M. Fayers and R.D. Hays (eds.), *Assessing Quality of Life* (2nd Edition). Oxford: Oxford University Press.

Bjorner, J.B., Rose, M., Gandek, B., Stone, A.A., Junghaenel, D.U., and Ware, J.E., Jr. (2014). Difference in method of administration did not significantly impact item response: An IRT-based analysis from the Patient-Reported Outcomes Measurement Information System (PROMIS) initiative. *Qual. Life Res.*, 23, 217–227.

Becker, J., Fliege, H., Kocalevent, R.D., Bjorner, J.B., Rose, M., Walter, O.B., et al. (2008). Functioning and validity of a computerized adaptive test to measure anxiety (A-CAT). *Depress Anxiety*, 25, E182–E194.

Campbell, D.T., and Fiske, D.W. (1959). Convergent and discriminant validation by the multitrait-multimethod matrix. *Psychol. Bull.*, 56, 81–105.

Cella, D., and Chang, C.H. (2000). A discussion of item response theory and its applications in health status assessment. *Med. Care*, 38, II66–II72.

Cella, D., Yount, S., Rothrock, N., Gershon, R., Cook, K., Reeve, B., et al. (2007). The Patient-Reported Outcomes Measurement Information System (PROMIS): Progress of an NIH roadmap cooperative group during its first two years. *Med. Care*, 45, S3–S11.

Choi, S.W., Schalet, B., Cook, K.F., and Cella, D. (2014). Establishing a common metric for depressive symptoms: Linking the BDI-II, CES-D, and PHQ-9 to PROMIS depression. *Psychol. Assess.*, 26, 513–527.

Cohen, Y., Ben-Simon, A., and Tractinsky, N. (1989). *Computerized Adaptive Test of English Proficiency*. Jerusalem, Israel: NITE.

Collins, D. (2003). Pretesting survey instruments: An overview of cognitive methods. *Qual. Life. Res.*, 12, 229–238.

Dockray, S., Grant, N., Stone, A.A., Kahneman, D., Wardle, J., and Steptoe, A. (2010). A comparison of affect ratings obtained with ecological momentary assessment and the day reconstruction method. *Soc. Indic. Res.*, 99, 269–283.

Drennan, J. (2003). Cognitive interviewing: Verbal data in the design and pretesting of questionnaires. *J. Adv. Nurs.*, 42, 57–63.

Edmondson, D., Shaffer, J.A., Chaplin, W.F., Burg, M.M., Stone, A.A., and Schwartz, J.E. (2013). Trait anxiety and trait anger measured by ecological momentary assessment and their correspondence with traditional trait questionnaires. *J. Res. Pers.*, 47, 843–852.

Embretson, S.E. (1996). The new rules of measurement. *Psychol. Assessment*, 8, 341–349.

Embretson, S.E, and Reise, S.P. (2000). *Item Response Theory for Psychologists.* London: Lawrence Erlbaum Associates.

Fliege, H, Becker, J., Walter, O.B., Bjorner, J.B., Klapp, B.F., and Rose, M. (2005). Development of a computer-adaptive test for depression (D-CAT). *Qual. Life Res.*, 14, 2277–2291.

Fisher, A.G. (1993). The assessment of IADL motor skills: An application of many-faceted Rasch analysis. *Am. J. Occup. Ther.*, 47, 319–329.

Fischer, G.H, and Molenaar, I.W. (1995). *Rasch Models—Foundations, Recent Developments, and Applications* (1st Edition). Berlin: Springer-Verlag.

Irwin, D.E., Varni, J.W., Yeatts, K., and DeWalt, D.A. (2009). Cognitive interviewing methodology in the development of a pediatric item bank: A patient reported outcomes measurement information system (PROMIS) study. *Health Qual. Life Outcomes*, 7, 3.

Fries, J.F., Witter, J., Rose, M., Cella, D., Khanna, D., and Morgan-DeWitt, E. (2014). Item response theory, computerized adaptive testing, and PROMIS: Assessment of physical function. *J. Rheumatol.*, 41, 153–158.

Garson, G.D. (2013). *Validity & Reliability.* Asheboro, NC: Statistical Associates Publishing.

Gulliksen, H. (1950). *Theory of Mental Tests.* New York: Wiley.

Kahneman, D., Krueger, A.B., Schkade, D.A., Schwarz, N., and Stone, A.A. (2004). A survey method for characterizing daily life experience: The day reconstruction method. *Scienc.*, 306, 1776–1780.

Kashdan, T.B., and Collins, R.L. (2010). Social anxiety and the experience of positive emotion and anger in everyday life: An ecological momentary assessment approach. *Anxiety Stress Coping*, 23, 259–272.

Kim, J., Keininger, D.L., Becker, S., and Crawley, J.A. (2005). Simultaneous development of the Pediatric GERD Caregiver Impact Questionnaire (PGCIQ) in American English and American Spanish. *Health Qual. Life Outcomes*, 3, 5.

Klare, G. (1976). A second look at the validity of readability formulas. *J. Reading Behav.*, 8, 129–152.

Klem, M., Saghafi, E., Abromitis, R., Stover, A., Dew, M.A., and Pilkonis, P. (2009). Building PROMIS item banks: Librarians as co-investigators. *Qual. Life Res.*, 18, 881–888.

Lord, F.M., and Norvick, M.R. (1968). *Statistical Theories of Mental Test Scores.* Reading: Addison-Wesley.

Lowe, B., Wahl, I., Rose, M., Spitzer, C., Glaesmer, H., Wingenfeld, K., et al. (2010). A 4-item measure of depression and anxiety: Validation and standardization of the Patient Health Questionnaire-4 (PHQ-4) in the general population. *J. Affect. Disord.*, 122, 86–95.

McHorney, C.A., and Tarlov, A.R. (1995). Individual-patient monitoring in clinical practice: Are available health status surveys adequate?. *Qual. Life Res.*, 4, 293–307.

McHorney, C.A., Ware, J.E., Jr., Lu, J.F., and Sherbourne, C.D. (1994). The MOS 36-item short-form health survey (SF-36): III. Tests of data quality, scaling assumptions, and reliability across diverse patient groups. *Med. Care*, 32, 40–66.

McHorney, C.A., Ware, J.E., Jr., and Raczek, A.E. (1993). The MOS 36-Item short-form health survey (SF-36): II. Psychometric and clinical tests of validity in measuring physical and mental health constructs. *Med. Care*, 31, 247–263.

Moosrugger, H., and Kelava, A. (2012). *Testtheorie udn Fragebogenkonstruktion.* Berlin: Springer.

Napoles-Springer, A.M., Santoyo, J., O'Brien, H., and Stewart, A.L. (2006). Using cognitive interviews to develop surveys in divers populations. *Med. Care, 44,* S21–S30.

Novick, M.R. (1966). The axioms and principal results of classical test theory. *J. Math. Psychol., 3,* 1–18.

Novak, J.D., and Canas, A.J. (2008). The Underlying Concept Maps and How to Construct and Use Them. Florida Institute for Human Machine Cognition. Technical Report IHMC Cmap0 Tools 2006-01 Rev 01-2008.

Pfaltz, M.C., Michael, T., Grossman, P., Margraf, J., and Wilhelm, F.H. (2010). Instability of physical anxiety symptoms in daily life of patients with panic disorder and patients with posttraumatic stress disorder. *J. Anxiety Disord., 24,* 792–798.

Rasch, G. (1960). *Probabilistic Models for Some Intelligence and Attainment Tests.* Chicago, IL: University of Chicago Press.

Rauchfleisch, U. (2005). *Testpsychologie. Eine Einführung in die Psychodiagnostik.* Göttingen, Germany: Vandenhoeck & Ruprecht.

Ravens-Sieberer, U., Devine, J., Bevans, K., Riley, A.W., Moon, J., Salsman, J.M., et al. (2014). Subjective well-being measures for children were developed within the PROMIS project: Presentation of first results. *J. Clin. Epidemiol., 67,* 207–218.

Rose, M., Bjorner, J.B., Becker, J., Fries, J.F, and Ware, J.E. (2008). Evaluation of a preliminary physical function item bank supported the expected advantages of the Patient-Reported Outcomes Measurement Information System (PROMIS). *J. Clin. Epidemiol., 61,* 17–33.

Rose, M., Bjorner, J.B., Gandek, B., Bruce, B., Fries, J.F., and Ware, J. (2014). The PROMIS physical function item bank was calibrated to a standarized metric and shown to improve measurement efficiency. J. Clin. Epidemiol., 67, 516–526.

Schalet, B.D., Cook, K.F., Choi, S.W., and Cella, D. (2014). Establishing a common metric for self-reported anxiety: Linking the MASQ, PANAS, and GAD-7 to PROMIS Anxiety. *J. Anxiety Disord., 28,* 88–96.

Selden, C., Zorn, M., Ratzan, S.C., and Parker, R.M. (2000). Health literacy (bibliography online). National Libary of Medicine, Bethesda, MD. Available from: www nlm nih gov/pubs/resources html [serial online].

Snaith, R.P. (2003). The hospital anxiety and depression scale. *Health Qual. Life Outcomes, 1,* 29.

Spearman, C. (1907). Demonstration of formulae for true measurement of correlation. *Am. J. Psychol., 18,* 161–169.

Spitzer, R.L., Kroenke, K., Williams, J.B., and Lowe, B. (2006). A brief measure for assessing generalized anxiety disorder: The GAD-7. *Arch. Intern. Med., 166,* 1092–1097.

Stone, A.A., Schwartz, J.E., Broderick, J.E., and Deaton, A. (2010). A snapshot of the age distribution of psychological well-being in the United States. *Proc. Natl. Acad. Sci. U S A, 107,* 9985–9990.

Tourengeau, R. (1984). Cognitive science and survey methods: A cognitive perspective. In: *Cognitive Aspects of Survey Design: Building a Bridge Between Disciplines* (pp. 73–100). Washington, DC: National Academic Press.

Tourangeau, R., Rips, L.J., and Rasinski, K. (2004). *The Psychology of Survey Response.* Cambridge, MA: Cambridge University Press.

U.S. Food and Drug Administration [FDA]. (2009). *Guidance for Industry—Patient-Reported Outcome Measures: Use in Medical Product Development to Support Labeling Claims.* Rockville, MD: FDA, 2009.

Valderas, J.M., and Alonso, J. (2008). Patient reported outcome measures: A model-based classification system for research and clinical practice. *Qual. Life. Res., 17,* 1125–1135.

van der Linden, W.J., and Hambleton, R.K. (1997). *Handbook of Modern Item Response Theory.* Berlin: Springer.

van der Linden, W.J., and Glas, C.A.W. (2000). *Computerized Adaptive Testing: Theory and Practice*. Dordrecht: Kluwer Academic Publishers.

Vos, T., Flaxman, A.D., Naghavi, M., Lozano, R., Michaud, C., Ezzati, M., et al. (2012). Years lived with disability (YLDs) for 1160 sequelae of 289 diseases and injuries 1990–2010: A systematic analysis for the Global Burden of Disease Study 2010. *Lancet*, *380*, 2163–2196.

Wahl, I., Lowe, B., Bjorner, J.B., Fischer, F., Langs, G., Voderholzer, U., et al. (2014). Standardization of depression measurement: A common metric was developed for 11 self-report depression measures. *J. Clin. Epidemiol.*, *67*, 73–86.

Wainer, H., Dorans, N.J., Eignor, D., et al. (2000). *Computerized Adaptive Testing: A Primer* (2nd Edition). Mahwah, NJ: Lawrence Erlbaum Associates.

Walter, O.B., Becker, J., Bjorner, J.B., Fliege, H., Klapp, B.F., and Rose, M. Development and evaluation of a computer adaptive test for 'Anxiety' (Anxiety-CAT). *Qual. Life Res.*, *16*(Suppl 1), 143–155.

Ware, J.E. (1993). Measuring patients' views: The optimum outcome measure. *BMJ*, *306*, 1429–1430.

Ware, J.E,, Jr. (2008). Improvements in short-form measures of health status: Introduction to a series. *J. Clin. Epidemiol.*, *61*, 1–5.

Ware, J.E., Jr., Bjorner, J.B., and Kosinski, M. (2000). Practical implications of item response theory and computerized adaptive testing: A brief summary of ongoing studies of widely used headache impact scales. *Med. Care*, *38*, II73–II82.

Ware, J.E., Jr., Kosinski, M., Bjorner, J.B., Bayliss, M.S., Batenhorst, A., Dahlöf, C.G., et al. (2003). Applications of computerized adaptive testing (CAT) to the assessment of headache impact. *Qual. Life. Res.*, *12*, 935–952.

Ware, J.E., Jr., and Sherbourne, C.D. (1992). The MOS 36-item short-form health survey (SF-36). I. Conceptual framework and item selection. *Med. Care*, *30*, 473–483.

Wild, D., Grove, A., Martin, M, Eremenco, S., McElroy, S., Verjee-Lorenz, A., et al. (2005). Principles of good practice for the translation and cultural adaptation process for patient-reported outcomes (PRO) measures: Report of the ISPOR task force for translation and cultural adaptation. *Value Health*, *8*, 94–104.

Willis, G.B. (1999). *Cognitive Interviewing: A "How To" Guide*. Rockville, MD: Research Triangle Institute.

Willis, G.B. (2005). *Cognitive Interviewing: A Tool for Improving Questionnaire Design*. Thousand Oaks, CA: Sage Publications.

Wilson, I.B., and Cleary, P.D. (1995). Linking clinical variables with health-related quality of life. A conceptual model of patient outcomes. *JAM.*, *273*, 59–65.

Zigmon, A., and Snaith, R. (1983). The hospital anxiety and depression scale. *Acta. Psychiatr. Scand.*, *67*, 361–370.

10 Alternative approaches to questionnaires in measuring health concepts: The example of measuring how patient actually performs activities in daily life

Wilfred F. Peter, Francis Guillemin, and Caroline B. Terwee

Rationale for developing a new instrument

In the permanent search of optimizing the way of measuring health-related phenomena, there might be a few good reasons for developing a new instrument. An emerging concept, some progresses in taxonomy, the redefinition of the paradigm in which a phenomenon has to be captured, or simply unsatisfactory measurement properties of existing measures are some of these reasons. A new development needs solid theory and conceptualization before starting. The adaptation to new technologies and particularly e-health technologies will increasingly offer such opportunities and favor such developments. We will show with an example that such technologies, by bridging new gaps and offering new interfaces, may offer innovative and attractive measures, though somewhat difficult to fully fit in existing conceptual framework.

A comprehensive assessment of activity limitations in daily activities is essential in the management of hip and knee osteoarthritis (OA). Ideally, one should know how patients actually perform their daily activities in routine daily life. However, this is not feasible because this would be highly time consuming. Alternatively, two types of outcome measures are generally used: Patient-Reported Outcome Measures (PROMs) and performance-based tests (Gandhi et al., 2009).

The constructs of PROMs and performance-based tests are fundamentally different (Kennedy et al., 2003; Wittink et al., 2003). PROMs rely on self-reporting and measure the extent to which patients perceive difficulty in performing daily activities (referred to as "performance" in the International Classification of Function, Disability and Health (ICF) World Health Organization, 2002), whereas performance-based tests aim to evaluate the ability to perform isolated tasks (often measured in terms of time) administered in a standardized environment (referred to as "capacity" in the ICF World Health Organization, 2002). Because of this difference in perspective, the present body of evidence advocates the complementary implementation of both PROMs and performance-based measures (Stratford and Kennedy, 2006; Wright et al., 2011).

Both methods, however, have advantages and disadvantages: Self-report questionnaires are easy to use and cheap. However, patients' responses on self-report questionnaires are not only determined by the severity of the disease but also by a number of personal and environmental factors. It has been shown that patients use different reference frames when they respond to questions such as: "What degree of difficulty do you have ascending stairs?" (a question from the Knee Injury and Osteoarthritis Outcome Score (KOOS); Groot et al., 2008). Their responses will depend on the comparison group they have in mind. Some patients compare themselves to how they performed before they got their disease, or how they performed some time ago, whereas others compare themselves to healthy peers (Fayers et al., 2007). Their responses will also depend on what kind of stairs they have in mind as well as the importance of stair climbing in their daily life (Marsh et al., 2011). Patients' responses are also influenced by the confidence patients have in their own ability to climb stairs (Marsh et al., 2011). Cognitive impairments (Watson and Pennebaker, 1989), cultural factors, comorbidity, age, and education level also play a role in answering these and other kind of self-report questions (Hoeymans et al., 1997; Elam et al., 1991; Sager et al., 1992). Finally, responses to self-report questions are determined by the patients' interpretation of the word "difficulty." Patients may consider limitations in performing daily activities but they may also consider other factors, like pain or fatigue. It has been shown that self-report questionnaires are more influenced by pain and fatigue than performance-based tests (Maly et al., 2006; Stratford and Kennedy, 2004, 2006; Terwee et al., 2006).

Performance-based tests are less influenced by personal and environmental factors, but they also have a number of disadvantages. They measure physical functioning in an artificial situation that may provide little information about how a patient performs in his/her own environment. Furthermore, they capture only a snapshot of what a patient can functionally do. Performance-based tests can be influenced by short-term impairments, observer bias, stimulation by the tester, and by the patient's motivation to perform the test (Myers et al., 1993; Sager et al., 1992). The greatest problem with performance-based tests, however, is that they require personnel, test facilities, and physical presence of patients, which means that they are time consuming, expensive, and a burden for patients. Performance-based tests are therefore often considered unsuitable for use in large studies.

Construct: Measure of activity limitations

To the authors' knowledge none of the existing measures strives to determine how the patient actually performs activities in daily life. In light of this, the computerized Animated Activity Questionnaire (AAQ) was developed. With the AAQ, patients watch animated videos on a computer, in which a dummy (an animation of a person) performs different activities, such as stair climbing and rising from a chair, in several ways (each way exposing a different level of difficulty for the patient). Patients are asked to select the video that best represents their way of performing the activity. The AAQ combines the advantages of PROMs and performance-based tests, without many of their limitations. By showing animations, the influence of the patient's own reference frame is minimized. And due to a standardized virtual reality, the impact of different environments is also minimized. Compared with performance-based tests, the AAQ is less exposed to observer bias, bias by different test instructors and the motivation of the participant to perform the test. And because the items refer to the average performance during the past week, the AAQ does not only cover a snapshot of reality. It is expected, therefore, that an animated activity questionnaire measures the same aspects of physical functioning as measured by performance-based tests but without the practical limitations of performance-based tests.

The construct of measurement can be summarized as follows: The aim of the AAQ is to measure how a person performs basic activities in their daily life.

Central to this purpose is the term "how," which indicates that the AAQ is a measure of the quality of performance of a certain task. All activities incorporated in the AAQ should meet the following three conditions:

1 The AAQ should comprise basic daily activities (e.g., walking, stair climbing, rising, and sitting down) and not more complex activities (e.g., shopping or domestic duties) (Sikkes et al., 2009).
2 The AAQ should contain activities of which different levels of limitations can be differentiated.
3 The AAQ items must be relevant for hip and knee OA patients in different countries to facilitate international implementation.

We intended to develop a disease-specific instrument, which means that the activities to be included should be activities that patients with hip or knee OA may find difficult to perform because of their hip or knee OA.

The aims of the AAQ are

1 To support the screening for activity limitations to find indications for treatment
2 To evaluate the effect of treatment at the individual patient level in daily clinical care
3 The effect of intervention in groups of patients within a research project

The AAQ was thus developed for discriminative and evaluative purposes.

To ensure that the items of the AAQ are suitable for these purposes, only activities that can be changed by the natural course of disease or improved by therapy were included.

Target population

The AAQ was developed for patients diagnosed with hip and knee OA according to the American College of Rheumatology (ACR) criteria and aged over 18 years.

Steps in the AAQ development

Development of the AAQ—Step 1

A pilot version of the AAQ was developed in 2009. For the pilot version seven activities were selected, which patients with hip of knee OA often consider difficult to perform and that are included in most self-report questionnaires on physical functioning: ascending and descending stairs, sitting down and standing up from a low couch, sitting down and standing up from a toilet, and walking. The pilot version of the videos showed a basic virtual environment. The results of construct validity showed promising results (Terwee et al., 2014; Peter et al., 2015).

The correlation of the total score of the AAQ with the total score of the performance-based test was >0.70, as expected (0.79 (0.61–0.89)). The total score of the AAQ correlated moderately as expected with the H/KOOS activities of daily living (ADL) score (0.60 (0.32–0.78)) and the H/KOOS sport score (0.68 (0.44–0.83)), but higher than expected with the total score of questionnaires regarding specific limitations (0.90 (0.81–0.95)).

The results of the pilot study suggested that the AAQ might be a good alternative for measuring physical functioning of patients with hip or knee OA. However, the content validity of the AAQ needed to be improved, by adding more levels of difficulty to some items and adding more activities that are relevant for OA patients. In this pilot version, only seven activities were included. More animations of important activities like walking on uneven ground, picking up items from the floor, and dressing needed to be developed. In addition, patients indicated that for some activities (e.g., rising and sitting down on the toilet), additional levels of difficulty (e.g., a level including support from a grip, wall, or sink) were required. And finally, the virtual environment could be improved in order to be more close to the real-life situation in which the activity is performed.

Development of the AAQ—Step 2

Item selection

In item selection COSMIN (Mokkink et al., 2010) standards were followed to optimize content validity. Subsequently, the ICF core set for hip and knee OA (Dreinhofer et al., 2004), items from existing self-reported questionnaires (Groot et al., 2008; de Groot et al., 2007), performance-based tests (Bennel et al., 2011; Dobson et al., 2013), and self-reported activity limitations (by use of the Patient-Specific Complaints [PSC] questionnaire) (Beurskens et al., 1999) were collected from 400 patients in the Amsterdam Osteoarthritis ("AMS-OA"). Cohorts in an outpatient center for rehabilitation and rheumatology (Reade, Amsterdam, the

Netherlands) (van der Esch et al., 2012) were used to compose a list of activities for the AAQ. Then two focus groups of 10 hip and knee OA patients each were composed. In the first group limited activities were discussed to add missing activities to the draft list. In the second focus group for each activity, different levels of difficulty in execution were selected, resulting in a final list of 17 activities and three to five levels of performance (Appendix A) (Peter et al., 2015).

Response options

Every item of the AAQ included between four and six response options, corresponding with different levels of functioning, including an additional option of "unable to perform." For a complete description of all items and corresponding response options, see Appendix A.

Developing animations

For all activities a detailed virtual environment was created. Two trained physical therapists experienced in the treatment of hip and knee OA (i.e., one male, one female) were referred to as actors. A special suit with 54 integrated motion sensors was used to record movement activity with 24 cameras from different angles, according to the motion capture technique. By the use of this technique the actors' actions were transferred into animated movements (Figures 10.1 through 10.3). A specialized three-dimensional production studio, MOTEK Entertainment, Amsterdam, the Netherlands, was involved in the development of the animations. In cooperation with, and feedback from, two patient research partners (one male with hip OA, one female with knee OA), the actors mimicked different levels of performance per selected activity representing different stages of functioning.

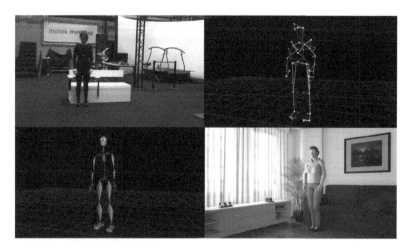

Figure 10.1 Making of an item of the Animated Activity Questionnaire (AAQ) by motion capture.

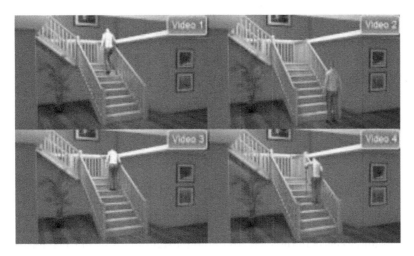

Figure 10.2 Ascending stairs by a male.

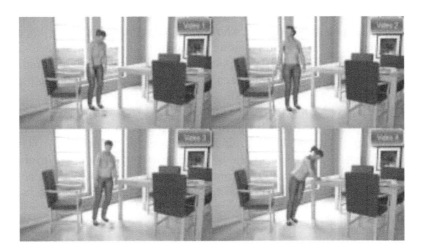

Figure 10.3 Picking up an object from the floor by a female.

Developing online questionnaire

The AAQ was embedded in an online survey software program "NetQuestionnaire." In the online survey, patients could watch all videos of one activity at the same time on one screen to facilitate comparison. All items were accompanied by the following instruction: "The video that best matches my own attempt is...." Patients were requested to select the video that provided the best representation of their average performance during the past 7 days. The videos could be repeated infinitely if considered necessary.

Scoring

Each activity was scored from 1 to 6 and summarized to a total score. The total score was then transformed into a score from 0 to 100 with higher scores corresponding to higher levels of functioning.

Psychometric properties of the AAQ

Content validity

Content validity was not formally evaluated but ensured through the development process, as described under item selection and in more detail available in the first publication regarding the AAQ (Peter et al., 2015). We think the AAQ has a good content validity because all included activities were considered relevant for the construct, the measurement aim, and the target population by patients and experts in the field, and no important items seem to be missing.

Internal consistency

A total of 1092 patients diagnosed with hip and knee OA according to the ACR criteria, aged over 18 years, and who received treatment for hip or knee OA during the past 3 years (including joint replacement surgery), were included in a validation study (Table 10.1). This study is part of an ongoing international validation study of the AAQ in seven European countries (Denmark, France, Italy, the Netherlands, Norway, Spain, and United Kingdom).

Cronbach's alpha and corrected item—total correlations were calculated to assess the degree to which the items in the AAQ are correlated. A high Cronbach's alpha of 0.95 was found with corrected item-total correlations ranging from 0.46 to 0.81. It should be noted, however, that a high Cronbach's alpha does not guarantee a good internal consistency because it has not yet been shown that the scale is unidimensional. Factor analysis needs to be performed to evaluate the internal structure of the AAQ.

Construct validity

Construct validity study 1

The preliminary results of construct validity in 110 patients were promising (Peter et al., 2015). In the continuing data collection from 1092 patients the AAQ, and the H/KOOS ADL subscale (Groot et al., 2008;de Groot et al., 2007) were completed. Subsequently, patients were requested to rate their average hip- or knee-related pain in the past week on an 11-point Numeric Rating Scale (NRS), with 0 corresponding to no pain and 10 to worst imaginable pain. No missing data were encountered because the applied computer program did not allow for any missing values.

A random subgroup of 231 patients was additionally invited to visit the outpatient clinic of a rehabilitation center to execute three performance-based tests after the AAQ and the self-reported questionnaire were completed. The stair climbing

Table 10.1 Patient characteristics

	Total group (n = 1092)	Subgroup reliability (n = 231)	Subgroup validity performance-based tests (n = 198)	Subgroup home-recorded videos (n = 22)
Sex, female (%)	788 (72.2%)	169 (73.2%)	142 (71.7%)	16 (72.7%)
Age, mean (standard deviation, SD)	64.1 (9.8)	64.1 (10.1)	64.9 (9.6)	65.3 (8.1)
Body mass index (BMI), mean (SD)	27.7 (6.3)	29.1 (6.8)	27.5 (5.5)	31.5 (7.2)
Current physical therapy treatment?	491 (45.0%)	94 (40.7%)	71 (35.9%)	5 (22.7%)
Animated Activity Questionnaire (AAQ) score (range 0–100), mean (SD)	76.4 (18.5)	77.5 (19.4)	77.5 (19.4)	73.1 (17.7)
H/KOOS ADL subscore, (range 0–100), mean (SD)	66.1 (20.6)	64.3 (19.4)	69.6 (19.2)	56.1 (17.1)
Numeric rating scale (NRS) pain score (range 0–10), mean (SD)	4.3 (2.6)	4.7 (2.5)	4.0 (2.5)	5.9 (2.3)

test (SCT) (Bennel et al., 2011; Dobson et al., 2013; Stratford et al., 2006; Steffen et al., 2002), the timed up and go test (TUG) (Bennel et al., 2011; Dobson et al., 2013; Steffen et al., 2002), and the 30-second chair stand test (CST) (Dobson, et al., 2013; Jones et al., 1999). Correlations between the AAQ, H/KOOS ADL subscale, the performance-based tests, and NRS pain scores were calculated by means of a Spearman correlation coefficient with 95% confidence intervals. To adequately average correlations of the three performance-based tests, scores were transformed into Fisher's Z-scores. After summarizing and averaging the three scores, the mean was transferred back into a correlation coefficient. Construct validity was determined by hypothesis testing (see below).

Table 10.2 shows Spearman's correlation coefficients between the AAQ score, H/KOOS ADL subscale score, home-recorded videos score (see *Construct*

Table 10.2 Spearman correlations (95% confidence interval [CI]) between the total scores of the Animated Activity Questionnaire (AAQ), Knee injury and Osteoarthritis Outcome Score (H/KOOS) ADL subscale, home-recorded videos, performance-based tests, and pain in 1092 patients with hips and knee osteoarthritis

	AAQ	H/KOOS ADL subscore	Home-recorded videos	Average score performance-based tests[a]	Stair climbing test (SCT)	Timed up and go test (TUG)	30 sec chair stand test (CST)	Pain
Animated Activity Questionnaire (AAQ)	1.00	0.73 (0.70–0.76)	0.83 (0.62–0.93)[b]	0.64 (0.55–0.71)[c]	0.68 (0.60–0.74)[c]	0.61 (0.52–0.69)[c]	0.35 (0.23–0.46)[c]	0.54 (0.50–0.58)
Knee injury and Osteoarthritis Outcome Score (H/KOOS) physical functioning		1.00		0.45 (0.35–0.55)[c]	0.41 (0.29–0.51)[c]	0.35 (0.23–0.46)[c]	0.51 (0.41–0.60)[c]	0.74 (0.71–0.76)
Home-recorded videos			1.00					
Average score performance-based t-tests*				1.00				
Stair climbing test (SCT)					1.00	0.87 (0.84–0.91)[c]	0.29 (0.16–0.40)[c]	0.43 (0.31–0.54)[c]

(Continued)

Table 10.2 Spearman correlations (95% confidence interval [CI]) between the total scores of the Animated Activity Questionnaire (AAQ), Knee injury and Osteoarthritis Outcome Score (H/KOOS) ADL subscale, home-recorded videos, performance-based tests, and pain in 1092 patients with hips and knee osteoarthritis (*Continued*)

	AAQ	H/KOOS ADL subscore	Home-recorded videos	Average score performance-based tests[a]	Stair climbing test (SCT)	Timed up and go test (TUG)	30 sec chair stand test (CST)	Pain
Timed up and go test (TUG)						1.00	0.31 (0.19–0.42)[c]	0.36 (0.24–0.47)[c]
30 sec chair stand test (CST)							1.00	0.42 (0.30–0.52)[c]
Pain								1.00

a   Scores based on transformation of separate performance-based tests scores into Fisher's Z scores, calculating the average and back transformation into an average correlation score.

b   Data analyses in a subgroup of 22 patients in which videos were taken in the patients home situation.

c   Data analyses in a subgroup of 231 patients.

Validity Study 2), performance-based tests scores, and NRS pain score. For comparisons between AAQ and H/KOOS ADL subscale and pain, the total group of 1092 patients was used, but comparisons with performance-based tests were done in a subgroup of 231 patients. Two out of four a priori set hypotheses were confirmed. The results in relation to our hypotheses were as follows:

1   The AAQ showed an average correlation of 0.64 with the SCT, TUG, and CST (0.68, 0.61, and 0.35, respectively), which confirmed the hypothesis (>0.60).
2   The correlation between the total score of the AAQ and H/KOOS score was 0.73 and higher than expected (0.30–0.60).
3   The average correlation of the total score of the AAQ with the scores of the performance-based tests (0.64) was 0.19 points higher than the average correlation of the scores of the H/KOOS ADL subscale with the scores of the performance-based tests (0.45), and the difference in correlation was almost as expected (>0.20).
4   The correlation between the total score of the AAQ and the NRS pain score (0.54) was weaker than the correlation between the H/KOOS ADL subscale and the NRS pain score (0.74), which confirmed the hypothesis (>0.10).

The results support our hypothesis that the AAQ would correlate highly with the results of performance-based tests. However, the high correlation between the AAQ and H/KOOS in this study (0.73) was unexpected because previous studies mostly found low to moderate correlations between performance-based tests and PROMs (Kennedy et al., 2003; Wittink et al., 2003; Stratford and Kennedy, 2006; Terwee et al., 2006). A possible explanation for the high correlation could be the fact that not all patients may be aware of their own movement patterns. This could mean that the patient's perception has an influence on the AAQ, although not as much as on the self-reported H/KOOS.

Construct validity study 2

The aim of this study (Peter et al., 2015) was to evaluate the validity of the AAQ by comparing the AAQ to home videos of daily activities in a subgroup of 22 patients. After completing the AAQ and the H/KOOS, home videos were taken from 11 basic daily activities: rising from a chair; sitting-down on a chair; walking 6 m after 15 minutes sitting-down; ascending stairs; descending stairs; sitting down on a couch; rising from a couch; rising from a toilet; sitting down on a toilet; picking something (i.e., a small coffee mug) up from the floor and rising from the floor. Finally, patients were asked to execute the three performance-based tests at home. The home-videos were scored from 1 to 5 according to the ICF (Dreinhofer et al., 2004): a score of 1 point indicated no problems; 2 points indicated mild problems; 3 points indicated moderate problems; 4 points indicated severe problems; and 5 points were scored if a subject was not able to perform the activity. Subsequently, the total score was transformed to a 0–100 scale for comparison with the other measurement instruments.

Based on the construct of the AAQ, a strong correlation between the AAQ and home videos was expected (>0.6) and found (0.83) (see Table 10.2). Also, the correlation between the AAQ and the performance-based tests was high (0.73) as expected (>0.6). However, unexpectedly the correlation between the AAQ and the H/KOOS was also high (0.79, as compared with an expected correlation of 0.3–0.6), but similar to the first construct validity study.

Test–retest reliability

A random sample of 198 of the 1092 patients included in construct validity study 1 were asked to complete the AAQ a second time in their own home after 7 days to assess test–retest reliability. The test–retest reliability of the AAQ was high with an intraclass correlation coefficient (ICC) of 0.92 (95% confidence interval 0.89–0.94).

Cross-cultural validity

The AAQ is easily trans-culturally applicable because only a minimal translation of instructions is required. This is a clear advantage over self-report questionnaires. In the development of the animations, we also tried to exclude cultural-specific aspects in the virtual reality environments. However, it is important to evaluate whether the difficulty of the activities is the same across countries. In an ongoing international study, we will examine whether patients from different countries with the same level of functional status have indeed the same probability of choosing a certain video (Differential Item Functioning).

Feasibility

The AAQ also has several practical advantages: It can be completed by patients at home. It is trans-culturally applicable and can be completed by nonnative speakers and patients with low literacy, making it suitable for health care and (international) research in a larger variety of patients than currently possible with PROMs. It is cheap and applicable in many settings.

Future perspectives

The AAQ was developed to assess activity limitations in hip and knee OA patients. It combines the advantages of PROMs and performance-based tests, without many of their limitations. Content validity was considered good, and the AAQ showed good test–retest reliability. Construct validity, however, needs further study. Continuing research will focus on assessing construct validity and cross-cultural validity in a larger study sample European wide. In addition, future studies will focus on responsiveness and minimal important change to examine whether the AAQ is able to measure change and to make scores more interpretable.

In an ongoing research item response theory (IRT) analyses will be performed on a data set of at least 1100 subjects to estimate the quality of the individual items of the AAQ, to see how well they measure activity limitations and how appropriate they are for the respondents. This analysis can also be used to examine whether the AAQ can be shortened for use in daily clinical practice and whether its items are suitable for the development of a computer adaptive test (CAT) version in the future. In a CAT version, items are administered in a sequence and length determined by a computer based on responses to previous questions. With CATs patients do not need to complete all items and items are tailored to the patient. There is increasing attention in the field of measurement for CATs (Cella et al., 2007; Reeve et al., 2007).

Another important next step is to make the AAQ ready for large-scale use in clinical practice and research. A web-based application will be developed through which the AAQ can be administered in all kinds of clinical and research settings. The aim of this application is that the AAQ can be downloaded on a local computer or will be provided as an online service.

Conclusion

With innovative potential of e-health technology, new ways of measuring health may become possible, implying individual participation, either actively or passively, through automated systems. This may generate a huge amount of data collected out of health professionals view, in real-life situations. Beyond increasing easiness of obtaining such data, the capacity of researchers to interpret them appropriately would be challenged. Such innovation may question the very nature of the phenomenon measured and will need to be anchored in solid theory and concept definition.

References

Bennel, K., Dobson, F., and Hinman, R. (2011). Measures of physical performance assessments; self-paced walk test (SPWT), stair climb test (SCT), six-minute walk test (6MWT), chair stand test (CST), timed up & go (TUG), sock test, lift and carry test (LCT), and car task. *Arthritis Care Res.*, 63(Suppl 11), S350–S370.

Beurskens, A.J., Vet HC de, Koke AJ, Lindeman E, van der Heijden, G.J., Regtop, W., et al. (1999). A patient-specific approach for measuring functional status in low back pain. *J. Manipulative Phys. Ther.*, 22(3), 144–148.

Cella, D., Gershon, R., Lai, J.S., Choi, S. (2007). The future of outcomes measurement: Item banking, tailored short-forms, and computerized adaptive assessment. *Qual. Life Res.*, 16(Suppl 1), 133–141. Epub 2007 Mar 31.

de Groot, I.B., Reijman, M., Terwee, C.B., Bierma-Zeinstra, S.M., Favejee, M., Rose E.M., et al. (2007). Validation of the Dutch version of the hip disability and Osteoarthritis Outcome Score. *Osteoarthritis Cartilag*, 15(104), 109.

Dobson, F., Hinman, R.S., Roos, E.M., Abbott, J.H., Stratford, P., Davis, A.M., et al. (2013). OARSI recommended performance-based tests to assess physical function in people diagnosed with hip or knee osteoarthritis. *Osteoarthritis Cartilag,* 21, 1042–1052.

Dreinhofer, K., Stucki, G., Ewert, T., Huber, E., Ebenbichler, G., Gutenbrunner, C., et al. (2004). ICF core sets for osteoarthritis. *J. Rehabil. Med.,* 44 (Suppl), 75–80.

Elam, J.T., Graney, M.J., Beaver, T., el Derwi, D., Applegate, W.B., and Miller, S.T. (1991). Comparison of subjective ratings of function with observed functional ability of frail older persons. *Am. J. Public Healt.,* 81, 1127–1130.

Fayers, P.M., Langston, A.L., and Robertson, C. (2007). Implicit self-comparisons against others could bias quality of life assessments. *J. Clin. Epidemiol.,* 60(10), 1034–1039.

Gandhi, R., Tsvetkov, D., Davey, J.R., Syed, K.A., and Mahomed, N.N. (2009). Relationship between self-reported and performance-based tests in a hip and knee joint replacement population. *Clin. Rheumatol.,* 28, 253–257.

Groot, I.B., de, Favejee, M.M., Reijman, M., Verhaar, J.A., and Terwee, C.B. (2008). The Dutch version of the knee injury and osteoarthritis outcome score: A validation study. *Health Qual. Life Outcome,* 6, 16.

Hoeymans, N., Wouters, E.R., Feskens, E.J., van den Bos, G.A., and Kromhout, D. (1997). Reproducibility of performance-based and self-reported measures of functional status. *J. Gerontol. A Biol. Sci. Med. Sci.,* 52, M363–M368.

Jones, C.J., Rikli, R.E., and Beam, W.C. (1999). A 30-s chair-stand test as a measure of lower body strength in community-residing older adults. *Res. Q. Exerc. Sport,* 70, 113e9.

Kennedy, D., Stratford, P.W., Pagura, S.M., and Gollish, J.D. (2003). The relationship between self-report and performance-related measures: Questioning the content validity of timed tests. *Arthritis Rheum.,* 49, 535–540.

Maly, M.R., Cosigan, P.A., and Olney, S.J. (2006). Determinants of self-report outcome measures in people with knee osteoarthritis. *Arch. Phys. Med. Rehabil.,* 87, 96–104.

Marsh, A.P., Ip, E.H., Barnard, R.T., Wong, Y.L., and Rejeski, W.J. (2011). Using video animation to assess mobility in older adults. *J. Gerontol. A Biol. Sci. Med. Sci.,* 66(2), 217–227.

Mokkink, L.B., Terwee, C.B., Knol, D.L., Stratford, P.W., Alonso, J., Patrick, D.L., et al. (2010). The COSMIN checklist for evaluating the methodological quality of studies on measurement properties: A clarification of its content. *BMC Med. Res. Methodol.,* 10, 22.

Myers, A.M., Holliday, P.J., Harvey, K.A., and Hutchinson, K.S. (1993). Functional performance measures: Are they superior to self-assessments? *J. Gerontol.,* 48, M196–M206.

Peter, W.F., Loos, M., de Vet, H.C.W., Boers, M., Harlaar, J., Roorda, L.D., et al. (2015). Development and preliminary testing of a computerized Animated Activity Questionnaire (AAQ) in patients with hip and knee osteoarthritis. *Arthritis Care Res. (Hoboken),* 67(1), 32–39.

Peter, W.F., Loos, M., van den Hoek, J., and Terwee, C.B. (2015). Validation of the animated activity questionnaire (AAQ) for patients with hip and knee osteoarthritis: Comparison to home-recorded videos. *Rheumatol. Int.,* 35(8), 1399–408.

Reeve, B.B., Burke, L.B., Chiang, Y.P., Clauser, S.B., Colpe, L.J., Elias, J.W., et al. (2007). Enhancing measurement in health outcomes research supported by Agencies within the US Department of Health and Human Services. *Qual. Life Res.,* 16(Suppl. 1), 175–186. Epub 2007 May 26.

Sager, M.A., Dunham, N.C., Schwantes, A., Mecum, L., Halverson, K., and Harlowe, D. (1992). Measurement of activities of daily living in hospitalized elderly: A comparison of self-report and performance-based methods. *J. Am. Geriatr. Soc.,* 40, 457–462.

Sikkes, S.A., de Lange-de Klerk, E.S., Pijnenburg, Y.A., Scheltens, P., and Uitdehaag, B.M. (2009). A systematic review of Instrumental Activities of Daily Living scales in dementia: Room for improvement. *J. Neurol. Neurosurg. Psychiatry,* 80(1), 7–12.

Steffen, T.M., Hacker, T.A., and Mollinger, L. (2002). Age- and gender-related test performance in community-dwelling elderly people: Six-Minute Walk Test, Berg Balance Scale, Timed Up & Go Test, and gait speeds. *Phys. Ther.*, *82*(2), 128–137.

Stratford, P.W., and Kennedy, D.M. (2004). Does parallel item content on WOMAC's pain and function subscales limit its ability to detect change in functional status? *BMC Musculoskelet. Disord.*, *5*, 17.

Stratford, P.W., and Kennedy, D.M. (2006). Performance measures were necessary to obtain a complete picture of osteoarthritic patients. *J. Clin. Epidemiol.*, (59), 160–167.

Stratford, P.W., Kennedy, D.M., and Woodhouse, L.J. (2006). Performance measures provide assessments of pain and function in people with advanced osteoarthritis of the hip or knee. *Phys. Ther.*, *86*(11), 1489–1496.

Terwee, C.B., Coopmans, C., Peter, W.F., Roorda, L.D., Poolman, R.W., Scholtes, V.A.B., et al. (2014). Development and validation of a computer-administered Animated Activity Questionnaire (AAQ) to measure physical functioning of patients with hip or knee osteoarthritis. *Phys. Ther.*, *94*(2), 251–261.

Terwee, C.B., van der Slikke, R.M.A., van Lummel, R.C., Bennink, J.B., Meijers, W.G.H., de Vet, H.C.W. (2006). Self-reported physical functioning was more influenced by pain than performance-based physical functioning in knee-osteoarthritis patients. *J. Clin. Epidemiol.*, *59*, 724–731.

van der Esch, M., Knoop, J., van der Leeden, M., Voorneman, R., Gerritsen, M., Reiding, D., Romviel, S., et al. (2012). Self-reported knee instability and activity limitations in patients with knee osteoarthritis: Results of the Amsterdam osteoarthritis cohort. *Clin. Rheumatol.*, *31*(10), 1505–1510.

Watson, D., and Pennebaker, J.W. (1989). Health complaints, stress, and distress: Exploring the central role of negative affectivity. *Psychol. Rev.*, *96*, 234–254.

Wittink, H., Rogers, W., Sukiennik, A., and Carr, D.B. (2003). Physical functioning: Self-report and performance measures are related but distinct. *Spine*, *28*(20), 2407–2413.

World Health Organization. (2002). *Towards a Common Language for Functioning*. Geneva: Disability and Health ICF.

Wright, A.A., Hegedus, E.J., David Baxter, G., and Abbott, J.H. (2011). Measurement of functioning in hip osteoarthritis: Developing a standardized approach for physical performance measures. *Physiother. Theor. Pract.*, *27*, 253.

Section 3

Interpretation of perceived health data

11 Interpretation of perceived health data

Dorcas Beaton

Introduction

There is a phrase, often attributed to Einstein, that says "Everything should be as simple as possible and no simpler" (http://quoteinvestigator.com/2011/05/13/einstein-simple/). The saying is fitting for the challenge of determining how to interpret the meaning of the numbers we obtain when assessing perceived health, where simplicity is the goal, but chapters like those that follow in this section suggest it may not be as simple as we would like. We must aim for as simple as possible ... but not simpler. In the last 25 years, the outcomes movement has made enormous gains in the inclusion of a wider variety of domains in an outcome assessment. Along with biomarkers of disease, advanced imaging, and the precise impact of an intervention on a target condition, this movement has advocated measures of the lived experience of the patient (side effects, symptoms, life impact) (Lohr and Zebrack, 2008; Boers et al., 2014; Testa and Simonson, 1996; Gabriel and Normand, 2012) advocating that we have an equal need to follow how a health condition or its treatment makes a person feel and perceive their health and well-being (Walton et al., 2015). Although these advances have been great and mirrored in the development of many instruments to address these needs (McHorney, 1999), many measurement standards to ensure their quality (Reeve et al., 2013; Lohr et al., 1996), and many methods to evaluate and synthesize evidence of their measurement properties (Terwee et al., 2016; Valderas et al., 2008), we are still faced with the need to make qualitative sense of the now quantified attribute of pain, quality of life (QoL), or perceived health. Ironically, the efforts we place on quantifying a qualitative attribute like health are now slipped and our efforts are now to being able to *qualify* the meaning of the *quantified* attribute. Interpretability has been recognized as a challenge since early efforts—the "crock of gold at the end of the rainbow" according to Kirwan (2001).

In the chapters that follow, we will read of some very specific challenges that are facing the interpretation of measures of health and health perceptions that will impact our use of them in future research, policy making, and clinical care of health conditions. Some may seem insurmountably difficult to overcome. Others show the progress that has been made over years of work. All will deepen our understanding of perceived health and the context in which it is being measured, so that we can improve our ability to interpret the scores meaningfully. We should enter into these chapters knowing that they improve our understanding and engage us in further improvements in the interpretation of measures of perceived health.

Engaging in the unsettling world of interpretability

Derived from the verb "interpret," interpretability means "ability to provide the meaning of" in our case scores on perceived health scales (http://www.oxford-dictionaries.com/definition/english/interpret). Interpretation or interpretability of measures of perceived health has often fallen to the tasks of minimally impor-tant differences or more recently thresholds depicting a patient-acceptable symp-tom state (acceptable/tolerable pain). And we see this in the work of Rat and Pouchot in Chapter 17. There is a long history of effort and controversy in this field (Hays and Woolley, 2000; Jaeschke et al., 1989; Wright, 1996; Wyrwich et al., 2013; Beaton et al., 2002; Guyatt et al., 2002), with challenges covered well in the issues raised by Rat and Pouchot. Establishing "THE" single threshold of universal meaning for an outcome measure has been described as being "ram-pant with controversy" (Gatchel and Mayer, 2010). Some in their frustration have thrown up their hands and questioned whether the pursuit of a minimal important change should be abandoned (Carragee, 2010). But the field persists in the struggle because it is so important to know when a change or a given state means something that we should pay a great deal of attention to and when it does not (i.e., trivial or unimportant change). The field is evolving to accept that there will unlikely be a single threshold of change with meaning for all persons using a given instrument.

Interpretation also moves us beyond the field of thresholds of meaning, to the essence of what good health is really about and how well our current approaches at interpretability capture it. Health and perceived health might be most easily measured at a functional status or task level—dressing, opening jars. But when we wish to see how people appraise that functional status in an overall perception of their health (so, how are you?), we are asking them to integrate their abilities into their lives (experienced and desired). People are sometimes "good enough" to consider themselves to have a good or fulfilling QoL as shown recently by Wiitavaara et al. in persons with chronic musculo-skeletal pain (Wiitavaara et al., 2016). Perceived health measurement means being open to individual experiences and identifying methods to represent them (interpret them, given them meaning) in our health research. In this sec-tion, Vanier et al.'s (2016) comprehensive review on response shift phenom-enon provides a model for how appraisals of health can shift within people as they experience a health condition or indeed adapt to ongoing residual effects of a chronic disease and challenge the use of change scores when the under-lying concept has shifted in meaning or appraisal. Alonso et al. (2016) offer insight into how the lived experience of the disease, captured in measures of disability, influence perceived health appraisals again broadening our sense of interpretability to include the individual's lived experience. This could lead one to question whether we can ascribe meaning to appraised health without first understanding how the individual has experienced the impact of the health condition in their own lives.

Our understanding of interpretability must, however, be expanded to also face the challenges posed by the work of Lang et al. (2016) and Jusot et al. (2016), who identify societal level factors that impact the way we should assign meaning to the scores obtained, not only because of the social/physical/economic opportunities of subgroups but also because of the different ways they appear to be thinking about and responding to the questions of perceived health. The groups have different truths; how we use our tools to represent those truths so that we can interpret measures of health status equitably and with integrity when comparing across these differences is important.

Compiling the issues we face in the accurate interpretation of health status indicators into one section of a textbook could create concern rather than confidence in the measurement of perceived health. However, this is the growing edge of health measurement. This is where the science is. Had we never measured health perceptions, we may not have encountered response shifts or differences in appraisal of health across socioeconomic strata. Why did we not just keep things simple? Perhaps because that was too simple. There is more to be learned by engaging in this body of work. Health perceptions are measured to move the field of clinical and population health forward, and sometimes that means relooking at the way we use and interpret our scale scores—maybe in their noise and variability they are trying to point us to something new. The insights gained by juxtaposing these works with each other in this book could open doors for the next group of learners to see the correct way through a challenge that we should not give up on.

Concept and context—Identifying and resolving tensions

It seems that a key factor in moving forward in the interpretation of measures of perceived health will be to be open to relooking at the concept and context of things like the minimal clinically important difference (MCID) or thresholds of meaning. Interpretability might best be considered in the same way we are setting up measurement needs: What do we need to be able to measure and in what context do we intend to use this information. If measurement properties are now accepted as being context specific, it seems imperative that interpretations of their scores are also considered in the same light. Matching how we want to be able to use this interpretability (change, threshold of score, trajectory) and knowing the context (chronic disease, comorbid conditions, culture, personal adaptation to disease, social situation) will help us narrow down what is useful from estimates of interpretability.

Often there seems to be a tension placed between the use of perceived health outcomes at a group level (mean differences in a population health or clinical trial setting for example) and their use at an individual level (for example in clinical care). However, shifts in the reporting of clinical trials to encourage responder analyses (proportion of patients who had a benefit) and advances in our capacity to model intraindividual differences in trajectory can offer more insights into our interventions than simpler approach (Chapman et al., 2011; Donaldson and Moinpour, 2002). For example, intraindividual differences in response, once a flag for significant concern, may teach us even more about our area of study—be it response to a drug treatment, or return to role functioning. Perhaps the polarities of individual versus group level analyses are converging in favor of efforts to improve the interpretability of our measures in individual patients, or groups of individuals concurrently (Lohr and Zebrack, 2008; Wyrwich et al., 2013).

When Barsky introduced his 1988 paradox of health, that is, declining health perceptions despite population level improvements in indicators of morbidity and mortality, he did not conclude that the perceived health was invalid or biased (error) but that "physicians should become more aware of these paradoxical consequences of medical progress" (Barsky, 1988, pp. 414). When we encounter tension between our measurement and its meaning, we can likely learn from that as well. Although it is challenging to be clear on the concept of interest, and the framework for testing the impact of the context of its measurement, the task is too important to abandon.

Conclusion

Opening the measurement of health perception up to the challenges of interpreting change, making valid cross national comparisons of health, and making health policy decisions risks rendering the perceptions of these instruments as of being of little value. However, not picking up the challenge of dealing with the issues posed by the context of use of the instruments with a full commitment to their ongoing use would be a far greater risk, that of losing the patient's perspective of their own health. This would return us to a model of care and public health that did not allow a person to say that they were okay with their current, though perhaps diminished, health state. The chapters that follow in this section may challenge our confidence in indicators of perceive health but should also be indicators of ways to improve our use of them and get better answers. We need to remember this when faced with Rat's work on the complexities of interpreting change (Rat and Pouchot, 2016), or the nature of social inequities posted by Lang et al. (2016) and Jusot et al. (2016), or the seemingly impossible hurdle of detecting and managing a response shift as outlined by Vanier et al. (2016). These complexities can lead us to improve what we do with these instruments as shown in Alonso's work on modeling the nature of the influence of disability experience (context) on perceived health in persons with chronic health conditions (Alonso et al., 2016).

King, in a paper on the complexities of interpreting QoL scores, reminded us that "simple messages resonate more readily in the research literature than complex ones" and that in dealing with interpretability the simplest answers, perhaps too simple, often stick (King, 2011, pp. 177). We might find ourselves in an uncomfortable place facing the challenges and in some cases without all the answers. But we need to continue. Ostelo, having completed a very thorough review and international consensus on the ways to interpret change in low back pain outcomes said: "These are not the final answers but offer a common starting point for future research" (Ostelo et al., 2008, p. 93). The following chapters open up the issues and become a starting point for advancing the interpretation of health outcomes in our work.

References

Alonso, J., Forero, C.G., Adroher, N.D., Vilagut, G., on behalf of the World Mental Health (WMH) Consortium. (2017). Chronic conditions, disability and perceived health: Empirical support of a conceptual model. In: Guillemin, F., Leplège, A., Briançon, S., Spitz, E., Coste, J. (eds.) *Perceived Health and Adaptation in Chronic Disease*. New York: Routledge, 155–174.

Barsky, A.J. (1988). The paradox of health. *N. Engl. J. Med.*, *318*(7), 414–418.

Beaton, D.E., Boers, M., and Wells, G.A. (2002). Many faces of the minimal clinically important difference (MCID): A literature review and directions for future research. *Curr. Opin. Rheumatol.*, *14*, 109–114.

Boers, M., Idzerda, L., Kirwan, J.R., Beaton, D., Escorpizo, R., Boonen, A., et al. (2014). Toward a generalized framework of core measurement areas in clinical trials: A position paper for OMERACT 11. *J. Rheumatol.*, *41*(5), 978–985.

Carragee, E.J. (2010). The rise and fall of the "minimum clinically important difference." *Spine J.*, 10(4), 283–284.

Chapman, C.R., Donaldson, G.W., Davis, J.J., and Bradshaw, D.H. (2011). Improving individual measurement of postoperative pain: The pain trajectory. *J. Pain*, *12*(2), 257–262.

Donaldson, G.W., and Moinpour, C.M. (2002). Individual differences in quality-of-life treatment response. *Med. Care*, 40(Suppl. 6), III-39–III-53.

Gabriel, S.E., and Normand, S.L. (2012). Getting the methods right—The foundation of patient-centered outcomes research. *N. Engl. J. Med.*, *367*(9), 787–790.

Gatchel, R.J., and Mayer TG. (2010). Testing minimal clinically important difference: Consensus or conundrum? *Spine J.*, *10*(4), 321–327.

Guyatt, G.H., Osoba, D., Wu, A.W., Wyrwich, K.W., Norman, G.R., and Clinical Significance Consensus Meeting Group. (2002). Methods to explain the clinical significance of health status measures. *Mayo. Clin. Proc.*, 77, 371–383.

Hays, R.D., and Woolley, J.M. (2000). The concept of clinically meaningful difference in health-related quality of life research. *PharmacoEconomics*, *18*(5), 419–423.

Jaeschke, R., Singer, J., and Guyatt, G.H. (1989). Measurement of health status. Ascertaining the minimal clinically important difference. *Control. Clin. Trials*, *10*, 407–415.

Jusot, F., Tubeuf, S., Devaux, M., Sermet, C. (2017). Social heterogeneity in self-reported health status and the measurement of inequalities in health. In: Guillemin, F., Leplège, A., Briançon, S., Spitz, E., Coste, J. (eds.) *Perceived Health and Adaptation in Chronic Disease*. New York: Routledge, 175–195.

King, M.T. (2011). A point of minimal important difference (MID): A critique of terminology and methods. *Expert Rev. Pharmacoecon. Outcomes Res.*, *11*(2), 171–184.

Kirwan, J. (2001). Minimum clinically important difference: The crock of gold at the end of the rainbow? *J Rheumatol.*, *28*, 439–444.

Lang, T., Delpierre, T., Kelly-Irving, M. (2017). Social heterogeneity of perceived health. In: Guillemin, F., Leplège, A., Briançon, S., Spitz, E., Coste, J. (eds.) *Perceived Health and Adaptation in Chronic Disease*. New York: Routledge, 196–201.

Lohr, K.N., Aaronson, N.K., Alonso, J., Burnam, M.A., Patrick, D.L., Perrin, E.B., et al. (1996). Evaluating quality-of-life and health status instruments: Development of scientific review criteria. *Clin. Ther.*, *18*(5), 979–992.

Lohr, K.N., and Zebrack, B.J. (2008). Using patient-reported outcomes in clinical practice: Challenges and opportunities. *Qual. Life Res.*, *18*(1), 99–107.

McHorney, C.A. (1999). Health status assessment methods for adults: Past accomplishments and future challenges. *Annu. Rev. Public Health*, *20*, 309–335.

Ostelo, R.W., Deyo, R.A., Stratford, P., Waddell, G., Croft, P., Von Korff, M., et al. (2008). Interpreting change scores for pain and functional status in low back pain towards international consensus regarding minimal important change. *Spine*, *33*(1), 90–94.

Rat, A.C., Pouchot, J. (2017). Interpretation of perceived health data in specific disorders. In: Guillemin, F., Leplège, A., Briançon, S., Spitz, E., Coste, J. (eds.) *Perceived Health and Adaptation in Chronic Disease*. New York: Routledge, 231–262.

Reeve, B.B., Wyrwich, K.W., Wu, A.W, Velikova, G., Terwee, C.B., Snyder, C.F., et al. (2013). ISOQOL recommends minimum standards for patient-reported outcome measures used in patient-centered outcomes and comparative effectiveness research. *Qual. Life Res.*, *22*(8), 1889–1905.

Terwee, C.B., Prinsen, C.A., Ricci Garotti, M.G., Suman, A., de Vet, H.C., Mokkink, L.B., et al. (2016). The quality of systematic reviews of health-related outcome measurement instruments. *Qual. Life Res.*, *25*(4), 767–779.

Testa, M.A., and Simonson, D.C. (1996 March 28). Assessment of quality-of-life outcomes. *N. Eng. J. Med.*, *334*, 335–340.

Valderas, J.M., Ferrer, M., Mendivil, J., Garin, O., Rajmil, L., Herdman, M., et al. (2008). Development of EMPRO: A tool for the standardized assessment of patient-reported outcome measures. *Value Health*, *11*(4), 700–708.

Vanier, A., Falissard, F., Sébille, V., Hardouin J.B. (2017). The complexity of interpreting changes observed over time in health-related quality of life: A short overview of 15 years of research on response shift theory. In: Guillemin, F., Leplège, A., Briançon, S., Spitz, E., Coste, J. (eds.) *Perceived Health and Adaptation in Chronic Disease*. New York: Routledge, 202–230.

Walton, M.K., Powers, J., Hobart, J., Patrick, D., Marquis, P., Vamvakas, S., et al. (2015). Clinical outcome assessments: Conceptual foundation—Report of the ISPOR clinical outcomes assessment—Emerging good practices for outcomes research task force. *Value Health*, *18*, 741–752.

Wiitavaara, B., Bengs, C., and Brulin, C. (2016). Well, I'm healthy, but...—Lay perspectives on health among people with musculoskeletal disorders. *Disabil. Rehabil.*, *38*(1), 71–80.

Wright, J.G. (1996). The minimal important difference: Who's to say what is? [see comment][comment]. *J. Clin. Epidemiol.*, *49*(11), 1221–1222.

Wyrwich, K.W., Norquist, J.M., Lenderking, W.R., Acaster, S., Industry Advisory Committee of International Society for Quality of Life Research (ISOQOL). (2013). Methods for interpreting change over time in patient-reported outcome measures. *Qual. Life Res.*, *22*(3), 475–483.

12 Chronic conditions, disability, and perceived health: Empirical support of a conceptual model

Jordi Alonso, Carlos G. Forero, Núria D. Adroher, Gemma Vilagut, on behalf of the World Mental Health (WMH) Consortium

Introduction

From a holistic perspective, perceived health (PH) is a crucial component of the concept of health status, conveying an overall valuation of the illness by the individual. There is clear evidence that PH ratings can predict survival, even after adjusting by the presence of disease severity and risk factors (Idler and Benyamini, 1997). PH is also an independent predictor of utilization and health-care costs (Lee and Shinkai, 2003), as well as future disability (Lee and Shinkai, 2003; Ashburner et al., 2011). All of these outcomes are very relevant from the health services point of view; thus PH is recognized as an important indicator of health (Rohrer et al., 2007; Perruccio et al., 2007) to monitor health trends of the general population (Heistaro et al., 1996) as well as to assess patient-centered outcomes in clinical studies (Alonso, 2000). Nevertheless, some criticisms have also been pointed out (Salomon et al., 2004; Sen, 2002).

PH is one of the components of Health-Related Quality of Life (HRQL). A number of definitions of HRQL have been proposed. One of them was proposed by Patrick and Erickson as "the value assigned by individuals, groups of individuals and the society lifespan modified by impairments, functional states, perceptions and social opportunities that are influenced by disease, injury, [medical] treatment or policy [health]" (Patrick and Erickson, 1993). Also, different models of HRQL exist. The one proposed by Wilson and Cleary (1995) depicts health as a continuum that can be assessed from biological and physiological variables to PH and overall quality of life. Between these extremes, symptoms and functional status are in the middle of a dominant causal association. A modification of this model was proposed by Ferrans et al. (2005), expanding the previous model to better explicate individual and environmental factors. A recent review includes the World Health Organization (WHO) International Classification of Functioning Disability and Health (ICF) (World Health Organization, 2001) as the third most popular model of HRQL (Bakas et al., 2012). Finally, a synthesis of all the Wilson and Cleary (1995) and the ICF models has been proposed, and it is depicted in Figure 12.1 (Valderas and Alonso, 2008).

According to the WHO's ICF, disability is a state of decreased functioning associated with disease, disorder, injury, or other health conditions, which in the contest of one's environment is experienced as an impairment, activity limitation, or participation restriction. And it has been defined as a difficulty in functioning at the body, the person, or the societal level, in one or more domains, as experienced by an individual with a health condition in interaction with contextual factors (Leonardi et al., 2006). We hypothesize that these functional limitations would influence the association between chronic conditions and PH.

Chronic diseases have an important negative influence on our own perception of health (Alonso et al., 2004; Damian et al., 2008; Leinonen et al., 2001; Saarni et al., 2006; Schultz and Kopec, 2003). There are many ways and factors by which disease can influence PH: disease symptoms (such as pain, shortness of breath or fatigue), disability associated with those symptoms or with other more complex disease constructs (such as limitations in basic daily activities or difficulties to achieve more complex roles and desired activities), and personal, social or environmental factors (from personality, health values, education, and socio-economic status (SES), to disease labeling, disease prognosis, cultural stereotypes and stigma associated to the condition).

The models by Wilson and Cleary (1995), and by Ferrans et al. (2005), indicate or suggest that disability would mediate the impact of chronic

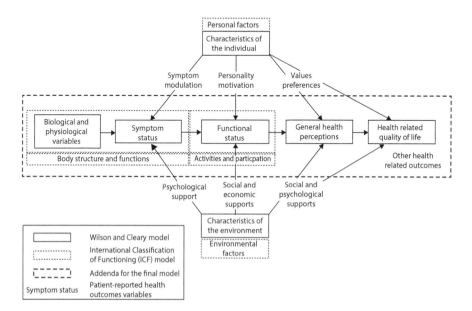

Figure 12.1 An integrated model for health outcomes. (From Valderas, J.M., and Alonso, J., *Qual. Life Res.*, 17, 1125–35, 2008. With permission.)

conditions on PH. That is, the influence on PH by chronic conditions would be to some extent explained by their disabling capacity, rather than only by a direct effect (Baron and Kenny, 1986; Pearl, 2012). Consistent with this model, mounting evidence shows that disability is significantly associated with PH both cross-sectionally (Damian et al., 2008; Lee et al., 2008) and longitudinally (Leinonen et al., 2001; Lee et al., 2008; Mavaddat et al., 2011). There is also evidence that chronic conditions are significantly associated with disability (Ormel et al., 2008; Blain et al., 2010; Boot et al., 2011). A few studies have assessed the mediating role of disability in the association of chronic conditions and mental health (Ormel et al., 1997; Buist-Bouwman et al., 2008). But we are not aware of an explicit evaluation of the mediating role of disability in the association between chronic conditions and PH in a large international general population sample.

Here we explore the extent to which a multidimensional assessment of disability mediates the associations of mental disorders and physical conditions on PH in surveys of the WHO World Mental Health (WMH) surveys initiative (Kessler and Ustun, 2008), a consortium of cross-sectional general population epidemiological surveys carried out in 22 countries throughout the world. We focus not only on the extent to which disability mediates the total effects of chronic conditions but also on the relative importance of individual disability dimensions. We had hypothesized that a significant proportion of the decrease in PH status associated to mental and physical conditions would be mediated by disability dimensions. We also anticipated that the pattern of disability mediation could be different for mental and physical conditions.

Methods

General empirical approach

Here we analyze data from a series of large international surveys of the general population in 22 countries. Based on personal interviews, participants were assessed about mental health disorders, physical conditions, PH, disability, and many other health-related variables. In this chapter, we assess the association between mental disorders and physical conditions with PH. In addition to their direct association, we consider the possible mediating role of disability in that association. Mediation consists on a relationship model between triads of variables. The mediation hypothesis states that changes of the independent variable affect the outcome but that the effect is not direct. Instead, the independent variable affects causally the mediator, which in turn has the causal effect on the outcome. When introduced into the model, the mediator diminishes the *direct* effect of the independent variable on the outcome, so that its effect is *indirect*, that is, it influences the outcome by means of the mediator (Alwin and Hauser, 1975). The simplest mediator model hypothesizes the relationships between just three variables and it is depicted in Figure 12.2. The simplest mediation model involves three variables and the mechanism of

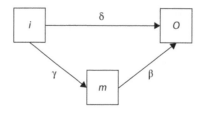

Figure 12.2 The simplest mediation model.

influence between (*i*) the independent variable, (*o*) outcome, and (*m*) mediator. The direct effect of the independent variable on the outcome is (δ); the indirect effects are the product between independent effect on the mediator (γ) and the mediator effect on the outcome (β). A multiple mediator model implies various mediated effects between a number of independent and mediator variables; however, the structures of the effects can be decomposed into several simple models acting simultaneously.

Sample

A total of 23 surveys were carried out in 22 countries, 6 classified by the World Bank (2009), at the time of data collection, as low and lower-middle income (Colombia, India [Pondicherry region], Iraq, Nigeria, Peoples' Republic of China [cities of Beijing/Shanghai and Shenzhen], and Ukraine), 5 upper-middle income countries (Brazil—Sao Paulo metropolitan area—Bulgaria, Lebanon, Mexico, and Romania) and 11 high income (Belgium, France, Germany, Israel, Italy, Japan, Netherlands, Northern Ireland, Portugal, Spain, and United States of America).

The weighted average response rate across countries was 72.0%, with country-specific response rates ranging from 45.9% (France) to 87.7% (Colombia). All surveys were based on probability samples of the country's adult household population that were either nationally representative (in the majority of countries) or representative of particular regions or areas of the country (in Brazil, People's Republic of China, Colombia, India, Japan, Mexico, and Nigeria). The age ranges of the sample varied across participating countries. Most countries had a minimum age of 18 years, whereas the minimum ages in Japan and Israel were 20 and 21, respectively. The upper age was unrestricted in most surveys but was 70 in China and 65 in Colombia and Mexico. Additional details about sampling and respondents are available elsewhere (Kessler et al., 2013).

Mental disorders

Mental disorders were assessed with Version 3.0 of the WHO Composite International Diagnostic Interview (CIDI 3.0), a fully structured lay-administered interview designed to generate diagnoses of mental conditions based on the *Diagnostic and Statistical Manual of the American Psychiatric Association*, IV edition (*DSM-IV*). The mental disorders considered here are depressive disorders (major depressive disorder, minor depressive disorder), bipolar disorder (mania, hypomania, bipolar I, bipolar II), panic disorder (panic disorder, agoraphobia without panic), specific phobia, social phobia, generalized anxiety disorder, posttraumatic stress disorder, alcohol abuse with or without dependence, and drug abuse with or without dependence. Only disorders present in the past 12 months are considered here. Generally, good concordance has been found between CIDI diagnoses of anxiety and depressive disorders and independent clinical assessment (Wittchen, 1994; Haro et al., 2006).

Chronic physical conditions

Physical conditions were assessed with a standard chronic conditions checklist that asked respondents if they had ever suffered from the given physical health condition, if they had the condition in the past 12 months, and if they had received any treatment. The 10 conditions considered here are arthritis, cancer, cardiovascular (heart attack, heart disease, hypertension, and stroke), chronic pain (chronic back or neck pain and other chronic pain), diabetes, frequent or severe headache or migraine, insomnia, neurological (multiple sclerosis, Parkinson's, and epilepsy or seizures), digestive (stomach or intestine ulcer or irritable bowel condition), and respiratory (seasonal allergies like hay fever, asthma, or chronic obstructive pulmonary disease (COPD) or emphysema). For the symptom-based conditions such as arthritis, chronic pain, and headache, heart attack or stroke respondents were asked to report whether they had experienced these conditions. For the remaining silent conditions, the question was prefaced by the phrase "have you ever been told by a doctor or health professional that you had any of these conditions?"

Perceived health

Overall PH was assessed using a numerical verbal rating scale based on the visual analog approach (Alonso et al., 2011). Respondents were asked to use a 0–100 scale where 0 represents the worst possible health a person can have and 100 represents perfect health to "describe your own overall physical and mental health during the past 30 days."

Disability

Disability was assessed with a modified version of the WHO Disability Assessment Schedule 2.0 (WHODAS) (Ustun et al., 2010; Von Korff et al., 2008). Questions were asked about difficulties in (a) understanding and communication (cognition), (b) moving and getting around (mobility), (c) attending personal hygiene, dressing , and living alone (self-care), and (d) interacting with other people (getting along). These four previous subscales were considered as latent variables (i.e., factors) as indicated from their respective items.

In addition, we assessed the number of days out of the past 30 that they were totally unable to carry out their normal activities or work, that they had to cut down in the activities, that they had to reduce their quality, or that they needed to exert an extreme effort to carry out their activities, due to physical or mental health problems or use of alcohol or drugs (role functioning). Respondents were also asked about the extent of embarrassment (stigma) and discrimination or unfair treatment (discrimination) they experienced due to their health condition, and finally, they were asked about the interference of their health condition on the day-to-day activities of their family members (family burden). Given that information on discrimination, stigma and family burden were based on just one indicator—they were treated as observed instead of latent. Scores on latent dimensions followed a standardized normal distribution (average = 0, standard deviation [SD] = 1), scaled so that higher values indicated higher degree of disability.

Statistical analysis

The 19 conditions were grouped in $p = 2$ groups of pathology (any mental disorder and any physical condition). Path analysis was used to estimate, through simultaneous regression mediation submodels, the total, the direct, and the indirect (i.e., mediated by disability) effects of each group of pathology in predicting PH scores. The direct effect of each group on PH score is the part of its total effect, which is not mediated via intervening variables.

The condition groups were included as independent variables through $k = 8$ disability dimensions, which acted as mediators, for a total of $p \times k$ ($2 \times 8 = 16$) simultaneous mediation paths in a structural equation modelling (SEM). The general structural model is depicted in Figure 12.3. The effect of each group of conditions can be decomposed in two paths: (1) PH regressed on condition groups (direct effects, δ_g, $g = \{1,2\}$), and (2) a causal set of mediation chains of PH regressed on mediators which in turn are regressed on mental and physical groups (indirect effects, I_g). The indirect effects of each group of conditions on PH, via WHODAS domains, were generated as the product of regression coefficients (the regression coefficient of PH score regressed on the WHODAS domain, β_j, ($j = \{1, ..., 8\}$) multiplied by the coefficient of the domain regressed on group of conditions, γ_{gi}). Note that mediators 1–4 (cognition, getting along, mobility, and self-care) are represented in circles (standing for the latent trait variables containing no measurement error) and indicated by items i via factor loadings λ. Mediators 5–8 (role functioning, discrimination, family burden, and stigma) are represented in squares (standing for observed indicators). The partial indirect effect of a condition group on PH through a mediator M_j is $\gamma_{ig} \times \beta_j$, whereas its total indirect effect I_g is the sum of the k products across mediators ($I_g = \sum_{j=1}^{k} \gamma_{jg} \times \beta$). Total effects for a disorder are the sum of direct and total indirect effect ($\delta_g + I_g$).

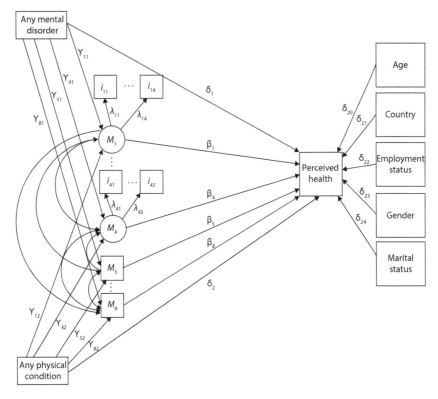

Figure 12.3 General mediation model used in the analysis of the association between mental and physical conditions and perceived health (PH). The World Mental Health (WMH) surveys. *Path-diagrammatic conventions:* The model depicts the impact of $p = 2$ groups of conditions (mental and physical conditions) on PH mediated by $k=8$ *disability dimensions* M_j. Notice that mediators 1–4 (cognition, getting along, mobility, and self-care) are represented in circles (standing for the latent trait variables) and indicated by items i, depending on them via factor loadings λ. Note that each latent trait has a different number of indicators (four for M_1, three for M_4, etc.). Mediators 5–8 (role functioning, discrimination, family burden, and stigma) are represented in squares (standing for observed indicators). Arrows represent regression slope parameters from independent variables to outcomes. The δ parameter stands for the direct effect regression from condition groups to the final outcome. The γ and β parameters indicate the two regression components of conditions indirect effects as mediated by M: (a) $p \times k$ regression parameters from disorders to M (γ_{ig}) and (b) k regression parameters from M to PH (β_j).

In our study, directionality cannot be assumed as a causal association but only as a causal hypothesis, due to its cross-sectional, observational nature. Also note that in the general model, the effect of each group of conditions on each mediator is adjusted by the direct effect of the other group (thus controlling for physical and mental comorbidity), whereas the impact of a group on

PH is controlled by the total effects of the other group. Disability is thus fully taken into account, even though it is decomposed in subscales. The effects on PH are also controlled for age, gender, marital status, employment status, and country.

The factor measurement model for latent mediators cognition, getting along, mobility, and self-care was incorporated so that each WHODAS subscale was indicated by its respective items, and all subscales were all intercorrelated. The factor model was held fixed across all countries and subgroups, and showed excellent fit (root mean square error of approximation [RMSEA] = 0.01, comparative fit index [CFI] = Tucker Lewis index [TLI] = 0.999), with factor loading over 0.94 and interfactor correlations between 0.53 and 0.81).

To test the stability of the model across different income countries, an additional multigroup model by income level (high, upper middle, and lower middle/low) was tested. We tested whether the same overall model sufficed for describing the overall sample by comparing the overall versus group effect models using robust χ^2 difference at a 5% significance level.

Model parameter estimation was conducted using a diagonally weighted least squares (DWLS) estimator, which allows robust estimation of parameter standard errors and fit indexes. We used SUDAAN® V11.0 Statistical Software for Analysing Correlated Data (RTI International, Durham, NC, USA) to generate estimates of condition prevalence and descriptive statistics for the distributions of the continuous variables. We used MPlus 7.1 (Muthén and Muthén, Los Angeles, CA) to conduct all multivariate analyses in parallel in the total sample and within three subsamples consisting of respondents low and lower-middle, upper-middle, and high-income countries. To account for the complex sample design, standard errors and statistical tests were calculated using a sandwich estimator implemented in M-Plus, which is equivalent to the Taylor series linearization method.

Results

A total of 51,344 respondents (Part 2 respondents) were assessed, of which 16,051 were from low/lower-middle income, 10,496 from upper-middle income, and 24,797 from high-income countries (Table 12.1). Individuals were an average of 42 years of age, and they were significantly younger as the income level decreased from an average of 46 years in high-income countries to an average of 37 years in low/lower-middle income countries. Almost 52% were female and just above a third (35.7%) were not married, with a higher proportion of married individuals in low-income countries. Overall, 41.6% of the sample was not working (41.9% in low/lower-middle income, 46.5% in upper middle income, and 39.3% in high-income countries). In the overall sample, the 12-month prevalence of either a mental or a physical condition was 55.8%. Physical chronic conditions were notably more prevalent than mental disorders (51.4% vs. 14.4%). Prevalence of conditions was higher among

Table 12.1 Overall sample characteristics, and according to country income level (the World Mental Health [WMH] surveys)

Country	Overall sample	Country income level			Group comparison: low, middle, high statistic (p-value)
		High	Upper middle	Low and lower middle	
N	51,344	24,797	10,496	16,051	
Mean age (SE)	42.3 (0.1)	46 (0.2)	41.5 (0.2)	37.0 (0.2)	633[a] (<.0001)
% Females (SE)	51.8 (0.3)	52.1 (0.4)	52.1 (0.7)	51.1 (0.6)	1.2[b] (.3)
% Not married (SE)	35.7 (0.3)	35.4 (0.5)	33.3 (0.7)	37.9 (0.6)	12.6[b] (<.0001)
% Not working (SE)	41.6 (0.3)	39.3 (0.5)	46.5 (0.7)	41.9 (0.6)	36.9[b] (<.0001)
% Any mental disorder (SE)	14.4 (0.2)	15.7 (0.3)	14.8 (0.4)	12.1 (0.3)	31.4[b] (<.0001)
% Any physical condition (SE)	51.4 (0.4)	56 (0.5)	49.3 (0.8)	45.6 (0.6)	85.5[b] (<.0001)
% Any mental or physical (SE)	55.8 (0.4)	60.5 (0.5)	53.6 (0.7)	49.8 (0.6)	89.6[b] (<.0001)

SE, standard error. [a] Wald's F statistic. [b] Wald's χ^2 (df = 2).

high income countries (60.5%) than among upper-middle (53.6%) and low (49.8%) income countries (Table 12.1).

Distribution of WHODAS and PH scores

Table 12.2 shows the distribution information of disability (WHODAS) and PH, by country income level. For the overall sample, the role functioning was the disability dimension most frequently affected (31.7%) followed by mobility and stigma (11.4% and 8.3%, respectively).

Table 12.2 also shows the PH scores distribution. The mean PH score was 81.0 in the overall sample, a value that did not change substantively across country income levels (range= 80.7–81.6). On average, respondents with mental conditions showed lower mean PH (72.2) than those with physical conditions (75.0), a trend that was consistent across all country income levels.

Effects of conditions on PH

The overall model for any physical and mental conditions showed excellent fit (RMSEA = 0.017; CFI = 0.99, TLI = 0.99) and explained a total of 36% of PH variance. Table 12.3 presents the association of groups of

Table 12.2 Distribution of disability (WHODAS) and perceived health scores, by country income level (the World Mental Health [WMH] surveys)

Scale	*Subscale*	*Statistic*	*Overall Sample*	*High*	*Upper middle*	*Low/lower middle*
WHODAS	Cognition	% with score > 0 (SE)	6.9 (0.14)	7.9 (0.2)	5.8 (0.3)	6.1 (0.27)
		Overall mean (SE)	0.8 (0.03)	1 (0.04)	0.8 (0.06)	0.6 (0.05)
	Mobility	% with score > 0 (SE)	11.4 (0.19)	14.6 (0.3)	7.8 (0.3)	8.7 (0.29)
		Overall mean (SE)	3.2 (0.07)	4.4 (0.13)	2.2 (0.11)	2.0 (0.09)
	Self-care	% with score > 0 (SE)	3.4 (0.1)	4.1 (0.15)	2.1 (0.17)	3.2 (0.2)
		Overall mean (SE)	1.0 (0.05)	1.3 (0.08)	0.7 (0.06)	0.7 (0.09)
	Getting along	% with score > 0 (SE)	3.9 (0.11)	4.8 (0.17)	2.2 (0.18)	3.5 (0.2)
		Overall mean (SE)	0.6 (0.03)	0.8 (0.04)	0.5 (0.06)	0.5 (0.05)
	Role functioning	% with score > 0 (SE)	31.7 (0.3)	42 (0.43)	18.3 (0.56)	24.6 (0.46)
		Overall mean (SE)	9.0 (0.14)	10.7 (0.21)	7.1 (0.27)	7.8 (0.23)
	Family burden	% with score > 0 (SE)	8.1 (0.15)	8.7 (0.22)	7.7 (0.27)	7.4 (0.28)
		Overall mean (SE)	3.7 (0.08)	3.7 (0.08)	3.5 (0.14)	3.3 (0.15)
	Stigma	% with score > 0 (SE)	8.3 (0.16)	7.6 (0.19)	9.1 (0.32)	8.9 (0.35)
		Overall mean (SE)	4.0 (0.08)	3.6 (0.1)	4.8 (0.18)	4.3 (0.18)
	Discrimination	% with score > 0 (SE)	3.5 (0.1)	2.8 (0.11)	4.3 (0.2)	4.3 (0.23)
		Overall mean (SE)	1.7 (0.05)	1.3 (0.06)	2.0 (0.11)	1.9 (0.11)

(continued)

Table 12.2 Distribution of disability (WHODAS) and perceived health scores, by country income level (the World Mental Health [WMH] surveys)*(continued)*

Scale	Subscale	Statistic	Country income level			
			Overall Sample	High	Upper middle	Low/lower middle
Perceived health (0–100)		Overall sample (SE)	81.0 (0.1)	80.7 (0.2)	81.0 (0.3)	81.6 (0.2)
		Any mental (SE)	72.2 (0.3)	72.6 (0.4)	71.6 (0.7)	71.9 (0.7)
		Any physical (SE)	75.0 (0.2)	76.0 (0.2)	73.2 (0.5)	74.3 (0.4)
		Any condition (SE)	75.5 (0.2)	76.4 (0.2)	73.8 (0.5)	74.9 (0.4)

SE, standard error; WHODAS, World Health Organization Disability Assessment Schedule.

conditions with PH score for the overall sample. Total effects are similar for both condition groups with a decrement of 8.5 and 8.2, respectively. They represent an effect size of about 0.43, as the standard deviation of PH scores is 19.89. The table also shows the proportions of the total effects that should be considered indirect (via WHODAS dimensions). More than 50% of these effects were mediated by the disability dimensions. The percentage of indirect effects was greater for the mental than for the physical condition groups (73.6% vs. 59.0%, respectively). This information is also presented in Figure 12.4.

Figure 12.5 and the second part of Table 12.3 show the relative importance of each disability dimension as a mediator (adjusted by comorbidity and the rest of dimensions) on PH, decomposing their relative contribution to the 100% of total overall indirect effects in mental and physical condition groups. As it can be seen, the relative contribution of the different mediators was substantively different for each group of conditions. The main mediators in mental disorders were role functioning (21%) and cognition (21%).

Mobility was the main one in physical conditions (29%), with cognition being, again, the second largest in contribution (19%), and role functioning a close third contributor (17%). In the case of mental disorders, mobility, stigma, and family burden had similar contributions (16%, 15%, and 12%, respectively), whereas self-care, getting along, and discrimination had lower mediating weights (<10%). For physical conditions, self-care and stigma had modest contributions (12% and 10%, respectively), with family burden, getting along, and discrimination contributing lowly to the overall effect.

Table 12.3 Effects (total, direct, and indirect via WHODAS dimensions) of chronic conditions on PH scores, and WHODAS dimension direct effects in the overall sample (the World Mental Health [WMH] surveys)

| | Total effects | Direct effects | Indirect effects via WHODAS | % Indirect over total effects | Direct effects via each WHODAS dimension[a] | | | | | | | |
| | | | | | Cognition | Getting along | Mobility | Self-care | Role functioning | Discrimination | Family burden | Stigma |
	Coefficient (SE)	Coefficient (SE)	Coefficient (SE)	Coefficient (SE)	Coefficient (SE)	Coefficient (SE)	Coefficient (SE)	Coefficient (SE)	Coefficient (SE)	Coefficient (SE)	Coefficient (SE)	Coefficient (SE)
Mental disorders	−8.5* (0.3)	−2.2* (0.2)	−6.24* (0.2)	73.7* (2.3)	−1.3* (0.2)	−0.3 (0.3)	−1.0* (0.2)	−0.6* (0.2)	−1.3* (0.1)	−0.1* (0.02)	−0.7* (0.04)	−0.9* (0.04)
Physical conditions	−8.2* (0.3)	−3.4* (0.3)	−4.84* (0.2)	59.0 (2.5)	−0.9* (0.2)	−0.2 (0.2)	−1.4* (0.2)	−0.6* (0.2)	−0.8* (0.1)	−0.1* (0.01)	−0.4* (0.03)	−0.5* (0.03)
Direct effects of WHODAS scales on PH	Cognition −0.6 (0.1)*; getting along −0.1 (0.1); mobility −0.5 (0.1)*; self-care −0.3 (0.1)*; role functioning −0.4 (0)*; discrimination −0.9 (0.2)*; family burden −2.8 (0.1)*; stigma −3.4 (0.1)*											

PH, perceived health; SE, standard error; WHODAS, World Health Organization Disability Assessment Schedule; WMH, World Mental Health.
* Significant at the .05 level, two-sided test.
a Only dimensions with statistically significant direct effect are included. "Getting along" and "discrimination" not statistically significant.

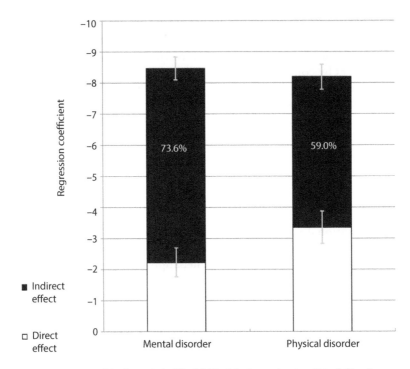

Figure 12.4 Direct and indirect (via World Health Organization Disability Assessment Schedule [WHODAS] dimensions) effects of group of conditions on perceived health (PH), overall sample. The World Mental Health (WMH) surveys.

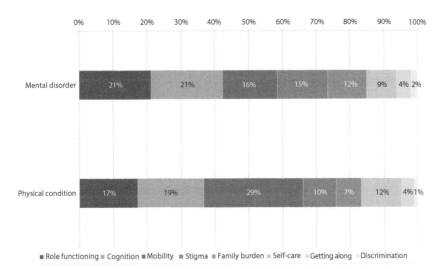

Figure 12.5 Relative contribution of World Health Organization Disability Assessment Schedule (WHODAS) dimensions to indirect (i.e., mediated by disability) effects of chronic conditions on perceived health (PH) by group of conditions, overall sample. The World Mental Health (WMH) surveys.

A unique model with effects fixed across all income levels showed adequate fit (RMSEA = 0.017, CFI = 0.99, TLI = 0.99), thus demonstrating a certain degree of invariance by income level. Nevertheless, a noninvariant model with free parameters by country income level showed a small but significant increment in absolute fit (χ^2 = 190.4, df = 52, p < .0001). However, the degree of noninvariance was very small: the income-level invariant model explained 41%, 29%, and 35% variance in high, upper-middle, and low income groups, respectively, whereas the noninvariant model explained 40%, 31%, and 37% in the same groups.

Discussion

In this international study, we found that the presence of mental disorders or physical conditions has a relevant negative impact on PH (on average, over an 8-point decrease in a 0–100 scale, approximately a 0.43 effect size). A large proportion of such decrement in PH is mediated by disabilities (73.7% for mental and 59.0% for physical conditions). Our results also suggest that relevant mediation of disability dimensions tend to differ depending on the condition group: Mobility is predominant for physical conditions, whereas role functioning and cognition are more important for mental disorders. Results are fairly consistent across the different country income levels. Taken together, these data confirm our a priori hypotheses and provide empirical support to the validity of the conceptual model proposed by Wilson and Cleary (Wilson and Cleary, 1995) and other models that suggest that disability is a causal component in the pathway between conditions and perception of health.

To our knowledge, the mediating role of disability on PH has never been reported for samples of the general population representing so many countries worldwide for the large range of conditions and disability dimensions assessed here. Certainly, many studies have previously shown an association between particular dimensions of disability and PH, in samples of patients with particular diseases. For instance, social functioning is an important determinant of PH among heart failure patients (Carlson et al., 2013), whereas physical ability has an important role on PH among spinal cord injury patients (Machacova et al., 2011). And for individuals with major depressive episode, cognition, and embarrassment seem to be very relevant disability dimensions (Buist-Bouwman et al., 2008). Our work represents a first systematic attempt to disentangle the association between a range of chronic conditions and PH considering a comprehensive range of disability indicators. Nevertheless, more research is needed for further understanding causality and the underlying process of PH and disability evaluations and how they may differ by different levels of health.

Mobility limitation is a frequent mediator of the effect of chronic physical conditions on PH (29% of the total effect), whereas it is a less important for mental disorders (16%). Many of the physical conditions considered in our study imply either pain (arthritis, back–neck pain), or impairment on the extremities and their functional performance (neurological conditions, cardiovascular, respiratory), or general weakness (cancer and others). All of these have an impact on the mobility function and modify the perception of health of the individual (Alonso et al., 2004, 2011; Garin et al., 2010). Interestingly, cognition is a similarly relevant mediator of PH for both mental and physical conditions (around 20%).

The empirical direct and indirect associations described here provide a textured picture of the ways health conditions impact on health perceptions, as well as the mediating role of disability. This should be important beyond description as it might help to guide therapeutic efforts toward particular disabilities. For instance, in a descriptive study of breast cancer survivors, it was estimated that potential interventions including physical mobility could prevent decreases in self-rated health among breast cancer survivors (Schootman et al., 2012). Also, the use of specific clinical problem-solving tools for physical and rehabilitation medicine could be liaised with assessments of PH (Steiner et al., 2002). Consistent with previous work (Buist-Bouwman et al., 2008), our data suggest that assessing stigma and family burden and trying to combat them can limit the decrements in PH of individuals with mental conditions. The types of relationships described here for the general adult population suggest that a systematic assessment of disability might help identifying areas of needed improvement for individuals with chronic conditions. Our results also suggest that effectively addressing disability should have a noticeable positive impact on the overall perception of health of the general population.

It is important to note that the overall results of our study tended to be fairly consistent across different country income levels, which differ in the prevalence of both disability and chronic conditions. Such prevalence differences are consistent with previous reports suggesting that cultural and work-related issues as well as differential access to health and social services could cause higher rates of disability in developed countries (Madan et al., 2008; Sokka et al., 2010). In contrast, PH levels were very similar across countries, both in the general population and among individuals with chronic conditions. When taking into account groups of disorders, the model describing PH fitted adequately across countries. This homogeneity does not mean, nevertheless, that local culture can be totally ignored, because the multigroup analysis showed minor departures from the overall pattern. Although role functioning was the main mediator of mental disorders and mobility was the most salient in physical disorders in the overall sample, the first had greater contributions to PH in high income countries. Noticeably, mobility had a major contribution to the effect of mental disorders on PH in middle to low income countries. Getting along was important for both types of disorders only in middle income countries, and cognition had a main role in the contribution of disorders to PH in low income countries. These results align with the well-established need to take into account ethnic, cultural, and social dimensions in combating disability (Lefley, 1990; Imrie, 1997).

Our results must be interpreted taking into account a number of limitations. First, we could not evaluate the overall conceptual model proposed by Wilson and Cleary (1995) because we have not collected all the necessary information, nor we have analyzed some important components of the model, such as symptoms or the personal and the environmental components. We nevertheless used some available information. When including pain as an additional mediator of the physical condition effects on PH, we found a nonsignificant 3% increase in PH explained variance. Neither total effects of physical conditions on PH nor indirect effects via disability dimensions differed significantly from the nonpain-mediated model. However, the pain-mediated model added significant amounts of explained variance to the disability dimensions, suggesting that pain explains disability but does not have a substantial direct contribution to PH. A more systematic testing of symptoms should be attempted in future work. We also simplified the data presented collapsing information on specific disorders in two broad categories of mental disorders and physical conditions. This was useful for facilitating the presentation and interpretation of results. But it is an oversimplification of reality. The same models for 19 different conditions or groups of conditions provide results that are very consistent with the aggregated results. At a microlevel, a model including all disorders across countries also showed excellent fit (RMSEA = 0.012, CFI = 0.98, TLI = 0.98), and explained 39.2% of PH variance, only a 3% increase than the model for grouped conditions (data not shown but available upon request).

Two other limitations are briefly mentioned below. One is that chronic physical conditions and mental conditions were differently assessed. The latter were measured with a standard diagnostic instrument, the CIDI, with high levels of reliability and acceptable validity for research purposes. Conversely, chronic physical conditions were self-reported by respondents. Although we used standardized questions that have shown acceptable validity levels (Kriegsman et al., 1996; Baumeister et al., 2010), misclassification cannot be ruled out, in particular, underreporting of physical health conditions in countries with lower access to health care. Also, we did not assess some particularly disabling brain conditions such as nonaffective psychotic conditions and dementia (Murray and Lopez, 1996). Our study, therefore, likely underestimates disability caused by mental and physical conditions.

Implications

A large proportion of the decrements in PH associated with chronic conditions is mediated by disability. This is well in agreement with predominant concepts of disability comprising the body impairments, the functional limitations, and the social restrictions associated with different health conditions. And our results should call attention to the importance of addressing disability to increase PH status among individual with common conditions. Although disability can be more or less obviously related with the index condition, a systematic evaluation of disability could be beneficial. Mobility is the disability most frequently mediating the effect of chronic physical conditions, but nevertheless role functioning and stigma are important mediators of the health effect of mental disorders. Thus, measuring stigma among individuals with mental disorders might improve the assessment and understanding of PH reports among those individuals. Addressing stigma effectively could translate in gains in PH of individuals with mental disorders, given that the associations described here are causal. Other implications of our results relate with a public health perspective, not only that of the individual with chronic conditions. The objective of healthier populations will be only achieved if disability is systematically assessed and monitored. Given the importance of contextual factors for disability, the factors associated with or causing more disability should be identified and addressed.

The findings described here also suggest that there is a need to learn more about the importance and ways of indirect association between chronic conditions and PH. In particular, evaluating whether interventions addressed to improve specific disabilities may improve PH of individuals with common chronic conditions beyond benefits that would be obtained with the usual treatment for these conditions. From a conceptual perspective, the model should be expanded to accommodate the full pathway between biology and health perceptions, in particular, by adding symptoms as well as the personal, economic, social, and environmental factors that are proposed as modifiers of the impact of medical conditions on health.

References

Alonso, J. (2000 March). The measurement of health related-quality of life in clinical research and practice. *Gac. Sanit.*, 14(2), 163–167.

Alonso, J., Ferrer, M., Gandek, B., Ware, J.E., Aaronson, N.K., Mosconi, P., et al. (2004). Health-related quality of life associated with chronic conditions in eight countries. Results from the International Quality of Life Assessment (IQOLA) project. *Qual. Life Res.*, 13, 283–298.

Alonso, J., Vilagut, G., Chatterji, S., Heeringa, S., Schoenbaum, M., Bedirhan, U.T., et al. (2011). Including information about co-morbidity in estimates of disease burden: Results from the World Health Organization World Mental Health Surveys. *Psychol. Med.*, 41(4), 873–886.

Alwin, D.F., and Hauser, R.M. (1975). The decomposition of effects in path analysis. *Am. Sociol. Rev.*, 40(1), 37–47.

Ashburner, J.M., Cauley, J.A., Cawthon, P., Ensrud, K.E., Hochberg, M.C., Fredman, L. (2011 April 15). Self-ratings of health and change in walking speed over 2 years: Results from the caregiver-study of osteoporotic fractures. *Am. J. Epidemiol.*, 173(8), 882–889.

Bakas, T., McLennon, S.M., Carpenter, J.S., Buelow, J.M., Otte, J.L., Hanna, K.M., et al. (2012). Systematic review of health-related quality of life models. *Health Qual. Life Outcomes*, 10, 134.

Baron, R.M., and Kenny, D.A. (1986 December). The moderator-mediator variable distinction in social psychological research: Conceptual, strategic, and statistical considerations. *J. Pers. Soc. Psychol.*, 51(6), 1173–1182.

Baumeister, H., Kriston, L., Bengel, J., and Harter, M. (2010 May). High agreement of self-report and physician-diagnosed somatic conditions yields limited bias in examining mental-physical comorbidity. *J. Clin. Epidemiol.*, 63(5), 558–565.

Blain, H., Carriere, I., Sourial, N., Berard, C., Favier, F., Colvez, A., et al. (2010 August). Balance and walking speed predict subsequent 8-year mortality independently of current and intermediate events in well-functioning women aged 75 years and older. *J. Nutr. Health Aging*, 14(7), 595–600.

Boot, C.R., Koppes, L.L., van den Bossche, S.N., Anema, J.R., and van der Beek, A.J. (2011 June). Relation between perceived health and sick leave in employees with a chronic illness. *J. Occup. Rehabil.*, 21(2), 211–219.

Buist-Bouwman, M.A., Ormel, J., de Graaf, R., de Jonge, P., van Sonderen, E., Alonso, J., et al. (2008 October 14). Mediators of the association between depression and role functioning. *Acta. Psychiatr. Scand.*, 118, 451–458.

Carlson, B., Pozehl, B., Hertzog, M., Zimmerman, L., and Riegel, B. (2013 May 2). Predictors of overall perceived health in patients with heart failure. *J. Cardiovasc. Nurs.*, 28(3), 206–215.

Damian, J., Pastor-Barriuso, R., and Valderrama-Gama, E. (2008). Factors associated with self-rated health in older people living in institutions. *BMC Geriatr.*, 8, 5–10.

Ferrans, C.E., Zerwic, J.J., Wilbur, J.E., and Larson, J.L. (2005). Conceptual model of health-related quality of life. *J. Nurs. Scholarsh.*, 37(4), 336–342.

Garin, O., Ayuso-Mateos, J.L., Almansa, J., Nieto, M., Chatterji, S., Vilagut, G., et al. (2010 May 19). Validation of the World Health Organization Disability Assessment Schedule (WHODAS-2) in patients with chronic diseases. *Health Qual. Life Outcomes*, 8, 51.

Haro, J.M., Arbabzadeh-Bouchez, S., Brugha, T.S., de Girolamo, G., Guyer, M.E., Jin, R,, et al. (2006 December). Concordance of the composite international diagnostic interview Version 3.0 (CIDI 3.0) with standardized clinical assessments in the WHO world mental health surveys. *Int. J. Methods Psychiatr. Res.*, 15(4), 167–180.

Heistaro, S., Vartiainen, E., and Puska, P. (1996 September). Trends in self-rated health in Finland 1972–1992. *Prev. Med.*, 25(5), 625–632.

Idler, E.L., and Benyamini, Y. (1997 March). Self-rated health and mortality: A review of twenty-seven community studies. *J. Health Soc. Behav.*, 38(1), 21–37.

Imrie, R. (1997 July). Rethinking the relationships between disability, rehabilitation, and society. *Disabil. Rehabil.*, 19(7), 263–271.

Kessler, R.C., Chatterji, S., Heeringa, S.G., Pennell, B.E., Petukhova, M.V., Vilagut, G., et al. (2013). Methods of the world mental health surveys. In: S.C.Y.H. Jordi Alonso (ed.), *The Burdens of Mental Disorders: Global Perspectives from the WHO World Mental Health Surveys* (pp. 7–38). New York: Cambridge University Press.

Kessler, R.C., and Ustun, T.B. (2008). *The WHO World Mental Health Surveys: Global Perspectives on the Epidemiology of Mental Disorders.* New York: Cambridge University Press.

Kriegsman, D.M., Penninx, B.W., van Eijk, J.T., Boeke, A.J., and Deeg, D.J. (1996). Self-reports and general practitioner information on the presence of chronic diseases in community dwelling elderly. A study on the accuracy of patients' self- reports and on determinants of inaccuracy. *J. Clin. Epidemiol.*, 49(12), 1407–1417.

Lee, H.Y., Jang, S.N., Lee, S., Cho, S.I., and Park, E.O. (2008 July). The relationship between social participation and self-rated health by sex and age: A cross-sectional survey. *Int. J. Nurs. Stud.*, 45(7), 1042–1054.

Lee, Y., and Shinkai, S. (2003 July). A comparison of correlates of self-rated health and functional disability of older persons in the Far East: Japan and Korea. *Arch. Gerontol. Geriatr.*, 37(1), 63–76.

Lefley, H.P. (1990 March). Culture and chronic mental illness. *Hosp. Community Psychiatry*, 41(3), 277–286.

Leinonen, R., Heikkinen, E., and Jylha, M. (2001 May). Predictors of decline in self-assessments of health among older people—A 5-year longitudinal study. *Soc. Sci. Med.*, 52(9), 1329–1341.

Leonardi, M., Bickenbach, J., Ustun, T.B., Kostanjsek, N., Chatterji, S., and MHADIE Consortium. (2006 October 7). The definition of disability: What is in a name? *Lancet*, 368(9543), 1219–1221.

Machacova, K., Lysack, C., and Neufeld, S. (2011). Self-rated health among persons with spinal cord injury: What is the role of physical ability? *J. Spinal. Cord. Med.*, 34(3), 265–272.

Madan, I., Reading, I., Palmer, K.T., and Coggon, D. (2008 October). Cultural differences in musculoskeletal symptoms and disability. *Int. J. Epidemiol.*, 37(5), 1181–1189.

Mavaddat, N., Kinmonth, A.L., Sanderson, S., Surtees, P., Bingham, S., and Khaw, K.T. (2011 September). What determines Self-Rated Health (SRH)? A cross-sectional study of SF-36 health domains in the EPIC-Norfolk cohort. *J. Epidemiol. Community Health*, 65(9), 800–806.

Murray, C.J., and Lopez, A.D. (1996). Evidence-based health policy. Lessons from the global burden of disease study (see comments). *Science*, 274(5288), 740–743.

Ormel, J., Kempen, G.I., Penninx, B.W., Brilman, E.I., Beekman, A.T., and van Sonderen, E. (1997 September). Chronic medical conditions and mental health in older people: Disability and psychosocial resources mediate specific mental health effects. *Psychol. Med.*, 27(5), 1065–1077.

Ormel, J., Petukhova, M., Chatterji, S., Aguilar-Gaxiola, S., Alonso, J., Angermeyer, M.C., et al. (2008 May). Disability and treatment of specific mental and physical disorders across the world. *Br. J. Psychiatry*, 192, 368–375.

Patrick, D.L, and Erickson, P. (1993). *Health Status and Health Policy. Allocating Resources to Health Care.* New York: Oxford University Press.

Pearl, J. (2012 August). The causal mediation formula—A guide to the assessment of pathways and mechanisms. *Prev. Sci.*, 13(4), 426–436.

Perruccio, A.V., Power, J.D., and Badley, E.M. (2007 December). The relative impact of 13 chronic conditions across three different outcomes. *J. Epidemiol. Community Health*, 61(12), 1056–1061.

Rohrer, J.E., Young, R., Sicola, V., and Houston, M. (2007 February). Overall self-rated health: A new quality indicator for primary care. *J. Eval. Clin. Pract.*, 13(1), 150–153.

Saarni, S.I., Harkanen, T., Sintonen, H., Suvisaari, J., Koskinen, S., Aromaa, A., et al. (2006 October). The impact of 29 chronic conditions on health-related quality of life: A general population survey in Finland using 15D and EQ-5D. *Qual. Life Res.*, 15(8), 1403–1414.

Salomon, J.A., Tandon, A., and Murray, C.J. (2004 January 31). Comparability of self rated health: Cross sectional multi-country survey using anchoring vignettes. *BMJ*, 328(7434), 258–263.

Schootman, M., Deshpande, A.D., Pruitt, S., Aft, R., and Jeffe, D.B. (2012 February). Estimated effects of potential interventions to prevent decreases in self-rated health among breast cancer survivors. *Ann. Epidemiol.*, 22(2), 79–86.

Schultz, S.E., and Kopec, J.A. (2003 August). Impact of chronic conditions. *Health Rep.*, 14(4), 41–53.

Sen, A. (2002 April 13). Health: Perception versus observation. *BMJ*, 324(7342), 860–861.

Sokka, T., Kautiainen, H., Pincus, T., Verstappen, S.M., Aggarwal, A., Alten, R., et al. (2010). Work disability remains a major problem in rheumatoid arthritis in the 2000s: Data from 32 countries in the QUEST-RA study. *Arthritis. Res. Ther.*, 12(2), R42.

Steiner, W.A., Ryser, L., Huber, E., Uebelhart, D., Aeschlimann, A., and Stucki, G. (2002 November). Use of the ICF model as a clinical problem-solving tool in physical therapy and rehabilitation medicine. *Phys. Ther.*, 82(11), 1098–1107.

Ustun, T.B., Kostanjsek, N., Chatterji, S., and Rehm, J. (2010). *Measuring Health and Disability: Manual for WHO Disability Assessment Schedule (WHODAS 2.0).* Generva: World Health Organization.

Valderas, J.M., and Alonso, J. (2008 October 3). Patient reported outcome measures: A model-based classification system for research and clinical practice. *Qual. Life Res.*, 17(9), 1125–1135.

Von Korff, M., Crane, P.K., Alonso, J., Vilagut, G., Angermeyer, M.C., Bruffaerts, R., et al. (2008 November). Modified WHODAS-II provides valid measure of global disability but filter items increased skewness. *J. Clin. Epidemiol.*, 61(11), 1132–1143.

Wilson, I.B., and Cleary, P.D. (1995). Linking clinical variables with health-related quality of life. A conceptual model of patient outcomes. *JAMA*, 273(1), 59–65.

Wittchen, H.U. (1994). Reliability and validity studies of the WHO—Composite International Diagnostic Interview (CIDI): A critical review. *J. Psychiatr. Res.*, 28(1), 57–84.

World Health Organization. (2001). *The International Classification of Functioning, Disability and Health: ICF*. Geneva: World Health Organization.

13 Social heterogeneity in self-reported health status and the measurement of inequalities in health

Florence Jusot, Sandy Tubeuf, Marion Devaux, and Catherine Sermet

Introduction

The reduction of health inequalities is one of the main targets of the National Health Strategy announced in 2013 by the French Ministry of Health. Indeed, many studies have shown very large social inequalities in health in comparison to other European countries (Leclerc et al., 2000; Mackenbach et al., 2008; Van Doorslaer and Koolman, 2004). Beyond the analysis of the determinants of these inequalities and the evaluation of policies aimed at their reduction, health inequality measurement remains an issue for the monitoring of health inequalities (CSDH, 2008; Haut Conseil de la Santé Publique, 2013).

In this context, questions remain regarding the measurement of socioeconomic inequalities in health. In particular, we wonder to what extent measurement tools and input variables influence the magnitude of socioeconomic inequalities in health. For example, France is the European country with the highest level of health inequality when measured by the relative risk of premature mortality of blue collar workers compared with white collar workers (Kunst et al., 2000; Mackenbach et al., 2008). Nevertheless, France's level of health inequality is average when inequalities are measured by a concentration index of self-assessed health (Van Doorslaer and Koolman, 2004). The measurement of health, the measurement of the social dimension, and the measurement tool used influence the magnitude of the socioeconomic inequalities in health (Couffinhal et al., 2004; Dourgnon and Lardjane, 2007; Girard et al., 2000). This chapter aims to study the influence of measurements of health on the extent of socioeconomic inequalities in health.

Health status can be measured by many indicators such as mortality, morbidity, and functional limitations. We shall limit ourselves to health indicators, which are distinct from mortality indicators because they measure both quality of life and vital status. The health indicators we chose refer to one of the three dimensions composing an individual health status: subjective, medical, or functional health (Blaxter, 1985; Sermet and Cambois, 2002). The subjective model gathers self-assessed health, symptoms, and quality of life indicators. According to the medical or biological model, health can be evaluated by diagnosed or reported diseases and information from clinical, physiological, or psychiatric examination. Finally, according to the functional and social model, health is evaluated by functional limitations or an inability to perform normal tasks. Thus, these indicators represent different dimensions of health status. Finally, in addition to differences due to the dimension of health itself, differences in the nature of the indicator, such as reported or diagnosed information, induce different measurements of health.

Nevertheless, all indicators do not similarly describe inequalities in health. For instance, data from the latest Health and Health Insurance Survey show that inequalities in health between education and income groups are more important when health is measured by self-assessed health or functional limitations compared with frequency of chronic diseases (Table 13.1). One interpretation of these differences recently proposed in the literature was to consider that each indicator is prone to a socioeconomic reporting heterogeneity, that is, differences in reporting rates according to socioeconomic status at a same "given health status."

Some recent studies thus focused on reporting heterogeneity related to self-assessed health, which is the most regularly collected measurement of health in household surveys. Even if this indicator is a good predictor of mortality (Idler and Benyamini, 1997) and health-care utilization (DeSalvo et al., 2005), it is also the result of a complex aggregation process of several elements that an individual knows about their own health status. Initially, self-assessed health integrates morbidity, which depends not only on diseases and on functional limitations but also on diagnosed health problems and, thus, on interactions with health professionals. This measurement is subjective, and it therefore integrates personal expectations of good health, which are influenced by social and cultural environments. Several studies have highlighted discordance between health perception and other health indicators considered to be more objective. The literature underlines four sets of factors that can affect individual health judgment and therefore self-assessed health. The first group is related to the nature of diseases that an individual suffers. For example, Van Doorslaer and Gerdtham (2003) observe that men with hypertension report better health than women for a given death risk. Age and gender also influence reports: Women report a poorer health status than men for similar levels of incapacity. Moessgaard Iburg et al. (2002) suggest that women would have higher expectations of good health. In addition, Baron-Epel and Kaplan (2001) show that older people more favorably judge their health status than younger people. Reporting heterogeneity related to socioeconomic status has also been found. In France, self-assessed health is affected by optimism overestimation for both rich people and the poorest people for a given clinical health (Etile and Milcent, 2006). Finally,

Table 13.1 Differences in the magnitude of health inequalities according to the health measures

	Fair and poor perceived health		Chronic diseases		Activity limitations	
	%	Age–gender standardized index	%	Age–gender standardized index	%	Age–gender standardized index
Monthly income per consumption unit						
1st quintile [0–926 €]	43.7	1.34	42.3	1.15	36.8	1.39
2nd quintile [926–1264 €]	38.3	1.09	41.2	1.05	30.3	1.06
3rd quintile [1264–1600 €]	36.4	1.06	39.2	1.02	28.0	1.01
4th quintile [1600–2120 €]	30.4	0.92	36.6	0.97	23.9	0.91
5th quintile [2120 €–Max]	22.4	0.68	34.9	0.92	19.2	0.74
Nonresponse	35.9	0.95	37.7	0.90	28.7	0.93
Highest degree obtained						
No diploma	54.2	1.27	50.3	1.09	44.3	1.24
Certificate of primary education	60.5	1.13	59.5	1.06	50.7	1.11
Certificate of general education (lower high school degree)	36.8	1.05	39.7	0.99	28.7	1.03
Baccalaureate (high school graduation)	29.9	0.98	34.6	0.99	21.6	0.90
Higher education degree	19.0	0.68	31.1	0.94	16.2	0.75
Ongoing schooling	7.9	0.54	15.0	0.78	7.2	0.66

Source: Célant, N., et al. (2014). The 2012 Health, Health Care and Insurance Survey (ESPS). First Results. Irdes, Paris. Available from http://www.irdes.fr/english/issues-in-health-economics/198-the-2012-health-health-care-and-insurance-survey-esps.pdf.

health perception seems to depend on cultural characteristics: An Australian study showed that the indigenous population declared being in better health than the general population, despite higher incidence rates of serious illnesses (Mathers and Douglas, 1998).

Other reported health indicators also suffer from cultural and social reporting heterogeneity. A traditional example is that of the Kerala region in India, where reported morbidity is higher than anywhere else in India, whereas at the same time, this region has the lowest mortality rate and the highest literacy rate (Murray and Chen, 1992). Several analyses highlight an underreport of diseases in less educated people, in lower income levels, and in lower social groups (Elstad, 1996; Mackenbach et al., 2008; Murray and Chen, 1992). In the same way, using the Israeli data, Shmueli (2002, 2003) showed heterogeneity in reporting health related to age, gender, education, ethnic origin, and religious faith for the following health indicators: analogical visual scale (AVS), health related quality of life (HRQoL) using the Medical Outcomes Study Short Form 36 items (SF36) questionnaire, self-assessed health, and chronic diseases.

These reportings of heterogeneity related to socioeconomic, demographic, pathological, or cultural characteristics are recognized as important obstacles for interindividual comparisons of reported health levels (Bound, 1990) and for the analysis of socioeconomic inequalities in health (Elstad, 1996; Etile and Milcent, 2006; Jusot et al., 2005; Mackenbach et al., 1996). In France, few studies have examined this question; only reporting heterogeneity in self-assessed health related to income has been studied (Etile and Milcent, 2006). Therefore, reporting heterogeneity affecting other health indicators needs to be studied, especially because recent articles stress their importance in national contexts (Bago d'Uva et al., 2008a,b; Dourgnon and Lardjane, 2007; Etile and Milcent, 2006; Jurges, 2007). The most widespread approach consists of assuming that some indicators are more objective than others and trying to measure "true health." Reporting heterogeneity corresponds then to the difference between health as measured by the indicator considered to be "subjective" and health as measured by the more "objective" indicator (Delpierre et al., 2009, 2012a,b; Elstad, 1996; Etile and Milcent, 2006; Mackenbach et al., 1996; Malmusi et al., 2012; Schneider et al., 2012; Tubeuf and Perronnin, 2008; Van Doorslaer and Gerdtham, 2003). As this approach requires assuming one or several indicators to be more objective, it fails in taking into account the multidimensional concept of health. An alternative approach[1] suggested by some authors (Jurges, 2007; Shmueli, 2002, 2003; Tubeuf et al., 2008; Tubeuf and Perronnin, 2008) consists of building a health score based on several indicators, ignoring their relative objectivity and then analyzing discordance between that score and each health indicator on which it relies. Shmueli (2003) underlines the need to reproduce this analysis with other health indicators to test the sensitivity of the results.

Following this second approach, this chapter proposes to analyze the reporting heterogeneity related to socioeconomic and demographic characteristics affecting several health indicators in France. It emphasizes differences in inequalities in health according to the latent health indicator. In addition, it suggests the existence of reporting heterogeneity. For a given latent health status, health reports will depend on household composition, demographic, and socioeconomic characteristics. This chapter shows that the four health indicators suffer from reporting heterogeneity but that the report of chronic diseases is the indicator that biases the measurement of socioeconomic inequalities in health the most.

The analysis relies on the 2002–2003 Institut national de la statistique et des études économiques (Insee) National Health Survey, which is described in "Data" section, followed by "Methodology" and "Results" sections, and finally, a comprehensive "Discussion" section ends this chapter.

Data

The data come from the French National Health Survey carried out by INSEE in 2002–2003. The survey is representative of the community-dwelling French population. For the purpose of this chapter, the sample was restricted to the 20,145 adults aged 18–85 years and having answered all of the health-related questions.

Measurement of health status

To measure the health status, we selected four health indicators able to cover the different health dimensions suggested by Blaxter (1985): the three health questions of the Mini European Health Module (MEHM) (EHEMU, 2010) concerning self-assessed health, chronic diseases, and functional limitations plus the SF-36 mental health (MH) indicator (McCabe et al., 1996).

The self-assessed health indicator of the MEHM corresponds to the question: "How is your health in general?" and the possible answers are: "very good," "good," "fair," "bad," and "very bad." This indicator is dichotomized by grouping people who rate their health as very poor, poor, or average health status versus good or very good; 22.3% of the sample report having a very poor, poor, or average health status.

The indicator of chronic diseases comes from the second question of the MEHM: "Do you have any longstanding illness or longstanding health problem?" A total of 39.8% of the sample gave a positive response to this question.

Functional health was measured using the third indicator of the MEHM. It corresponds to the question: "For at least the past six months, to what extent have you been limited because of a health problem in activities people usually do?" A total of 11.4% of the individuals reported limitations.

The indicator of MH is generated from the SF-36 score of MH. Individuals had an average score of 66.7 out of 100. Individuals scoring lower than 56 (first quartile) are considered to have poor MH.

Measurement of socioeconomic status

In addition to age and gender, we considered five socioeconomic status indicators in our analysis: household composition, education level, household income, social occupation, and activity status. Ages are grouped into six classes: 18–24 years, 25–39 years, 40–49 years, 50–59 years, 60–74 years, and 75–85 years. Education level is measured by the highest diploma obtained and is separated into four categories: people without a diploma, people having a diploma lower than general or technical A-level, people having a diploma equivalent to the general or technical A-level, and people having a higher education diploma. Equivalized household income corresponds to the total household income (resulting from an exact report or an imputed amount from income categories) divided by the number of consumption units in the household. The equivalence scale used is the Organisation for Economic Co-operation and Development (OECD) scale, which gives a weight of 1 to the first member of the household, a weight of 0.5 for any other adult, and a weight of 0.3 for any child under 14 years of age. Equivalized household income is categorized into four income quartiles.

Social occupation is measured by either the current occupation or the last occupation. Six social classes are distinguished: farmers, self-employed workers, managers, clerks, employees, and workers and unknown occupation. Activity status is derived as a six-group variable as follows: employed, unemployed, student, retired, homemaker, and inactive.

Table 13.2 shows some descriptive statistics of the sample.

Table 13.2 Sample description

Variables	Freq.	Prop.
Gender		
Female	10,662	52.9%
Male	9483	47.1%
Age classes		
18–24	2326	11.5%
25–39	5879	29.2%
40–49	4261	21.2%
50–59	3586	17.8%
60–74	3153	15.7%
75–85	940	4.7%
Household composition		
Single	2725	13.5%
Couple without children	6144	30.5%
Couple with children	9407	46.7%
Single-parent family	1097	5.4%
Nonnuclear family	772	3.8%
Education level		
No diploma	2709	13.4%
Diploma lower than A-level	8677	43.1%
A-level	3445	17.1%
Diploma higher than A-level	5314	26.4%

(*Continued*)

Table 13.2 Sample description (*Continued*)

Variables	Freq.	Prop.
Household income		
1st income quartile	4224	21.0%
2nd income quartile	4983	24.7%
3rd income quartile	5286	26.2%
4th income quartile	5652	28.1%
Social occupation		
Farmer	667	3.3%
Self-employed	1047	5.2%
Manager	2853	14.2%
Clerk	4410	21.9%
Employee	5355	26.6%
Worker	4207	20.9%
Unknown occupation	1606	8.0%
Activity status		
Employed	11,898	59.1%
Unemployed	1246	6.2%
Student	1253	6.2%
Retired	3879	19.3%
Homemaker	1417	7.0%
Inactive	452	2.2%
Self-assessed health		
Reported poor self-assessed health (MEHM)	4486	22.30%
Poor general health status (SF-36 General Health score)	5143	25%
Reported morbidity		
Reported chronic disease problem (MEHM)	8022	39.80%
At least one reported chronic disease	12,551	62.3%
Functional health		
Reported functional limitations (MEHM)	2292	11.40%
At least one reported activity limitation	4979	24.20%
MH		
Poor MH (SF-36 MH score)	5143	25%
Having a depression risk (Center for Epidemiologic Studies-Depression [CES-D] scale score)	5143	25%

Source: Insee. Health Survey in 2002–2003. (2011). Paris. Available from https://www.insee.fr/en/metadonnees/source/s1101 (January 2017).

Methodology

We used a Multiple Indicators Multiple Index Causes (MIMIC) model, which is a structural equation model, as suggested by Shmueli to explore social heterogeneity affecting various health indicators (Shmueli, 2002, 2003). If we assume the existence of a latent "true health" status that explains individual responses to health indicators, we can build a synthetic health score based on a set of selected health indicators that provides an estimate of the "true health." Therefore, sociodemographic variation in each health indicator can be separated into variation in the true health and measure-specific variation, holding true health constant. The latter variation is referred to as "reporting heterogeneity." The variation in the estimated latent health status represents the true social health inequalities.

Construction of a synthetic health score

The construction of this model initially requires a factor data analysis to generate a continuous health score using the four selected health indicators as described in the "Data" section. The factor analysis empirically determines the number of relevant factors summarizing the information of these four health indicators, that is, the number of subjacent latent variables that influence responses to health indicators. The eigenvalue minimum criteria (i.e., the factor must have an eigenvalue equal at least to 1 to be selected) is used to identify the number of factors to be selected.

The exploratory factor analysis shows the existence of a unique latent factor behind the four health indicators, representing 62% of the total inertia. The confirmatory factor analysis confirms the good adequacy of the data with one latent factor model as the root mean square error of approximation[2] (RMSEA) criterion equals 0.031. The estimated latent variable, also called the true latent health, corresponds to a continuous synthetic indicator measuring poor health.

Analysis of report heterogeneity

In the second step of this study, we estimated a simultaneous equations model. Equation 13.1 estimates the effects of socioeconomic characteristics on the estimated latent health summarized by the health score. Equation 13.2 explains reports to the health indicators according to the latent health. The health score is thus used both as a dependent variable explained by various determinants of health in (Equation 13.1) and as an explanatory variable of reports to the health indicators in (Equation 13.2). Testing the existence of the social reporting heterogeneity of health is therefore equivalent to testing the existence of an effect of socioeconomic variables on individual reports to indicators, independent of their effect on the latent health variable. Direct effects on the health indicators are called "reporting bias," as it is usually done in this literature.

More formally, the MIMIC model with only one latent factor can be formalized as follows:

$$\eta = \Gamma'Z + z \tag{13.1}$$

$$Y = \Lambda\eta + \beta'Z + \varepsilon \tag{13.2}$$

The synthetic health score (η) is a continuous variable. The vector ($Y' = (Y_1, Y_2, Y_3, Y_4)$) is composed of four dichotomous health indicators: Y_1 is an indicator of poor self-assessed health, Y_2 is an indicator of reported chronic diseases, Y_3 is an indicator of reported activity limitations, and Y_4 is an indicator of poor MH. Socioeconomic characteristics are represented by ($Z = (Z_1, Z_2 \ldots)$). The vector ($\Lambda' = (\lambda_1, \lambda_2 \ldots)$) corresponds to contributions of the synthetic health indicator (η) to reports of health indicators (Y_i). The vector (G) represents the effects of socioeconomic variables (Z) on latent health (η), which can be interpreted as determinants of "true" health. The vector (β) corresponds to direct effects of socioeconomic variables (Z) on health indicators (Y), which are apparent to social reporting heterogeneity. Finally, we assume that the two error terms (ζ) and (ε) are uncorrelated, but measurement errors ($\varepsilon = (\varepsilon_1, \varepsilon_2 \ldots)$) are such that ($\varepsilon_i$) and ($\varepsilon_j$) with ($i, j = 1, 2 \ldots$ and $I \neq j$) can be correlated. The potential correlation of the measurement errors (ε_i) and (ε_j) permits incorporating reporting heterogeneity that could be common to some indicators and independent from socioeconomic characteristics.

This modeling strategy can be schematically represented as shown in Figure 13.1.

Equations 13.1 and 13.2 are simultaneously estimated using the M-Plus software. The estimated parameters in Equation 13.1 are linear regression coefficients, the health score being a continuous variable, and the coefficients of Equation 13.2 are coefficients from a probit model because Y_i are categorical variables. The adjustment of the model to the data is evaluated using the RMSEA criterion in which the satisfaction threshold is below 0.05.

Results

The MIMIC model is estimated and leads to a satisfactory adjustment with an RMSEA criterion equal to 0.007. Two series of results are shown; the first is

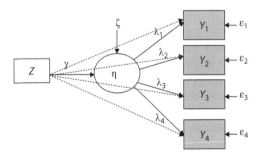

Figure 13.1 Multiple Indicators Multiple Index Causes model.

related to the determinants of latent health, and the second concerns reporting heterogeneity affecting reports of the four health indicators.

The column "poor latent health" in Table 13.3 presents the linear regression estimates of the latent health variable as explained by several individual socioeconomic characteristics. The four other columns present the Probit estimates associated with the four health indicators while adjusting for latent health. In this table, a negative coefficient shows a positive impact on good health. Gender, age, household composition, education level, income, and social status significantly influence latent health. Poor health increases with age, and men are in better health than women. People living alone are in poorer health than couples without children, but couples without children are in poorer health than those with children. Poor health decreases with higher education level, with higher income level and higher social position. Finally, unemployed people, retired people, inactive people, and homemakers are in poorer health than employed people.

The second series of results is related to the determinants of the four health indicators (columns 3–10 of Table 13.3). Only statistically significant coefficients have been reported in Table 13.3. Coefficients associated to the "latent health" show that latent health significantly contributes to the way health indicators are reported. True latent health contributes more to self-assessed health (coef = 1 by construction) compared with the other three indicators (chronic diseases reports [coef. = 0.609], activity limitations reports [coef. = 0.756], and MH [coef. = 0.54]).

Our results also shed light on the existence of various reporting heterogeneity affecting health indicators. On the one hand, the negative and significant correlation of the measurement errors attached to MH and chronic disease suggests a specific reporting bias related to these two health indicators independent of sociodemographic characteristics. On the other hand, the direct effects of some characteristics on health indicators for a given latent health suggest the existence of reporting heterogeneity related to demographic, economic, and social characteristics. Hence, for a given latent health, women report more chronic diseases and more MH problems than men. Older people report more chronic diseases and better MH. People living alone or in single-parent families report more MH problems compared with couples; they also self-assess a poorer health status. Conversely, nonnuclear families report fewer chronic diseases than couples. Education and income levels significantly influence health variables for a given latent health. A-level or less than A-level education is significantly related to better self-assessed health. In parallel, individuals with a diploma higher than A-level report more chronic diseases and activity limitations. Income level has a direct and positive effect on the chronic disease indicator: the higher the income, the more likely chronic diseases are reported. As for the social activity, clerks or managers report more chronic diseases and activity limitations than others for a given latent health. Finally, students report less general health problems than employed people, whereas retired and inactive people report more activity limitations.

Table 13.3 Determinants of poor latent health and the probability of reporting a poor health status with regard to each indicator

Individual characteristics	Poor latent health		Poor self-assessed health		Chronic disease		Activity limitation		Poor MH	
	Estim.	t-test	Estim.	t-test	Estim.	t-test	Estim.	t-test	Estim.	t-test
Gender										
Male	Ref.	Ref.			Ref.	Ref.			Ref.	Ref.
Female	0.087	3.734			0.05	2.293			0.296	13,371
Age classes										
18–24	−0.262	−5.697								
25–39	Ref.	Ref.	Ref.	Ref.	Ref.	Ref.	Ref.	Ref.	Ref.	Ref.
40–49	0.284	9.911			0.113	3.666			−0.07	−2429
50–59	0.503	15.227			0.335	6.22			−0.174	−5289
60–74	0.53	9.51			0.301	4.427			−0.31	−5426
75–85	0.88	13.32							−0.273	−3979
Household composition										
Single	0.071	2.336							0.204	6662
Couple without children	Ref.	Ref.	Ref.	Ref.	Ref.	Ref.	Ref.	Ref.	Ref.	Ref.

(Continued)

Table 13.3 Determinants of poor latent health and the probability of reporting a poor health status with regard to each indicator (*Continued*)

	Poor latent health		Poor self-assessed health		Chronic disease		Activity limitation		Poor MH	
	Estim.	t-test	Estim.	t-test	Estim.	t-test	Estim.	t-test	Estim.	t-test
Individual characteristics										
Couple with children	−0.054	−2.157								
Single-parent family	−0.088	−1.466	0.149	2.401					0.243	4748
Nonnuclear family	0.024	0.456			−0.145	−2.804				
Education level										
No diploma	Ref.		Ref.		Ref.		Ref.		Ref.	
Diploma lower than A-level	−0.1	−2.993	−0.119	−3.682						
A-level	−0.237	−5.469	−0.108	−2.498						
Diploma higher than A-level	−0.468	−11.477			0.185	4.691	0.18	3.48		
Household income										
1st income quartile	Ref.		Ref.		Ref.		Ref.		Ref.	
2nd income quartile	−0.074	−2.563			0.068	2.443				
3rd income quartile	−0.194	−6.452			0.124	4.226				
4th income quartile	−0.23	−6.981			0.156	4.839				

(*Continued*)

Table 13.3 Determinants of poor latent health and the probability of reporting a poor health status with regard to each indicator (*Continued*)

Individual characteristics	Poor latent health		Poor self-assessed health		Chronic disease		Activity limitation		Poor MH	
	Estim.	t-test	Estim.	t-test	Estim.	t-test	Estim.	t-test	Estim.	t-test
Social occupation										
Farmer	-0.1	-1.918								
Self-employed	-0.149	-3.332								
Manager	-0.298	-6.754			0.163	3.946	0.112	2.093		
Clerk	-0.171	-4.995			0.124	3.802	0.112	2.786		
Employee	-0.077	-2.723								
Worker	Ref.		Ref.	Ref.	Ref.	Ref.	Ref.	Ref.	Ref.	Ref.
Unknown occupation	-0.199	-3.046								
Activity status										
Employed	Ref.		Ref.	Ref.	Ref.	Ref.	Ref.	Ref.	Ref.	Ref.
Unemployed	0.314	7.849								
Student	0.251	2.769	-0.357	-3.521						
Retired	0.246	5.155					0.198	3.605		

(*Continued*)

Table 13.3 Determinants of poor latent health and the probability of reporting a poor health status with regard to each indicator (*Continued*)

Individual characteristics	Poor latent health		Poor self-assessed health		Chronic disease		Activity limitation		Poor MH	
	Estim.	t-test	Estim.	t-test	Estim.	t-test	Estim.	t-test	Estim.	t-test
Homemaker	0.173	4.214								
Inactive	0.942	14.875								
							0.547	8.898		
Threshold/intercept			0.709	14.816	0.567	13.122	1.367	24.345	0.592	13.252
Latent health			1	0	0.609	36.355	0.756	39.859	0.54	33.692
R^2	0.246		0.888		0.402		0.568		0.314	
Chi-square (weighted least square mean and variance adjusted [WLSMW])	73.244									
p-value	0.0005									
Root mean square error of approximation (RMSEA)	0.007									
Correlation between chronic disease and MH	−0.051	−4.012								

Source: National Health Survey, INSEE, 2002–2003, data analysis by IRDES.

Discussion

The objective of this chapter was to analyze social heterogeneity affecting health reporting and potentially affecting the measurement of social inequalities in health. All our results confirm social differences in latent health. Moreover, our results show reporting heterogeneity for a given latent health. Women and older people more often report chronic diseases than other for a comparable latent health status. MH problems are overreported by women and single people and are underreported by older people. Inactive people, retired people, and clerks more frequently report activity limitations. Finally, the most educated people, people with higher incomes, clerks, and managers more frequently report chronic diseases, whereas less educated people underreport poor self-assessed health, for a comparable latent health status.

The approach suggested by Shmueli (2002, 2003) has allowed us to generate a synthetic latent health indicator using four health indicators and to disentangle the association between sociodemographic characteristics and health indicators into (1) the contribution of these characteristics to the latent true health and (2) their direct contribution to reports of each health indicator considered as reporting bias. However, the methodology and the way to interpret results have some limitations that can be discussed in four points.

First, this method relies on the assumption of the existence of a single latent health variable explaining individual reports of various health indicators. The exploratory factor analysis on the four health indicators shows a unique latent factor summarizing health and thus confirms that health could satisfactorily be represented by a unique variable. However, this factor represents only 62% of total inertia. Therefore, the latent variable generated by this method does not permit having a complete representation of health, which is largely multidimensional concept.

Second, this first assumption implies to interpret the direct effects of sociodemographic characteristics on health indicators as health reporting biases. However, these effects can represent either reporting heterogeneity or effects of individual characteristics on some specific health dimensions, and thus determinants of health. For example, the particular effect of gender on the SF-36 MH score can be due to overreporting of MH problems by women, but it can also result from a strong association between gender and this dimension of health with regard to the other dimensions. Indeed, there is a strong difference in the prevalence of depression between women and men (Grigoriadis and Robinson, 2007). Similarly, inactive people have certainly specific risks for functional limitations but not necessarily higher risks of chronic disease. Thus, as various health indicators do not refer to the same dimension of health, they could lead to a different measurement of social health inequalities even in the absence of social reporting heterogeneity if socioeconomic differences in health do change according to the considered dimension of health.

Third, this method allows us to identify specific heterogeneity affecting each indicator, but does not allow us to identify common heterogeneity affecting the full set of health indicators. Therefore, an optimistic or pessimistic over- or underestimation affecting reports of the four indicators and correlated to a particular sociodemographic characteristic will not be identified as a bias, but will be mistaken for the effect of this characteristic on latent health. However, a potential correlation in measurement errors of two indicators was found between MH and chronic disease, suggesting a common reporting error.

Fourth, the latent health variable has been generated from information common to the four health indicators and may thus vary with changes in these indicators. To test the stability of our results, we have changed each of the four indicators by another indicator available in the survey, which refers to the same dimension of health: Self-assessed health of the MEHM has been replaced by self-assessed health of the SF-36, chronic diseases by a list or reported chronic diseases, activity limitations of the MEHM by reports of incapacities and deficiencies, and finally SF-36 MH score by the CES-D score, which is a validated depression scale (Radloff, 1977). Results were found to be stable since most of the heterogeneity situations highlighted in our model remained unchanged (results not shown, available in Tubeuf et al., 2008). In particular, the sensitivity analysis has confirmed underreporting of poor self-assessed health by students and overreporting by single-parent families; higher reporting of chronic diseases by older people, more educated people and the richer; higher reporting of functional problems by retired people, inactive people, and more educated people; and finally, overreporting of MH problems by women, single or single-parent families and underreporting by older people.

Nevertheless, this analysis provides consistent results with the literature. First, in line with many previous studies, social inequalities in health are found showing a deterioration of health with social status, education level, and income when health is measured by the latent health indicator (Mackenbach et al., 2008; Van Doorslaer and Masseria, 2004). We also found evidence of reporting heterogeneity affecting health reports according to four indicators: chronic diseases, activity limitations, self-assessed health, and the SF-36 MH score. A large number of direct effects affect the chronic diseases indicator, suggesting that this indicator provides a particularly biased health measurement according to individual sociodemographic characteristics. In line with Moessgaard Iburg et al. (2002), we show that women overreport—or men underreport—chronic diseases. Gender differences in diseases report may come from a more frequent use of health care for the same health status, a greater attention paid to health problems and a better knowledge of health problems that can be partly explained by the poorer latent health in women compared with men. Our results on over-reporting by the elderly support previous findings by Shmueli (2003); social differences by education level, income, and occupation are also confirmed by Mackenbach et al. (1996) and Elstad (1996). Again these findings can be explained by better medical information related to more frequent health-care utilization or by greater attention paid to health by higher social groups. Besides, one can wonder whether the concept of chronic diseases is well understood in any social group.

The activity limitations indicator also reveals reporting heterogeneity related to education level and activity status. Individuals having a diploma higher than A-level, clerks, and managers report more activity limitations than those in the working classes, even though they have a better latent health. This overreporting may be explained by a lower tolerance toward functional limitations and activity restrictions for these social groups. Moreover, we observe overreporting of activity limitations by retired and inactive people. This result may correspond to a justification bias as proposed by Bound (1990) according to which people would justify their exit from the labor market because of their poor health. However, one can also argue that inactive or early retired people experience a specific risk of suffering from activity limitations, which mainly explains their anticipated exit (Barnay and Debrand, 2006). The results related to the SF-36 MH score suggest overreporting of this type of health problem by women, in accordance with the results of the analysis carried out in Israel by Shmueli (2003). However, this finding can be due to a specific gender effect on this dimension of health, the risk of depression or anxiety being more widespread among women (Grigoriadis and Robinson, 2007). We also confirm the underreporting of MH problems by older people shown by Shmueli (2003). This effect may be explained by lower expectations in terms of the MH of old people because of the numerous health problems related to aging. Nevertheless, this effect may rather be related to a less marked age effect on MH than on other dimensions of health. Finally, we show overreporting of MH problems by single or single-parent families, which is undoubtedly partly due to the specific influence of isolation on this dimension of health (Wang, 2004).

The few direct effects observed with self-assessed health suggest that this indicator is less affected than the other health indicators. In opposition to Etilé and Milcent (2006), no evidence of heterogeneity related to income or occupation was found. Nevertheless, people having an intermediate education level less frequently report poor health compared with people without a diploma and to the most educated people for a given latent health status. This optimistic estimation compared with the most educated individuals could be explained by higher expectations for health when people are more educated as suggested by Mackenbach et al. (1996), Elstad (1996), or Delpierre et al. (2009, 2012a,b). However, students report better self-assessed health, whereas they have a poorer latent health than employed people possibly due to allergies, depression, and anxiety. Perhaps this optimism overestimation suggests that they do not take into account chronic health problems or MH in their appreciation of their general health status. Finally, single-parent people more frequently report a poor self-assessed health for a given latent health status. This overreporting may reflect health complaints or express a social difficulty through health problem reporting. Similarly, the higher probability of reporting a poor health status for people without a diploma for a given health status in comparison to individuals having an intermediate education level may be interpreted as a pessimistic estimation, but could also reflect specific health problems, distress, pain, or burden of pathologies that are not fully taken into account by the other health indicators.

This analysis thus underlines the existence of reporting heterogeneity related to sociodemographic characteristics affecting the set of considered health indicators. Among these indicators, chronic disease reporting suffers from many biases and particularly from a pessimism bias related to education, social status, and income. Consequently, this indicator cannot be regarded as a good measurement tool for social inequalities in health, as it would underestimate their magnitude. In contrast, self-assessed health, activity limitations, and MH seem to be the more relevant indicators. These indicators represent various dimensions of health; they can thus advantageously be used according to the objectives of the analysis. Aiming for an overall monitoring of social inequalities in health, self-assessed health finally seems to be a good health measurement tool.

Notes

1 Rather than comparing self-assessed health to more or less objective indicators, another methodology consists of examining variation in the evaluation of given health states represented by hypothetical case vignettes, called anchoring vignettes. However, this approach does not apply to self-rated health (Bago d'Uva et al., 2008a,b; King, 2004).
2 See the RMSEA definition in "Analysis of Report Heterogeneity" on page 182.

Acknowledgments

Financial support from the research program "Inégalités sociales de santé," supported by Mission de la Recherche (MiRe) of the Direction de la recherche, des études, de l'évaluation et des statistiques (Drees), Institut national de la santé et de la recherche médicale (Inserm), Direction Générale de la Santé (DGS), Institut national de la Veille Sanitaire (InVS), Institut National du Cancer (INCa), and Caisse Nationale d'Assurance Maladie des professions indépendantes (CANAM) is gratefully acknowledged.

Disclaimer

The content of this chapter does not necessarily reflect the views of the OECD or the governments of its member countries.

References

Bago d'Uva, T., O'Donnell, O., and Van Doorslaer, E. (2008a). Differential health reporting by education level and its impact on the measurement of health inequalities among older Europeans. *Int. J. Epidemiol.*, 37(6), 1375–1383.

Bago d'Uva, T., Van Doorslaer, E., Lindeboom, M., and O'Donnell, O. (2008b). Does reporting heterogeneity bias the measurement of health disparities?. *Health Econ.*, *17*(3), 351–375.

Barnay, T., and Debrand, T. (2006). L'impact de l'état de santé sur l'emploi des seniors en Europe L'impact de l'état de santé sur l'emploi des seniors en Europe. *Questions D'Economie de la Sante*. Paris: Irdes. 209, 1–6.

Baron-Epel, O., and Kaplan, G. (2001). General subjective health status or age-related subjective health status: Does it make a difference?. *Soc. Sci. Med.*, *53*(10), 1373–1381.

Blaxter, M. (1985). *A Comparison of Measures of Inequality in Morbidity*. Aldershot: Health Inequalities in European Countries Gower.

Bound, J. (1990). Self-reported versus objective measures of health in retirement models. *J. Hum. Resour.*, *26*, 107–137.

Célant, N., Dourgnon, P., Guillaume, S., Pierre,A., Rochereau, T., Sermet, C. (2014). The 2012 Health, Health Care and Insurance Survey (ESPS). First Results. Paris: Irdes. Available from http://www.irdes.fr/english/issues-in-health-economics/198-the-2012-health-health-care-and-insurance-survey-esps.pdf (January 2017).

Couffinhal, A., Dourgnon, P., and Tubeuf, S. (2004). Outils de mesure des inégalités de santé : Quelques débats d'actualité. *Sante Societe et Solidarite: Revue de L'Observatoire Franco-Quebecois*, (2), 163–171.

CSDH. (2008). Closing the gap in a generation: Health equity through action on the social determinants of health. In: *Final Report of the Commission on Social Determinants of Health*. Geneva: World Health Organization.

Delpierre, C., Datta, G.D., Kelly-Irving, M., Lauwers-Cances, V., Berkman, L., and Lang, T. (2012a). What role does socio-economic position play in the link between functional limitations and self-rated health: France vs. USA?. *Eur. J. Public Health*, *22*(3), 317–321.

Delpierre, C., Kelly-Irving, M., Munch-Petersen, M., Lauwers-Cances, V., Datta, G.D., Lepage, B, et al. (2012b). SRH and HrQOL: Does social position impact differently on their link with health status?. *BMC Public Health*, *12*, 19.

Delpierre, C., Lauwers-Cances, V., Datta, G.D., Berkman, L., and Lang, T. (2009). Impact of social position on the effect of cardiovascular risk factors on self-rated health. *Am. J. Public Health*, *99*(7), 1278–1284.

DeSalvo, K.B., Fan, V.S., McDonell, M.B., and Fihn, S.D. (2005). Predicting mortality and healthcare utilization with a single question. *Health Serv. Res.*, *40*(4), 1234–1246.

Dourgnon, P., and Lardjane, S. (2007). *Les Comparaisons Internationales D'état De Santé Subjectif Sont-Elles Pertinentes? Une Evaluation Par La Méthode Des Vignettes-Etalons*. Paris: Irdes.

EHEMU. (2010). *The Minimum European Health Module: Background Documents*. European Health Expectancy Monitoring Unit (Ed.), (pp. 1–29).

Elstad, J. (1996). How large are the differences—Really? Self-reported long standing illness working class and middle class men. *Sociol. Health Iln.*, *18*(4), 475–478.

Etile, F., and Milcent, C. (2006). Income-related reporting heterogeneity in self-assessed health: Evidence from France. *Health Econ.*, *15*(9), 965–981.

Girard, F., Cohidon, C., and Briançon, S. (2000). *Les Indicateurs Globaux De Santé. Les Inégalités Sociales De Santé*. Paris: La Découverte/INSERM.

Grigoriadis, S., and Robinson, G.E. (2007). Gender issues in depression. *Ann. Clin. Psychiatry*, *19*(4), 247–255.

Haut Conseil de la Santé Publique. (2013). Indicateurs de suivi de l'évolution des inégalités sociales de santé dans les systèmes d'information en santé. La Documentation Française.

Idler, E.L., and Benyamini, Y. (1997). Self-rated health and mortality: A review of twenty-seven community studies. *J. Health Soc. Behav.*, *38*(1), 21–37.

Jurges, H. (2007). True health vs response styles: Exploring cross-country differences in self-reported health. *Health Econ.*, 16(2), 163–178.

Jusot, F., Rochaix, L., and Tubeuf S. (2005). Income-related health inequalities in France between 1998 and 2002: Comparing trends with alternative health indicators. Ecuity III Worskhop, Bonn.

Kunst, A.E., Groenhof, F., Mackenbach, J.P., and EU Working Group on Socio-economic Inequalities in Health. (2000). Inégalités sociales de mortalité prématurée: La France comparée aux autres pays européens. In: *Les Inégalités sociales de Santé*. Paris: La Découverte/INSERM.

Leclerc, A., Fassin, D., Grandjean, H., Kaminski, M., and Lang, T. (2000). *Les Inégalités Sociales de Santé*. Paris: La découverte/INSERM.

Mackenbach, J.P., Looman, C.W., and van der Meer, J.B. (1996). Differences in the misreporting of chronic conditions, by level of education: the effect on inequalities in prevalence rates. *Am. J. Public Health*, 86(5), 706–711.

Mackenbach, J.P., Stirbu, I., Roskam, A.J.R., Shaap, M.M., Menvielle, G., Leinsalu, M, et al. (2008). Socioeconomic inequalities in health in 22 European countries. *N. Engl. J. Med.*, 358(23), 2468–2481.

Malmusi, D., Artazcoz, L., Benach, J., and Borrell, C. (2012). Perception or real illness? How chronic conditions contribute to gender inequalities in self-rated health. *Eur. J. Public Health*, 22(6), 781–786.

Mathers, C., and Douglas, R. (1998). Measuring progress in population health and well-being. In R. Eckersley (ed.), *Measuring Progress: Is Life Getting Better?* Clayton, Australia: CSIRO Publishing.

McCabe, C.J., Thomas, K.J., Brazier, J.E., and Coleman, P. (1996). Measuring the mental health status of a population: A comparison of the GHQ-12 and the SF-36 (MHI-5). *Br. J. Psychiatry*, 169(4), 516–521.

Moessgaard Iburg, K., Salomon, J., Tandon, A., and Murray, C. (2002). Cross-population comparability of physician-assessed and self-reported measures of health. In C. Murray, J. Salomon, C. Mathers, and C. Murray (eds.), *Summary Measures of Population Health: Concepts, Ethics, Measurement and Applications*. Geneva: World Health Organisation.

Murray, C., and Chen, J.T. (1992). Understanding morbidity change. *Popul. Dev. Rev.*, 18, 481–503.

Radloff, L. (1977). The CES-D Scale: A self-report depression scale for research in the general population. *Appl. Psychol. Assess.*, 1, 385–401.

Schneider, U., Pfarr, C., Schneider, B.S., and Ulrich, V. (2012). I fell good! Gender differences and reporting heterogeneity in self-assessed health. *Eur. J. Health Econ.*, 13(3), 251–265.

Sermet, C., and Cambois, E. (2002). Mesurer l'état de santé. In G. Caselli, and C. Sermet (eds.), *Démographie: Analyse et Synthèse. III - Les Déterminants De La Mortalité*. Paris: INED.

Shmueli, A. (2002). Reporting heterogeneity in the measurement of health and health-related quality of life. *Pharmacoeconomics*, 20(6), 405–412.

Shmueli, A. (2003). Socio-economic and demographic variation in health and in its measures: The issue of reporting heterogeneity. *Soc. Sci. Med.*, 57(1), 125–134.

Tubeuf, S., Jusot, F., Devaux, M., and Sermet, C. (2008). *Social Heterogeneity in Self-Reported Health Status and Measurement of Inequalities in Health*. Paris: Irdes.

Tubeuf, S., and Perronnin, M. (2008). *New Prospects in the Analysis of Inequalities in Health: A Measurement of Health Encompassing Several Dimensions of Health*. University of York. Health-Econometrics and data group.

Van Doorslaer, E., and Gerdtham, U.G. (2003). Does inequality in self-assessed health predict inequality in survival by income? Evidence from Swedish data. *Soc. Sci. Med.*, 57(9), 1621–1629.

Van Doorslaer, E., and Koolman, X. (2004). Explaining the differences in income-related health inequalities across European countries. *Health Econ.*, 13(7), 609–628.

Van Doorslaer, E., and Masseria, C. (2004). Income-related inequality in the use of medical care in 21 OECD countries. In A. Couffinhal (ed.), *Towards High-Performing Health Systems* (pp. 109–165). Paris: OCDE.

Wang, J.L. (2004). The difference between single and married mothers in the 12-month prevalence of major depressive syndrome, associated factors and mental health service utilization. *Soc. Psychiatry Psychiatr. Epidemiol.*, 39(1), 26–32.

14 Social heterogeneity of perceived health

Thierry Lang, Cyrille Delpierre, and Michelle Kelly-Irving

Perceived health (PH) is an interesting indicator for different reasons. From a conceptual point of view, PH is multidimensional and includes mental, physical, and social health. In an attempt to capture personal health needs, PH closely reflects the needs and perceptions of the individual. In these respects, PH is highly coherent with the 1946 World Health Organization (WHO) definition of health: "a state of complete physical, social and mental well-being." Its relation to health has been validated in several cohort studies, where it has been shown to be a good predictive measure of mortality, even years later and after adjusting for a diversity of factors. As a health indicator, PH is easy to collect in epidemiological or statistical studies, requiring only that individuals answer a simple question, without the need for biological or clinical examination.

However, the results obtained with self-assessed health in international comparisons are intriguing. As far as mortality is concerned, the relative index of inequality in France is the highest among Western European countries, twice the level observed in Italy or Spain. When self-reported health is concerned, using the same measure of inequality, France is among the countries with a low level of health inequalities, approximately at the same level of Italy and Spain (Mackenbach et al., 2008). In addition, the predictive value of PH regarding mortality has been shown to differ according to socioeconomic position (Singh-Manoux et al., 2007).

To understand these discrepancies, we can hypothesize that according to comparison processes theory, people compare themselves to others to whom they bear a social resemblance. Socially advantaged groups, such as the well-educated, may have the highest expectations about their quality of life (QoL) and health. Therefore, in the presence of the same illness, people with a higher educational level may experience a greater negative impact on their PH than those with a lower level of education whose health expectations are lower. This phenomenon could lead to an underestimation of the health inequalities existing between socioeconomic groups when using self-rated health (SHR) as an indicator of health (Delpierre et al., 2009a,b; Lang and Delpierre, 2009).

To test this hypothesis, our team analyzed studies on representative samples in France (Enquête décennale santé) and the United States (National Health and Nutrition Examination Survey). PH was compared with chronic diseases as reported by the individual and to biologically measured cardiovascular risk factors. For one disease or risk factor, the level of PH was more reduced for upper class social groups than for lower social groups. Using functional limitation (FL) as a measure of physical health in France and in the United States, the impact of an FL on PH was higher among highly educated men and women in both countries. These results were in accordance with the assumption of underestimation of social inequalities in health by using self-reported health as a health indicator. In contrast, the impact of health conditions on QoL was lower for socially advantaged people. QoL is a broader concept compared with PH. Several dimensions of life are important, such as subjective well-being, happiness, life satisfaction, and social relationships and networks. The notion of resources is probably in part at the origin of this contrast between the two indicators. If PH varies based on expectations and in relation to one's peers, the distribution of QoL is related to resources, which allow social functioning. Indeed, financial, social, and cultural resources become essential to cope with health conditions. In this context, a high level of resources could limit the impact of a disease on QoL.

To summarize our findings, the relationship between subjective health and health conditions was found to be influenced by socioeconomic position. Compared with people with a low socioeconomic position, health conditions seem to have a greater impact on PH among socially advantaged people, but lesser impact on or decreased QoL. Therefore, when aiming to analyze social inequalities in health, the use of subjective health indicators could underestimate (PH) or overestimate (QoL) the magnitude of health inequalities existing between socioeconomic groups. These subjective health indicators are, therefore, not equivalent measures and cannot be used interchangeably (Delpierre et al., 2009a,b; 2012a,b).

We would like to raise concerns regarding the use of PH as a tool to conduct policies, particularly with regard to international comparisons or to policies aiming at reducing inequalities in health.

According to the model used by Jusot et al. (2017), a "true health" is defined as a latent variable obtained from a combination of several dimensions of health. Indeed, the score is obtained by a statistical combination of measurement of health: SF-36 mental score, reported chronic diseases and reported functional limitations and self-assessed health. A "true" latent state of health would thus be measured by various indicators and one could observe *bias* for each indicator as compared with the "true" health. The goal here is thus to statistically test which of the perceived measure of health is less biased when taking the true health as a gold standard. The result of this analysis highlights that PH is the least biased health indicator. This finding suggests that PH is the best measure and self-reported illness the most biased indicator among the three they tested. However, merely being better than a poor indicator is not a proof of validity.

The conceptual assumption made by Jusot et al. (2017) that health has one dimension leads to a limitation to action unless an action on perception per se is a way of reducing inequalities. The interaction between socioeconomic position and PH or QoL, being in opposite direction, is an additional argument in favor of this multidimensionality.

Because indicators in epidemiology and public health also inform policy making, the question that may arise is the meaning of perceived measures of health, particularly when health inequalities are concerned. In addition to monitoring health inequalities, the indicators should provide elements to guide the action. With interventions ultimately in mind, the huge differences observed between PH or reported chronic diseases and external assessment of health have to be discussed.

Empirical evidence has shown the difficulties of interpretation as soon as PH is concerned. From 1989 to 2000 in the Netherlands, life expectancy increased. In parallel, life expectancy without chronic disease has decreased regularly (Perenboom et al., 2005). In an Australian study, aboriginal populations report to be in better health than the rest of the population, whereas the incidence of severe chronic diseases in this group is higher than in the rest of the population (Mathers and Douglas, 1998). Similar empirical evidence is provided by Sen (2002). Comparing reported morbidity and longevity, he observed that the lowest rates of reported morbidity were found in the Indian state of Bihar, where life expectancy was the shortest. In contrast, in Kerala, where life expectancy is the highest in India, the reported morbidity is the highest.

The relationship between external measures of health and PH is highly complex. It would be simplistic to oppose PH to a "true" measure of health, as assessed by mortality or morbidity. Indeed, the diagnostic tools and lists of causes of death are in constant evolution and redefinition. Similarly, illness, sickness, as well as disease that measure morbidity are also social constructs, which evolve in relation to society, history, culture, or medical thinking. However, from a theoretical point of view, the construction of PH is such a complex process that, as a measure of health, it should be used extremely cautiously for public health comparisons and decisions.

Figure 14.1 shows the theoretical relationships between different measures of morbidity. The frontier between silent morbidity and perceived morbidity is related to public health or medical activities (screening) or the biological and clinical evolution of the disease. In contrast, expressed morbidity and diagnosed morbidity depend on sociocultural factors as well as the nature of the health-care system. For a given disease, the relative proportion of one type of morbidity compared with the other, and thus the public health intervention, very much depends on social factors. If we examine the relationship between these types of morbidity and PH (Figure 14.1b), there is no relationship between silent morbidity as assessed by the most sophisticated tests and PH, because this morbidity is by definition silent. The relation with other types of morbidity (perceived, expressed, diagnosed) is influenced again by sociocultural, economic factors, as well as by the health-care system. Moreover, perceived, expressed, and diagnosed morbidity will impact PH differently according to social, cultural, economic factor or the nature of the health-care system.

Thus, we tend to agree with the following conclusion, proposed by one of Jusot's coauthors (Jusot et al., 2017) related to the analysis of French data concerning PH: "Between 1996 and 2008, it looks like PH has become poorer [...]. This evolution of PH cannot be interpreted directly as a decrease in health.

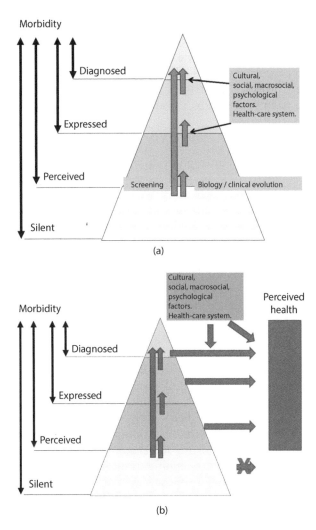

Figure 14.1 (a) Relationships among different types of morbidity and the factors involved. (b) Relationships between types of morbidity, and perceived health and the factors involved.

Medical knowledge of the population, increased access to care, improved treatment strategies, and expectations for well-being and QoL are factors, which may have influenced the way persons rate their health without modifying the health status" (Sermet, 2012). This conclusion emphasizes the difficulty of interpreting PH and drawing conclusions for public health policies.

To quote Sen, it seems wise to observe that "Recent reports suggest that using PH in a given country could be misleading and result in an underestimation of social health inequalities, with severe consequences on public health policies [...] Should we have a second thought before using PH for planning public health policies? The question is open to discussion" (Sen, 2002). These remarks do not concern randomized controlled trials. In this case, the randomization of the groups tends to discard the role of sociocultural factors. Due to the randomization process, they would be balanced between the treatment and the placebo group. The exact meaning of PH remains unclear, but we can assume that it is the same in both groups, thus allowing the comparisons.

Conclusions

Statements, perceptions, and reports on health status by an individual are variable according to time as well as demographic, socioeconomic, and social characteristics. The relation between health status and PH is modified by level of education and the association between health conditions and PH is greater among more highly educated individuals. Using vignettes has been proposed as a method to adjust perceptions of health (Salomon et al., 2004). In this case, theoretically, one could measure individual perceptions using a relative measure defined by the PH of another individual in the vignette. This technique has not yet shown great developments. Although PH is theoretically extremely important, because it reflects the values and preferences of the individual, we suggest that it is a "dynamic" indicator, the meaning of which is unstable across cultures and time, thus insufficiently understood to be used *alone* for planning public policies. Any comparison between social or cultural groups using PH should be made with great caution, because using PH as a general measure of health in this way could lead to an underestimation of the magnitude of health inequalities existing between socioeconomic groups. Sen's (2002) eloquent call for prudence on this matter still stands true, "there is a strong need for scrutinizing the statistics on self-perception of illness in a social context by taking note of levels of education, availability of health facilities, and public information on illness and remedy" (Sen, 2002). We propose that PH should be used along with another externally indicator (mortality, morbidity,...) before drawing any conclusions. Concordant levels or tendencies observed with both indicators would be rather simple to understand. In contrast, opposite relative levels or tendencies assessed by a perceived and an external indicator would require careful analysis for health policy planning.

References

Delpierre, C., Datta, G.D., Kelly-Irving, M., Lauwers-Cances, V., Berkman, L., and Lang, T. (2012a). What role does socio-economic position play in the link between functional limitations and self-rated health: France vs. USA?. *Eur. J. Public Health*, 22, 317–321.

Delpierre, C., Kelly-Irving, M., Munch-Petersen, M., Lauwers-Cances, V., Datta, G.D., Lepage, B., et al. (2012b). SRH and HrQoL: Does social position impact differently on their link with health status?. *BMC Public Health*, 12, 19.

Delpierre, C., Lauwers-Cances, V., Datta, G., Berkman, L.F., and Lang, T. (2009a). Impact of social position on the effect of cardiovascular risk factors on self-rated health. *Am. J. Public Health*, 99, 1278–1284.

Delpierre, C., Lauwers-Cances, V., Datta, G., Lang, T., and Berkman, L.F. (2009b). Using self-rated health in epidemiological studies: A risk for underestimating the gap between social classes?. *J. Epidemiol. Community Health*, *63*, 426–432.

Jusot, F., Tubeuf, S., Devaux, M., Sermet, C. (2017). Social heterogeneity in self-reported health status and the measurement of inequalities in health. In: Guillemin, F., Leplège, A., Briançon, S., Spitz, E., Coste, J. (eds.), *Perceived Health and Adaptation in Chronic Disease*. New York: Routledge, 175–195.

Lang, T., and Delpierre, C. (2009). How are you?: What do you mean?. *Eur. J. Public Health*, *19*(4), 353.

Mackenbach, J.P., Stirbu, I., Roskam, A.J., Schaap, M.M., Menvielle, G., Leinsalu, M., et al. (2008 June 5). Socioeconomic inequalities in health in 22 European countries. *N. Engl. J. Med.*, *358*, 2468–2481.

Mathers, C.D., and Douglas, R.M. (1998). Measuring progress in population health and wellbeing. In: R. Eckersley (ed.), *Measuring Progress: Is Life Getting Better?* (pp. 125–155). Collingwood Victoria: CSIRO Publishing (cited by Jusot).

Perenboom, R.J., van Herten, L.M., Boshuizen, H.C., and van den Bos, G.A. (2005). Life expectancy without chronic morbidity: Trends in gender and socioeconomic disparities. *Public Health Rep.*, *120*, 46–54.

Salomon, J.A., Tandon, A., and Murray, C.J. (2004 January 31). Comparability of self rated health: Cross sectional multi-country survey using anchoring vignettes. *BMJ*, *328*(7434), 258.

Sen, A. (2002). Health: Perception versus observation. *Br. Med. J.*, *324*, 860–861.

Sermet, C. (2012). Evolution de l'état de santé depuis 20 ans. *Actualités et Dossiers en Santé Publique*, *80*, 6–12.

Singh-Manoux, A., Dugravot, A., Shipley, M., Ferrie, J.E., Martikainen, P., Goldberg, M., et al. (2007). The association between self-rated health and mortality in different socioeconomic groups in the GAZEL cohort study. *Int. J. Epidemiol.*, *36*, 1222–1228.

15 The complexity of interpreting changes observed over time in health-related quality of life: A short overview of 15 years of research on response shift theory

Antoine Vanier, Bruno Falissard, Véronique Sébille, and Jean-Benoit Hardouin

Introduction

Patient-reported outcomes (PROs) are now widely used in health-related research to assess, for instance, health-related quality of life (HRQoL), often with self-administered questionnaires (Fayers and Machin, 2007). The emphasis on assessing HRQoL alongside clinical outcomes is related, in part, to the rise in the prevalence of chronically ill patients suffering from diseases that cannot be cured. In medical areas such as oncology and palliative care, HRQoL is measured over time to add relevant information on patients' subjective experiences in the course of treatment, to counterbalance objective data such as survival time (Leplège and Hunt, 1997). The increasing interest in collecting data on individuals' HRQoL also highlights the recognition that patients should have a say in the choice of their therapy (Fayers and Machin, 2007). To enable this, it is necessary to assess other outcomes than health status or symptom levels, because their improvement or deterioration is not always correlated with patients' subjective experiences (Wilson and Cleary, 1995).

Usually, HRQoL measures are based on the assumption that the meaning of concepts and measurement scales remain stable in individuals' minds over time (Ahmed et al., 2009). Thus HRQoL scores are assumed to be directly comparable for a given individual over time (Schwartz and Rapkin, 2004). However, a growing body of literature developed since the mid-1990s has pointed out that these assumptions can be oversimplistic, especially when a person experiences a salient health-related event, or has to adapt to living with a chronic disease. Numerous studies have suggested that the occurrence of a salient event can have an effect on one's representation of the concepts being measured (e.g., HRQoL), which can have an impact on changes observed (Schwartz et al.,

2006). Thus HRQoL is now more viewed as a dynamic concept in nature (Allison et al., 1997). To put it simply, the above-mentioned findings were interpreted as evidence that respondents understand the same questions differently over time (Sprangers and Schwartz, 1999; McClimans, 2010). This whole process, from the occurrence of the event, to the effect on HRQoL scores (via the changes in meaning of the concepts being measured in individuals' minds), is now known as the *response shift (RS) theory* (Rapkin and Schwartz, 2004).

The objective of this chapter is to provide an overview of the works conducted because RS is investigated in health-related research.

First occurrences of the notion of RS in psychology and health-related research

Within the field of educational training

Historically, the term "response shift" was introduced by Howard and Dailey in 1979 in the field of educational training (Howard and Dailey, 1979). Their aim was to experimentally assess the efficacy of various training interventions proposed by psychologists in college and work environments, like improving leadership and performance appraisal or reducing dogmatism.

The typical approach to assess training interventions involves collecting pretest and posttest data on subjects exposed to the intervention, and comparing them with an appropriate control group. In line with usual assumptions on self-report instruments, Howard et al. (1979) have posited that for pretest and posttest scores to be comparable, a common metric has to exist between the two sets of scores (Cronbach and Furby, 1970). Thus in the case of self-report, researchers assume subjects have an internalized perception of their level of functioning and this internalized standard would not change from one testing to the next (Howard and Dailey, 1979).

Nonetheless, Howard et al. published what they called a somewhat paradoxical finding (Howard et al., 1979). In a study, many subjects self-reported a higher level of dogmatism after the training despite clients' and therapists' perception that training had been beneficial (Howard et al., 1979). They interpreted these results as evidences that the intervention had the ability to improve one's insight or awareness of his or her own level of dogmatism (Howard et al., 1979). This led to a change of one's internal standard of measurement over time (Howard et al., 1979). Therefore, Howard et al. hypothesized that whenever such a shift occurs, conventional pretest/posttest self-reporting is unable to accurately gauge treatment effect (Howard et al., 1979). So, they claimed that the pretest measurement was inaccurate (Howard et al., 1979). Thus they developed a new experimental design, incorporating a retrospective self-assessment of pretest level (also called *then-test*) immediately after posttest assessment (Howard et al., 1979). The *difference between the then-test and the posttest* assessment was supposed to assess more accurately *changes induced by training* regarding the concept of interest. The *difference between pretest and then-test* self-report ratings has been referred to as *RS* (Howard and Dailey, 1979).

Within the field of management sciences

In 1976, in the field of organizational changes, Golembiewski et al. (1976) introduced a typology of within-individuals changes over time related to self-reports, in an article about the measurement of change and persistence in human affairs (Golembiewski, 1976).

They defined three types of changes (Golembiewski, 1976):

1 *Alpha change* involves a variation in the level of some existential state, given a constantly calibrated measuring instrument related to a constant conceptual domain.
2 *Beta change* involves a variation in the level of some existential state, complicated by the fact that some intervals of the measurement continuum associated with a constant conceptual domain have been recalibrated.
3 *Gamma change* involves a redefinition or reconceptualization of some domain, a major change in the perspective or frame of reference within which phenomena are perceived and classified, in what is taken to be relevant in some slice of reality.

Within the field of health-related research

One of the first occurrences of the concept of RS in health-related research can be found in a paper published in 1991 by Breetvelt and Van Dam (Breetvelt and Van Dam, 1991). The introduction of the notion was an attempt to explain what they called underreporting regarding HRQoL assessment in cancer patients despite frequently reporting a high level of physical complaints, some results suggested no differences in terms of psychological complaints or overall HRQoL between cancer patients and healthy people) (Breetvelt and Van Dam, 1991). In respect to Howard et al.'s definition, RS viewed as a change in internal standard of measurement was one of the proposed explanations (Breetvelt and Van Dam, 1991).

Breetvelt and Van Dam concluded that self-reported HRQoL outcomes should be approached with caution, and proposed a then-test design to assess more carefully changes in HRQoL related to the occurrence of cancer. In 1996, Sprangers proposed one of the first applications of the then-test on two measurement occasions of HRQoL data in cancer patients (Sprangers, 1996).

Definition and theoretical model

Current definition of RS

In 1999, Sprangers and Schwartz (1999) translated the notion of RS into the field of HRQoL . They proposed that the introduction of the RS concept could be relevant to interpret some paradoxical and counterintuitive findings

(Sprangers and Schwartz, 1999) like reporting of stable HRQoL by patients with a life-threatening disease (Andrykowski et al., 1993) or discrepancies between clinical measures of health and patients' own evaluations of their health (Daltroy et al., 1999).

Thus, RS has been defined as a change in the meaning of one's self-evaluation of a target construct over time (Sprangers and Schwartz, 1999). Grounded in the typology of changes introduced by Golembiewski et al. (1976), RS was operationalized in three forms (Sprangers and Schwartz 1999):

- *Recalibration*, which is a change in the respondent's internal standards of measurement (e.g., a person suffering from chronic pain and rating it on a pain scale as 7/10 will later rate it as 5/10 after experiencing acute pain, despite the chronic pain being the same as before), corresponds to Golembiewski et al.'s (1976) definition of *beta change*.
- *Reprioritization*, which is a change in the respondent's values (i.e., the relative importance of component domains in the target construct—e.g., an athletic person who considers physical functioning as an important part of his or her HRQoL may later place emphasis on social functioning after sustaining permanent physical injury), corresponds, in part, to Golembiewski et al.'s (1976) definition of *gamma change*.
- *Reconceptualization*, which is the redefinition of a target construct (e.g., an item of a multidomain questionnaire initially assessing the domain of mental health, will be later understood by the respondent as assessing another domain, like social functioning), also corresponds, in part, to Golembiewski et al.'s (1976) definition of *gamma change*.

First theoretical model proposed

The first theoretical model designed to address how RS may affect HRQoL after changes in health status was published by Sprangers and Schwartz in 1999 (Figure 15.1).

The model was designed to address relationships between five major components. Indeed, it includes

1 *The catalyst:* A salient event leading to a change in the respondent's health status.
2 *Antecedents:* Stable or dispositional characteristics of the individual. They have both direct and indirect effects on potentiating RS. They affect the kind of mechanisms engaged, magnitude, and type of RS.
3 *Mechanisms:* Behavioral, cognitive, and affective processes to accommodate the catalyst, like the use of coping strategies or upward or downward social comparisons.
4 *Perceived HRQoL:* A multidomain concept with frequently at least three broad domains (e.g., physical, psychological and social functioning) (Sprangers and Schwartz 1999).

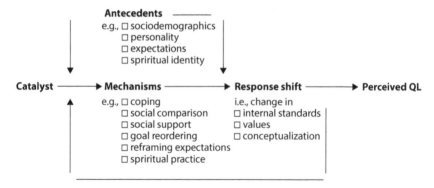

Figure 15.1 First theoretical model of response shift and perceived health-related quality of life (HRQoL) proposed by Sprangers and Schwartz. (From Sprangers, M.A.G., and Schwartz, C.E., *Soc. Sci. Med.*, 48, 1507–1515, 1999.)

The feedback loop included in the model illustrates that the process is thought of as iterative and dynamic: Perceiving a suboptimal HRQoL may lead the individual to reinitiate established or new mechanisms (Sprangers and Schwartz 1999).

According to Sprangers and Schwartz (1999), RS was isolated both from mechanisms and perceived HRQoL as it conceptualizes aspects that are likely to help understanding changes observed in HRQoL over time. The isolation of RS was therefore conceived as a pragmatic approach to explain some aspects of changes in HRQoL. As such, RS was not thought as a replacement to other theories like *adaptation theories* (Helson, 1964), *discrepancy theories* (Calman 1984), *uncertainty in illness theories* (Mishel, 1988), or *stress-coping theories* (Lazarus and Folkman, 1984), but rather as a concept that can be incorporated in such existing theories (Sprangers and Schwartz 1999).

Update of the theoretical model

In 2004, Rapkin and Schwartz (2004) extended the first theoretical model. One of the main reasons was that Rapkin and Schwhartz (2004) noticed that the formulation of the model could be criticized as it presented some issues of circular reasoning. In the first model, they pointed out that RS was not sufficiently differentiated from both mechanisms and outcomes. Therefore, the concept of RS overlapped with the psychological mechanisms leading to the RS effect and the outcome affected by the RS effect. So, there was a need to clearly distinguish mechanisms and outcomes from RS (Figure 15.2).

The main new idea behind this updated model is that RS is now thought of as a phenomenon occurring when there is a change in *appraisal* (Rapkin and Schwartz, 2004). Indeed, Rapkin and Schwartz supposed that any response to a HRQoL item can be understood as a function of an appraisal process. Rapkin and Schwartz posited at least four cognitive processes to account in an individual HRQoL assessment.

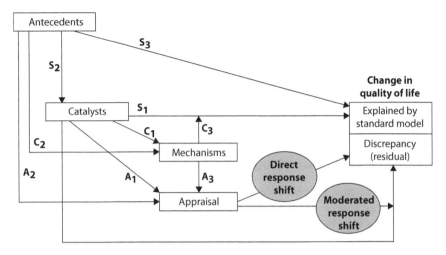

Figure 15.2 Updated theoretical model of response shift and changes in health-related quality of life (HRQoL) proposed by Rapkin and Schwartz. Accounting for changes in standard influences (S), coping processes (C), and appraisal variables (A). (From Rapkin, B.D., and Schwartz, C.E., *Health Qual. Life Outcomes*, 2, 14, 2004.)

These four processes are

1 A *frame of reference* comprising one or more subsets. These subsets can be understood as categories of experiences or events that individuals consider relevant to a particular HRQoL scale at the time of the assessment.
2 A *sampling strategy* to extract from categories within a frame of reference specific experiences used to make a HRQoL assessment (e.g., in assessing pain an individual can sample—recent instances of pain or—times when pain interfered with my activities).
3 A *standard of comparison* as a reference point to evaluate the specific experiences sampled (e.g., pain experiences may be compared with—worst pain I have ever had or to —what my doctor told me to expect).
4 A *combinatory algorithm* used to edit the responses by combining the evaluations into a summary of appraisal of HRQoL. It describes how people can use different subjective weights to increase or decrease the relative importance of different experiences (Rapkin and Schwartz, 2004).

Thus, RS can be equated neither to mechanisms nor to the outcome (observed scores). Rather, it is an effect triggered by psychological mechanisms, mediated through a change in appraisal, leading into changes in observed HRQoL scores that cannot be explained by standard influences (direct effect of the catalyst, and direct and indirect effect of antecedents: S pathways in Figure 15.2) (Rapkin and Schwartz, 2004).

The three forms of RS proposed by Sprangers and Schwartz were related to the aforementioned appraisal processes:

1   Change(s) in the frame of reference relate to reconceptualization
2   Change(s) in the sampling strategy or the combinatory algorithm relate to reprioritization
3   Change(s) in the standard of comparison relate to recalibration (Rapkin and Schwartz, 2004)

Debate and controversies about the concept of RS

Initially, in the field of educational training, RS, equated to recalibration, was interpreted as a measurement bias obscuring the appropriate assessment of the efficacy of an intervention (Howard and Dailey, 1979).

However, in the model proposed by Sprangers and Schwartz (1999) the RS effect is a consequence of the initiation of psychological mechanisms triggered by the catalyst, and it is viewed as one of the path explaining changes in perceived HRQoL.

Thus, RS is a concept that can be related to issues in psychology (explaining how people deal with life changes) and also to issues in experimental designs and psychometrics. This has resulted in an ongoing debate about the meaning of RS (Schwartz and Rapkin, 2004; Schwartz et al., 2005; Ubel et al., 2010; Sprangers and Schwartz, 2010; Reeve, 2010; Boyer et al., 2014; Ubel and Smith, 2010; Eton, 2010). This debate often opposes two views on RS:

1   A view where RS is interpreted more as a measurement characteristic and therefore a bias that needs to be corrected
2   A view where RS is interpreted more as a subject characteristic and therefore seen as a phenomenon leading to meaningful changes worth investigating (Schwartz et al., 2005)

This debate has been emphasized in a commentary by Ubel et al. (2010), which proposed to abandon the term RS. They argued that the use of the term RS does not help to disentangle two different phenomena. To them, the occurrence of recalibration is a threat to the validity of self-reports (i.e., a measurement bias), obscuring an appropriate assessment of *true change* (i.e., a change in the latent targeted construct itself, which corresponds to Golembiewski et al. (1976) *alpha change*). However, they view reprioritization and reconceptualization as processes by which people emotionally adapt to circumstances, leading to true change in HRQoL. Thus to them, the indistinct use of the term RS has led researchers to think of RS as mainly an issue of measurement bias. Therefore, they proposed to dichotomize RS by using the term "scale recalibration" when referring to recalibration RS, and using a term such as "emotional adaptation" or "hedonic adaptation" when referring to reprioritization and reconceptualization RS (Stanton et al., 2007; Carver and Scheier, 1982, 2000).

Nonetheless, this commentary has led to a rebuttal by Sprangers and Schwartz (2010). If they have agreed with Ubel et al. that the RS concept is the lumping together different phenomena, they have argued that the dichotomy proposed by Ubel et al. could be too restrictive. Indeed, Sprangers and Schwartz proposed that scale recalibration can also be a process leading to adaptation to illness, whereas reprioritization and reconceptualization can also be a psychometric issue (i.e., adding complexity to the measure of true mean change of an invariant construct) but only when HRQoL scores are compared, either within individuals over time, or between individuals who have different perspectives on HRQoL. Thus, according to Sprangers and Schwartz, adaptation is a psychological mechanism and the different types of RS are consequences of this mechanism.

Thus, if recent studies investigating changes in HRQoL put more emphasis on RS as one of the outcomes of interest (Barclay-Goddard et al., 2009a), the different hermeneutics that are subsumed under the RS theory are still debated (Boyer et al., 2014). In that regard, some authors have proposed it is needed to be more accurate about the purpose of an empirical study and the use of the RS concept when reporting results (Reeve, 2010; Schwartz et al., 2013).

Nonetheless, the debate on what RS is has helped to define what RS is not. Indeed, RS cannot be called anytime there is a difficulty in interpreting changes over time in observed HRQoL scores (Schwartz et al., 2005). Thus, RS cannot be equated to measurement error (Oort, 2005b). It also cannot be equated to other types of processes that may induce changes in observed HRQoL scores, like response tendencies such as social desirability or acquiescence, effort justification, or cognitive dissonance reduction (Sprangers and Schwartz, 1999).

Methodological approaches to address RS

Because of the occurrence of the first theoretical model of RS in health-related research, numerous methods have been designed and used to detect the RS effect. These methods can be partitioned into two groups (Table 15.1) (Barclay-Goddard et al., 2009a):

1 Methods based on specific study design: These approaches are based on a specific design or on the use of specific measurement tools. Therefore, they are used when RS is anticipated as one of the main outcome of interest.
2 Statistical methods: These approaches are based on the use of statistical tools to search for evidence of RS on data sets. Therefore, they can be used without the need of a specific design.

Methods based on specific study design

Retrospective rating or the then-test approach

The then-test approach is based on the same design used by Howard et al. (1979) in the field of educational training . Usually, changes in PRO observed scores, regarding the occurrence of a salient event (e.g., diagnosis of a disease, initiation

Table 15.1 A summary of some of the key characteristics of the different methods developed to detect response shift (RS)

Method	Level at which RS is detected	Forms of RS investigated	Quantitative assessment of RS	Number of time points investigated	True change estimate	Note
Methods based on specific study design						
Then-test (Howard et al., 1979; Sprangers, 1996)	Individual	Recalibration	Yes	2	RS adjusted change	Most used but criticized since
PGI-SEIQOL (Ring et al., 2005; O'Boyle et al., 2000)	Individual	Reprioritization, Reconceptualization	Possible, but complex	At least 2	Possible, but complex	Each person can define what HRQoL means for him/her
HEI-Q (Osborne et al., 2006)	Individual	Recalibration	Yes	2	RS adjusted change	Suppose awareness of the RS process
Vignette ratings (Korfage et al., 2007)	Individual	Reprioritization	No	At least 2	No	
Quality of life appraisal profile (QoLAP) (Rapkin and Schwartz, 2004)	Individual	All forms	Not directly	At least 2	Not directly	Provide an in-depth analysis of changes in appraisal processes
Qualitative interviews (Korfage et al., 2006; Elliott et al., 2014)	Individual	All forms	No	At least 2	No	Provide an in-depth analysis of changes observed over time in HRQoL

(Continued)

Table 15.1 (Continued) A summary of some of the key characteristics of the different methods developed to detect response shift (RS)

Statistical methods

Method	Level at which RS is detected	Forms of RS investigated	Quantitative assessment of RS	Number of time points investigated	True change estimate	Note
SEM (Schmitt's technique) (Schmitt, 1982; Ahmed et al., 2005)	Group analysis	All forms	Yes	2, more possible but complex	No	Rely on Golembiewski et al. (1976) typology of changes
SEM (OP) (Oort, 2005; Oort et al., 2005, 2009)	Group analysis	All forms	Yes	2, more possible but complex	Yes	Can assess RS from a measurement and a conceptual perspective. Currently used at domain level
Latent trajectory analysis of residuals (Mayo et al., 2008)	Identify subgroups with similar patterns of RS	Cannot distinguish which forms are detected	Possible	At least 3	Not directly	Can identify subgroups with similar patterns of RS along with the group which did not experienced RS
Relative importance analysis (Lix et al., 2012)	Group analysis	Reprioritization	Possible	Multiple times point	Not directly	Relative analysis: One group is compared with another
CART (Li and Schwartz, 2011)	Group analysis	All forms	No	2	No	Data mining technique: infer complex patterns of RS over time between different investigated groups

(Continued)

Table 15.1 (Continued) A summary of some of the key characteristics of the different methods developed to detect response shift (RS)

Method	Level at which RS is detected	Forms of RS investigated	Quantitative assessment of RS	Number of time points investigated	True change estimate	Note
CART + Random Forest (Boucekine et al., 2013)	Group analysis	Reprioritization	No	At least 2	No	Assess complex evolution of reprioritization RS over multiple times point
IRT (LLRA) (Anota et al., 2014)	Group analysis	Recalibration	Yes	2	No	Model retrospective assessment data, assumes absence of true change
IRT (ROSALI) (Guilleux et al., 2015)	Group analysis	Recalibration, reprioritization	Yes	2	Yes	Could be an interesting choice for detection of RS at item-level Reconceptulization would require multidimensional IRT modeling

HEI-Q, Health Education Impact Questionnaire; PGI, Patient Generated Index; SEIQOL, Schedule for the Evaluation of Individual Quality of Life; SEM, structural equation modeling; CART, Classification and Regression Trees; IRT, item response theory; LLRA, Linear Logistic with Relaxed Assumptions; ROSALI, RespOnse Shift ALgorithm in Item response theory.

of a therapy, etc.), are estimated by the difference between a baseline assessment (pretest, before the event) and a follow-up assessment (posttest, after the event). The then-test is a retrospective assessment of the baseline assessment, performed at the same time as the posttest (Schwartz and Sprangers, 1999). Therefore, it is assumed that posttest and then-test are sharing the same internal standards of HRQoL within individuals, thus accounting for recalibration of RS (Barclay-Goddard et al., 2009a). The difference between the then-test and the pretest assessment is assumed to be an estimate of the magnitude of the recalibration effect. The difference between the posttest and the then-test is used as a measure of recalibration-adjusted change (Figure 15.3) (Barclay-Goddard et al., 2009a).

The then-test has been the most used method for assessing recalibration effect (Schwartz et al., 2006). Since 1996, it has been used with a variety of PRO instruments and patient populations. However, it has been criticized since (Schwartz and Sprangers, 2010). First of all, the basic premise that the then-test and posttest share the same internal standards has been questioned (Nolte et al., 2009). Then, as the then-test asks respondents to provide a retrospective assessment, it implies that individuals can access the evaluated previous state in their minds appropriately without recall bias, although the effect of this bias has been shown in empirical studies (Schwartz et al., 2004). Third, there is a potential contamination due to other response biases, such as social desirability effect of effort justification (Howard and Dailey, 1979). Finally, the then-test implies that the retrospective assessment is achieved by directly extracting appropriate data about the health state being assessed and rating it accordingly. However, some authors have argued that the actual cognitive

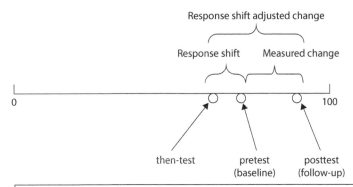

This figure represents a measure of HRQL on a 0–100 scale with a traditional pretest at baseline, posttest at follow-up, and a then test of baseline health occuring also at follow-up.

Example of a typical then-test question: Please remember when you last filled out this questionnaire 1 month ago. Please provide a new judgement about your quality of life at the time you last filled out this questionnaire 1 month ago. Rather than try to recall your prior responses, please offer a renewed judgement of your quality of life then, given what your perspective is today.

Figure 15.3 The then-test approach to detect response shift (RS). (From Barclay-Goddard, R. et al., *Qual. Life Res.*, 18, 335–346, 2009.)

mechanism engaged can be more understood as an *implicit theory of changes*, where people think about past times starting from the present and reconstruct their baseline state inferring what they think they were at that time (Norman, 2003). If true, it would threaten the possibility of a retrospective assessment. Thus, the use of the then-test as an adequate method to detect recalibration RS is currently heavily questioned (Schwartz and Sprangers, 2010).

Specific questionnaire assessing the magnitude of recalibration
for a specific intervention

The Health Education Impact Questionnaire (HEI-Q) was developed to identify recalibration among individuals participating in an arthritis self-management course (Osborne et al., 2006). Each of the nine items is rated using a seven-point scale to estimate if recalibration has occurred and at which magnitude. Recalibration is described as negative when people realize that they were worse than they thought at a prior point, positive when they were better than thought at a previous point, or absent (Osborne et al., 2006). This type of questionnaire has been designed to be used to assess the efficacy of a specific intervention whose purpose is to induce recalibration. Nonetheless, it seems that the heuristic of the questionnaire is based on the assumption that people are aware their internal standard of measurement has changed over time, which implies that recalibration is thought here as a conscious process only.

Questionnaires assessing how HRQoL is conceptualized by individuals

Using these questionnaires, an individual is asked to select and rate the value of different domains of HRQoL (Schwartz and Sprangers, 1999). Two PRO instruments have been used to detect reprioritization and reconceptualization RS: the Patient Generated Index (PGI) and the Schedule for the Evaluation of Individual Quality of Life (SEIQOL) (Ring et al., 2005; O'Boyle et al., 2000). Both instruments, if different in presentation, are close in process. First, a person is asked to select five life areas that are supposed to match his or her individual definition of HRQoL. Then, this person rates his or her ability in these areas and is asked to provide weights reflecting the relative importance according to each of the five areas. Over time, reprioritization can be inferred by a change in the weights of the different domains (Ahmed et al., 2005b) and reconceptualization by a change in the choice of the domains (Schwartz and Sprangers, 1999).

Those methods have the advantages of being very individualized procedures: Each individual can choose what domains best represent HRQoL for him or her. However, it is hard to provide a numerical value estimating the magnitude of the reprioritization and/or reconceptualization effect (Barclay-Goddard et al., 2009a).

Vignette ratings

When this design is used, patients are asked to read brief vignettes describing in a few sentences different hypothetical health states. For example, each vignette can briefly describe a side effect of prostate cancer treatment (Korfage et al., 2007). Before and after treatment (i.e., surgical removal of the cancer), patients rate how each state described by the vignettes appears to be detrimental by their own values. Reprioritization of RS can be detected when the rating of a vignette is significantly different before and after the treatment (Korfage et al., 2007).

Use of the quality of life appraisal profile

This questionnaire was designed to assess the four aforementioned cognitive appraisal processes engaged when respondents are asked to take a survey (Rapkin and Schwartz, 2004). The purpose of the questionnaire is to get a precise description of each of the processes (frame of reference, sampling strategy, standard of comparison and combinatory algorithm) for each respondent when asked about their level of HRQoL using a validated PRO instrument (Rapkin and Schwartz, 2004). Therefore, the occurrence of the RS effect can be inferred when there are changes in these appraisal processes over time for a given respondent. Each form of RS can be inferred as each appraisal processes have been linked to different forms of RS (Rapkin and Schwartz, 2004).

Qualitative Interviews

Qualitative interviews can be conducted to generate an in-depth knowledge of how a person is experiencing changes in HRQoL over time. Content analyses using specific tools can then be used to analyze the verbatim of the interviews and help eliciting occurrences of RS (Korfage et al., 2006; Elliott et al., 2014).

Statistical methods

Using structural equation modeling: The Schmitt technique

Historically, detecting account various types of within-individual changes over time a targeted construct using factor analysis has been proposed even before RS was defined in health-related research. Indeed, a method designed to detect the aforementioned types of changes introduced by Golembiewski et al. (1976) has been developed by Schmitt (1982).

The Schmitt technique relies on an operationalization of Golembiewski et al. (1976) typology of changes as change(s) in the value of structural equation modeling (SEM) parameters between two times of measurement.

This method has been used several times in the field of health-related research to detect RS when measuring changes observed over time in HRQoL scores (Gandhi et al., 2013a; Ahmed et al., 2005a, 2009; Visser et al., 2005).

Nonetheless, as the typology of changes on which it relies is not strictly equivalent to the typology of RS proposed by Sprangers and Schwartz, there was, since the late 2000s, a shift in use in favor of another method for detecting RS using SEM: the Oort's Procedure (OP).

Using structural equation modeling: The OP

The OP was first proposed in 2005. It relies on an operationalization of the different forms of RS (as proposed by Sprangers and Schwartz) as change(s) in the value of SEM parameters between two times of measurement (Oort, 2005b).

As OP proposes certain interesting features, it has been used to detect RS on several clinical data sets (Oort et al., 2005; Visser et al., 2005; Ahmed et al., 2009, 2014; Barclay-Goddard et al., 2009b, 2011; King-Kallimanis et al., 2011; Schwartz et al., 2011; Nagl and Farin, 2012; Fokkema et al., 2013; Gandhi et al., 2013a; Barclay and Tate, 2014). When used to model observed HRQoL scores of a multidomain questionnaire (RS detection at domain-level), it allows assessing for each domain whether it is affected by one or several specific form(s) of RS (and if so, by which magnitude), together with estimating true change in HRQoL after taking into account RS. It also allows indicating the respective contribution of true change and RS in explaining changes in each observed HRQoL domain scores (Oort et al., 2005).

The development of the OP has also been helpful as a framework to help clarify a formal definition of what is RS (in terms of models and psychometrics) (Oort, 2005a). Indeed, in 2009, Oort et al. proposed to formally define RS from two different perspectives (a *measurement perspective* and a *conceptual perspective*) (Oort et al., 2009; Tables 15.2 and 15.3). According to Oort et al. (2009), RS from a measurement perspective is a special case of measurement bias, where changes over time of the level of a latent attribute of interest A (e.g., true change in HRQoL itself) cannot fully determine changes of test scores X (e.g., observed HRQoL scores). However, RS from a conceptual perspective is a special case of explanation bias where a change over time of an attribute of

Table 15.2 Measurement perspective, conceptual perspective, measurement bias, explanation bias in health-related quality of life (HRQoL) according to Oort et al.

Bias	Measurement perspective	Conceptual perspective
Bias introduction	Measurement bias is bias in the measurement of the target construct (i.e., the attribute of interest). Differences between respondents in observed test scores cannot be fully explained by true differences between respondents in the attribute of interest. Variance in test scores does not fully represent true variance in the attribute.	Explanation bias is bias in the explanation (or prediction) of the target construct (i.e., the attribute of interest). In addition to the acknowledged explanatory variables, there are other variables that also explain part of the variance in the attribute of interest, possibly confounding the effects of the acknowledged explanatory variables.

(Continued)

Table 15.2 (Continued) Measurement perspective, conceptual perspective, measurement bias, explanation bias in health-related quality of life (HRQoL) according to Oort et al.

Bias	Measurement perspective	Conceptual perspective
Bias definition	Measurement bias is formally defined as a violation of measurement invariance,	Explanation bias can be formally defined as a violation of explanation invariance,
	$F(X\|A = a, V - v) - g(X\|A = a)$	$f(A\|E = e, V - v) - g(A\|E = e)$
	for all values of a and v, where X are observed variables (measurements of A), A are the attributes of interest, and V are possible violators of invariance. Function f is the distribution function of X given a and v, and function g is the distribution function of X given just a.	for all values of e and v, where A are the attributes of interest, E are acknowledged explanatory variables (i.e., causes or predictors) of A, and V are possibly confounding variables. Function f is the distribution function of A given e and v, and function g is the distribution function of A given just e.
Bias in HRQoL research	In HRQoL research, measurements X are observed scores on an HRQoL test, attributes A are HRQoL itself and a are true HRQoL values, and V are all other variables in HRQoL studies. With measurement bias in an HRQoL test, differences between patients in observed test scores cannot be fully explained by differences in their true HRQoL. As a result, test scores also represent something else besides HRQoL.	In HRQoL research, A are HRQoL values, E are causes or predictors of HRQoL, such as biological and physiological factors, physical and psychological symptoms, and V are all other variables that may also affect HRQoL but are not taken into account. The explanation of patients' HRQoL may be confounded by variables other than the acknowledged predictors or causes of HRQoL.
Note	In the measurement perspective, all variables other than A are considered potential violators of measurement invariance. We do not distinguish between acknowledged explanatory variables and other, possibly confounding variables; all such variables are subsumed under V.	In the conceptual perspective, we do distinguish between acknowledged explanatory variables E and possibly confounding variables V, but we do not distinguish between the attribute of interest itself A and its operationalization X; that is, A and X are assumed to coincide.

Source: Oort, F.J. et al., *J. Clin. Epidemiol.*, 62, 1126–1137, 2009.

Table 15.3 Response shift in measurement and conceptual perspective according to Oort et al.

Response shift	Measurement perspective	Conceptual perspective
Response shift introduction	In measurement perspective, response shift can be understood as bias in the measurement of change in attribute A: It explains observed change (in X) that cannot be fully explained by true change (in A). Hence, response shift is measurement bias that varies with time of measurement.	In conceptual perspective, response shift can be understood as bias in the explanation of change in attribute A: It explains (true) change in A that cannot be fully explained by the acknowledged explanatory variables E. Hence, response shift is explanation bias that varies with time of measurement.
Response shift definition	Response shift can be formally defined as measurement bias, with X representing the respondents' observed scores on repeatedly administered tests, A representing the true attribute values of the respondents at the times of measurement, and V being the time of measurement itself or other variables with effects on X that vary with time of measurement.	Response shift can be formally defined as explanation bias, with A representing (true) attribute values on repeated test administrations, E representing values for acknowledged explanatory variables (causes or predictors) of A, and V being the time of measurement itself or other variables with effects on A that vary with time of measurement.
Response shift in HRQoL research	In HRQoL research, X are observed scores on repeatedly administered HRQoL tests, A are true HRQoL values at the times of measurement, and V is (a coding for) the time of measurement itself, e.g., before or after a health-state change, or V are individual characteristics that interact with the time of measurement, or occur or change between the measurement occasions (e.g., adaptation, coping, social comparison). With response shift, observed changes in test scores cannot be fully explained by true changes in HRQoL.	In HRQoL research, A are HRQoL values at different measurement occasions, E are causes or predictors of changes in HRQoL (e.g., health-state change, medical diagnosis, medical treatment), and V is (a coding for) the time of the measurement occasion, or individual characteristics (other than E) that interact with the time of measurement (e.g., adaptation, coping, social comparison). With response shift, variables other than the acknowledged explanatory variables also affect changes in HRQoL.

(*Continued*)

Table 15.3 (Continued) Response shift in measurement and conceptual perspective according to Oort et al.

Response shift	Measurement perspective	Conceptual perspective
Response shift in terms of Sprangers and Schwartz (1999)	X are test scores and A are true values for HRQoL or other patient-reported "outcomes" at different measurement occasions. V can be "catalysts," e.g., health-state change, diagnosis, medical treatment, "mechanisms," e.g., adaptation, coping, social comparison, "antecedents," i.e., (other) individual and environmental characteristics, or any other variable that might be relevant. The "mechanisms" affect the observed test scores through recalibration, reprioritization, or reconceptualization of test items and response scales (but not true HRQoL). As a result, observed change does not reflect true change, and follow-up scores cannot be compared with previous (baseline) scores.	A are HRQoL variables or other patient-reported "outcomes" at different measurement occasions. E are "catalysts," e.g., health-state change, diagnosis, medical treatment, and possibly "antecedents," i.e., any individual and environmental characteristics that are commonly acknowledged as explanatory of A. V are "mechanisms," e.g., adaptation, coping, social comparison. The "mechanisms" affect true HRQoL through recalibration, reprioritization, or reconceptualization of true HRQoL. As a result, observed change still reflects true change, but effects of "catalysts" on HRQoL are possibly confounded by co-occurring effects of "mechanisms."

HRQoL, health-related quality of life.

Source: Oort, F.J. et al., *J. Clin. Epidemiol.*, 62, 1126–1137, 2009.

interest A cannot be fully explained by observed variables E representing standard influences on HRQoL but also by other variables V representing mechanisms (e.g., coping mechanisms, social comparisons, etc.) (Oort et al., 2009) (Figure 15.4). Thus, Oort et al. proposed in 2009 an extended revision of the OP, which allows detecting and accounting for RS from the two aforementioned perspectives. The measurement part of the SEM is used to detect RS from a measurement perspective, and the structural part of the SEM, including different variables (i.e., variables representing standard influences on HRQoL, but also psychological mechanisms) susceptible to explain changes in HRQoL itself, is used to detect RS from a conceptual perspective (Oort et al., 2009; King-Kallimanis et al., 2009) (Figure 15.4).

The main drawback of OP is the fact that this procedure implies analyses at the group level (Oort, 2005b). Therefore, when performing detection of RS using OP, it is assumed that a substantial part of the sample has experienced RS of a similar form(s), direction, and magnitude. In some study settings, this is probably a strong assumption (Mayo et al., 2008).

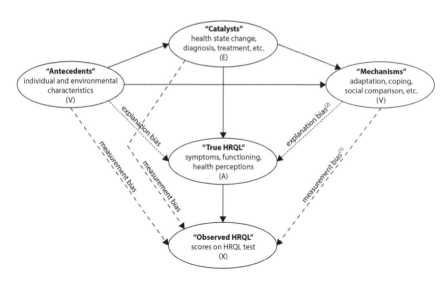

Figure 15.4 Measurement bias and explanation bias in health-related quality of life (HRQoL) according to Oort et al. In a longitudinal design with repeated measurements of HRQoL, this measurement bias (1) can be considered as a response shift in the measurement of change; and this explanation bias (2) can be considered as a response shift in the explanation of change. (From Oort, F.J. et al., *J. Clin. Epidemiol.*, 62, 1126–1137, 2009.)

Using longitudinal regression modeling and latent trajectory analysis

This method has been proposed to overcome the fact that OP is group-level analysis. Therefore, this method is suited when the purpose of the analyses is to identify subgroups of subjects exhibiting different patterns of RS over time or a subgroup having not experienced RS over time (Schwartz et al., 2011; Mayo et al., 2008; Ahmed et al., 2011).

Subgroups of patients exhibiting similar fluctuations of centered residuals over time (from a longitudinal regression model predicting changes of HRQoL over time using various predictors representing health status, background characteristics, and levels of symptoms) are supposed to be individuals exhibiting a similar pattern of RS over time. Thus, subgroups of individuals exhibiting different patterns of negative and/or positive RS can be identified along with the group of individuals supposed to have not experienced RS (the group with centered residuals close to zero over time) (Mayo et al., 2008). The timing of the occurrence of RS can also be hypothesized if appropriately spaced time points are modeled. Nonetheless, this method cannot identify the forms of RS and does not strictly provide a measure of true change.

Relative importance analysis using discriminant analysis and/or logistic regression

This method has been proposed to detect specifically reprioritization RS and therefore is suited when a researcher wants to test if reprioritization RS has occurred when HRQoL is measured with a large number of domain scores (Lix et al., 2012; Schwartz et al., 2013). It relies on the use of discriminant analysis and/or logistic regression to predict group membership (e.g., active versus inactive disease over a specific period of time) by the difference over time of various HRQoL domains scores. The occurrence of reprioritization over time is inferred in one group of individuals by comparison to another group (Lix et al., 2012). Thus, the method is useful when one hypothesizes a different evolution between two groups of individuals.

Using machine learning technique such as recursive partitioning tree analysis

This method has been proposed for inferring complex and nonlinear patterns of RS between two time points in a data set. It relies on a data-mining technique (i.e., Classification and Regression Trees [CART]) (Schwartz et al., 2011; Li and Schwartz, 2011). A graphical model, in the form of a decision tree, explaining the difference in HRQoL score is constructed by recursively splitting the data set into two groups on the basis of various predictors in such a way the heterogeneity of the obtained subsamples is minimized regarding HRQoL score. A model is fitted on various groups of the study based on disease trajectory. The occurrence of each form of RS can be hypothesized by searching for differences in the way the various predictors explain the differences in HRQoL score in each group.

A variant of this method has also been proposed specifically for detecting patterns of reprioritization RS over multiple time points by adding the use of random forest method to CART (Boucekine et al., 2013, 2015). This addition allows estimating the importance of each HRQoL domains in explaining overall HRQoL scores over time. Complex patterns of evolution of reprioritization RS can therefore be inferred by observing changes in importance of the HRQoL domains over time.

Using item response theory models

The use of item response theory (IRT) models to detect RS has sometimes been evoked, as they possess some interesting measurement properties (Barclay-Goddard et al., 2009a). Thus, the use of the Linear Logistic with Relaxed Assumptions (LLRA) model has been tested once for detecting recalibration RS (Anota et al., 2014). However, this method imposes specifying the model on retrospective assessment data and assumes an absence of true change. Nonetheless, recently, a method specifically designed to detect different forms of RS and estimating true change using IRT model was proposed: the RespOnse Shift ALgorithm in Item response theory (ROSALI) (Guilleux et al., 2015).

ROSALI relies on an operationalization of nonuniform and uniform recalibration, and reprioritization as change(s) in the value of polytomous IRT models between two times of measurement (Guilleux et al., 2015).

The use of IRT could be an interesting alternative for RS detection compared with OP, as it could beneficiate some properties of IRT models, in particular, the possibility to estimate a latent trait with interval scale property (Wang and Chyi 2004). In addition, as IRT directly models responses to items as a function of a latent trait, it could be a method of choice for RS detection at item level (i.e., with categorical responses to items as variables used to estimate a unidimensional concept).

However, ROSALI is currently based on unidimensional IRT models and does not yet include the possibility of reconceptualization detection, which would require multidimensional IRT modeling (Guilleux et al., 2015).

A brief overview of some results from studies investigating the occurrence of RS effect

Since the introduction of the first theoretical model of the RS effect on perceived HRQoL in 1999, a growing body of studies has investigated the occurrence of RS, in a variety of clinical settings, using various methods (although, most of the times the then-test approach was used; Schwartz et al., 2006). Thus, evidence of the RS effect (recalibration and/or reprioritization and/or reconceptualization) have been suggested in a wide range of diseases, including acute events like occurrence of cancer (Sprangers, 1996; Jansen et al., 2000; Bernhard et al., 1999; Hagedoorn et al., 2002), stroke (Barclay-Goddard et al., 2011; Ahmed et al., 2004, 2005), coronary artery disease (Gandhi et al., 2013a), hearing loss (Joore et al., 2002; Timmerman et al., 2003), different types of surgeries (Ring et al., 2005; Schwartz et al., 2013; Finkelstein et al., 2009; Razmjou et al., 2009, 2010), or chronic diseases like multiple sclerosis (King-Kallimanis et al., 2011; Ahmed et al., 2011), chronic back pain (Nagl and Farin, 2012), diabetes (Postulart and Adang, 2000), or end-renal stage disease (Elliott et al., 2014). The occurrence of RS has been investigated, not only as a consequence of the beginning of a salient disease but also when patients are recovering from a health-related event susceptible to leading to chronic disabilities (e.g., being handicapped after a stroke; Ahmed et al., 2005a), or after the beginning of a major treatment course (e.g., initiation of radiotherapy to treat cancer; Sprangers, 1996). Evidences of the RS effect have also been suggested after the initiation of a self-management course to help overcome difficulties related to a particular disease (Osborne et al., 2006; Ahmed et al., 2009). Finally, the occurrence of the RS effect has been documented in various populations, from children to elderly people (Barclay and Tate, 2014; Timmerman et al., 2003).

One of the many questions that were investigated in studies about RS was the magnitude of such an effect on changes in scores. In terms of magnitude, the RS effect on changes in observed scores is usually reported as a small effect. Nonetheless, the issue of the magnitude of the RS effect on HRQoL observed scores is related to the issue of the clinical importance of taking into account RS effect when assessing changes in—true HRQoL. Indeed, the possibility of missing a clinically important change in HRQoL if RS is not appropriately taken into account has been pointed out (Barclay-Goddard et al., 2009a).

In line with this point of view, studies have shown that changes in HRQoL can be underestimated when RS was not taken into account (Ring et al., 2005; Oort et al., 2005; Ahmed et al., 2004; Gandhi et al., 2013b).

As stated before, some statistical methods (e.g., Oort's Procedure) that can be used to detect RS make the assumption that a substantial part of the sample has demonstrated RS in the same direction and magnitude (Oort, 2005b). However, the results of some studies have challenged this assumption. Indeed, estimates of the prevalence of RS vary greatly across studies. Within individuals at 6 months poststroke, using a variety of methods to detect RS, it has been estimated that 28%–78% of the individuals have demonstrated RS (Ahmed et al., 2004, 2005b, c). In contrast, in two studies (on patients poststroke and on patients with multiple sclerosis respectively), it was suggested that most of the individuals did not exhibit RS (Mayo et al., 2008; Ahmed et al., 2011).

RS, as a psychological phenomenon, is theoretically often viewed as a process of adaptation: i.e., as a phenomenon triggered by psychological mechanisms helping people to adapt to negative circumstances and helping them to feel themselves as good as possible despite experiencing a deteriorating health (Sprangers and Schwartz, 1999; Barclay-Goddard et al., 2009a). Nonetheless, it has been hypothesized that RS could be, in some circumstances, a maladaptive process (Sprangers and Schwartz, 2008). Thus, it can be noted that some studies have pointed out that within a sample of individuals experiencing the same health-related event, RS can be detected as having an effect on HRQoL scores in opposite directions across subgroups (Osborne et al., 2006; Mayo et al., 2008).

The occurrence of the RS effect is often investigated in explaining changes in observed HRQoL pre-and postoccurrence of an acute event, or in explaining changes related to dealing with a chronic disease. Nonetheless, the possibility that RS can be a phenomenon occurring only with the mere passage of time has been postulated (Schwartz et al., 2005). Currently, results have been reported supporting the idea that RS can occur without strong evidences of the occurrence of an acute health-related event (Barclay and Tate, 2014). But, in a recent study investigating changes in HRQoL within individuals living with chronic diseases, but with reported stable health, little evidences for RS effect was found over a year of follow-up (Ahmed et al., 2014).

Last, it has been proposed that RS can be anticipated as a positive effect of interventions such as self-management and psychosocial programs, rehabilitation, and palliative care. Inducing RS may be a desired outcome of such interventions, when proposed to people suffering from a chronic disease, where symptoms and functions may not be dramatically improved, but better HRQoL is desired. Some studies have shown evidences that interventions designed to facilitate RS can help to improve HRQoL over time (Osborne et al., 2006; Ahmed et al., 2009; Schwartz and Sendor, 1999; Schwartz, 1999).

Conclusion

The development of the RS theory has been helpful in highlighting that when individuals are asked to rate their level of HRQoL, their appraisal of the construct being measured can change over time, leading to changes in perceived HRQoL. So, interpreting observed changes in HRQoL scores over time, especially when a salient health-related event has occurred can be more complex than initially thought. Thus, RS theory has provided a pragmatic theoretical framework, which was translated into different methods designed to help assessing changes over time of a targeted construct. It was used in various empirical settings.

Nonetheless, the research field about RS in health-related research is still a young field and there is a lot of room for improvement.

On a theoretical level, if the first theoretical model has been empirically tested once (Visser et al., 2012), the updated theoretical model proposed by Rapkin and Schwartz has never been tested on data with statistical methods designed to test linear structural relationships (Li and Rapkin 2009). Such studies should be conducted. In addition, there is still the need of pursuing the debate on the meaning of RS effect, to clarify what is the hermeneutic of RS in various study settings. A needed related discussion can also be the debate on interpreting the RS effect as a phenomenon linked to subjects' characteristics as opposed as a phenomenon linked to the characteristics of a PRO instrument (Schwartz et al., 2005). Indeed, if RS is currently often interpreted as an effect highlighting how individuals adapt to life changes, some authors have also pointed out that the characteristics of a questionnaire can also participate in enhancing RS. For example, it has been postulated that RS can be more susceptible to occur when a concept is measured by means of evaluation-based items (i.e., rating experiences compared with an internal standard, e.g., how difficult is it to walk up a flight of stairs?), as opposed to performance-based items (e.g., time to walk up a flight of stairs) or perception-based items (e.g., how often do you walk up stairs?) (Schwartz and Rapkin, 2004). It has also been postulated that RS could occur because HRQoL scales assumed that people are weak evaluators (i.e., people would rate their level of HRQoL in regards to contingent circumstances, like current physical condition), although people could probably be strong evaluators instead (i.e., people would rate their level of HRQoL in regards to how a condition have an impact on higher-level individuals' motivations or purposes) (McClimans et al., 2013). In addition, it has been hypothesized recently that the occurrence of RS could be linked with the semantic complexity of concepts and items (Vanier et al., 2015a).

On a methodological level, if various methods have been developed to detect and take into account for RS, there are still issues. Currently, each method has drawbacks. The then-test approach has been the most used, but it is currently less recommended (Schwartz and Sprangers, 2010). OP allows detecting all forms of RS along with an estimate of true change, but it currently implies group-analysis, which can be a strong assumption (Oort, 2005b; Oort et al., 2009). Latent trajectory analysis allows identifying subgroups of subjects with different RS patterns over time, but it cannot assess the form of RS and does not provide directly an estimate of true change (Mayo et al., 2008). Relative importance analysis can be useful when focusing on differences between two groups, but it can only detect reprioritization in one group compared with another (Lix et al., 2012). CART and random forest method can be useful for inferring complex patterns of RS over time, but they do not provide a quantitative assessment of RS (Li and Schwartz, 2011; Boucekine et al., 2013). ROSALI shares the advantages of OP along with some interesting measurement properties because of the use of IRT models, but it cannot be currently used with multidimensional constructs (Guilleux et al., 2015). In addition, there is the need to clarify what is RS at item level as opposed to RS at domain level (Ahmed et al., 2014; Vanier et al., 2015b). To provide a method, or a combination of methods, that could allow detecting subgroups of subjects with different patterns of RS, detecting each form of RS in each group, on multiple time points, both for item and/or domain level, along with a direct estimate of true change will be a challenge.

Finally, when investigating the occurrence of RS as a phenomenon of interest in empirical settings, there are still a lot of questions that need future developments or clarifications. For example, little is currently known about the subjects' characteristics that are susceptible to explain why some individuals will experience RS after the occurrence of a catalyst, whereas others will not (Barclay-Goddard et al., 2009a). There are still questions about the timing RS, or about the interrelationships between each of the components (from the catalyst to perceived HRQoL) when explaining occurrence, direction, and magnitude of RS.

Future researches conducted altogether in the three aforementioned areas (i.e., theoretical level, methodological level, and empirical level) will be needed to assess if RS theory will be one of the most heuristic framework in explaining observed changes in HRQoL, useful either in studies dealing with the assessment of interventions or in large epidemiological settings.

References

Ahmed, S., Bourbeau, J., Maltais, F., and Mansour, A. (2009). The Oort structural equation modeling approach detected a response shift after a COPD self-management program not detected by the Schmitt technique. *J. Clin. Epidemiol.*, 62, 1165–1172. DOI:10.1016/j.jclinepi.2009.03.015

Ahmed, S., Mayo, N., Scott, S., Kuspinar, A., and Schwartz, C. (2011). Using latent trajectory analysis of residuals to detect response shift in general health among patients with multiple sclerosis article. *Qual. Life Res.*, 20, 1555–1560. DOI:10.1007/s11136-011-0005-6

Ahmed, S., Mayo, N.E., Corbiere, M., Wood-Dauphinee, S., Hanley, J., and Cohen, R. (2005a). Change in quality of life of people with stroke over time: True change or response shift?. *Qual. Life Res.*, 14, 611–627.

Ahmed, S., Mayo, N.E., Wood-Dauphinee, S., Hanley, J.A., and Cohen, S.R. (2005b). Using the patient generated index to evaluate response shift post-stroke. *Qual. Life Res.*, 14, 2247–2257.

Ahmed, S., Mayo, N.E., Wood-Dauphinee, S., Hanley, J.A., and Cohen, S.R. (2004). Response shift influenced estimates of change in health-related quality of life post-stroke. *J. Clin. Epidemiol.*, 57, 561–570. DOI:10.1016/j.jclinepi.2003.11.003

Ahmed, S., Mayo, N.E., Wood-Dauphinee, S., Hanley, J.A., and Cohen, SR. (2005c). The structural equation modeling technique did not show a response shift, contrary to the results of the then test and the individualized approaches. *J. Clin. Epidemiol.*, 58, 1125–1133. DOI:10.1016/j.jclinepi.2005.03.003

Ahmed, S., Sawatzky, R., Levesque, J-F., Ehrmann-Feldman, D., and Schwartz, C.E. (2014). Minimal evidence of response shift in the absence of a catalyst. *Qual. Life Res.*, *23*, 2421–2430. DOI:10.1007/s11136-014-0699-3

Ahmed, S., Schwartz, C., Ring, L., and Sprangers, M.A.G. (2009). Applications of health-related quality of life for guiding health care: Advances in response shift research. *J. Clin. Epidemiol.*, *62*, 1115–1117. DOI:10.1016/j.jclinepi.2009.04.006

Allison, P.J., Locker, D., and Feine, J.S. (1997). Quality of life: A dynamic construct. *Soc. Sci. Med.*, *45*, 221–230.

Andrykowski, M., Brady, M., and Hunt, J. (1993). Positive psychosocial adjustment in potential bone narrow transplant recipients: Cancer as a psychosocial transition. *Psychooncology*, *2*, 261–276.

Anota, A., Bascoul-Mollevi, C., Conroy, T., Guillemin, F., Velten, M., Jolly, D, et al. (2014). Item response theory and factor analysis as a mean to characterize occurrence of response shift in a longitudinal quality of life study in breast cancer patients. *Health Qual. Life Outcomes*, *12*, 32. DOI:10.1186/1477-7525-12-32

Barclay, R., and Tate, R.B. (2014). Response shift recalibration and reprioritization in health-related quality of life was identified prospectively in older men with and without stroke. *J. Clin. Epidemiol.*, *67*, 500–507. DOI:10.1016/j.jclinepi.2013.12.003

Barclay-Goddard, R., Epstein, J.D., and Mayo, N.E. (2009a). Response shift: A brief overview and proposed research priorities. *Qual. Life Res.*, *18*, 335–346. DOI:10.1007/s11136-009-9450-x

Barclay-Goddard, R., Lix, L.M., Tate, R., Weinberg, L., and Mayo, N.E. (2009b). Response shift was identified over multiple occasions with a structural equation modeling framework. *J. Clin. Epidemiol.*, *62*, 1181–1188. DOI:10.1016/j.jclinepi.2009.03.014

Barclay-Goddard, R., Lix, L.M., Tate, R., Weinberg, L., and Mayo, N.E. (2011). Health-related quality of life after stroke: Does response shift occur in self-perceived physical function?. *Arch. Phys. Med. Rehabil.*, *92*, 1762–1769. DOI:10.1016/j.apmr.2011.06.013

Bernhard, J., Hürny, C., Maibach, R., Herrmann, R., Laffer, U. (1999). Quality of life as subjective experience: Reframing of perception in patients with colon cancer undergoing radical resection with or without adjuvant chemotherapy. *Ann. Oncol.*, *10*, 775–782.

Boucekine, M., Boyer, L., Baumstarck, K., Millier, A., Ghattas, B., Auquier, P, et al. (2015). Exploring the response shift effect on the quality of life of patients with schizophrenia: An application of the random forest method. *Med. Decis. Making.*, *35*, 388–397. DOI:10.1177/0272989X14559273

Boucekine, M., Loundou, A., Baumstarck, K., Minaya-Flores, P., Pelletier, J., Ghattas, B, et al. (2013). Using the random forest method to detect a response shift in the quality of life of multiple sclerosis patients: A cohort study. *BMC Med. Res. Methodol.*, *13*, 20.

Boyer, L., Baumstarck, K., Michel, P., Boucekine, M., Anota, A., Bonnetain, F, et al. (2014). Statistical challenges of quality of life and cancer: New avenues for future research. *Expert Rev. Pharmacoecon. Outcomes Res.*, *14*, 19–22. DOI:10.1586/14737167.2014.873704

Breetvelt, I.S., and Van Dam, F.S. (1991). Underreporting by cancer patients: The case of response-shift. *Soc. Sci. Med.*, *32*, 981–987.

Calman, K. (1984). Quality of life in cancer patients: An hypothesis. *J. Med. Ethics.*, *10*, 124–127.

Carver, C.S., and Scheier, M.F. (1982). Control theory: A useful conceptual framework for personality, social, clinical and health psychology. *Psychol. Bull.*, *92*, 111–135.

Carver. C.S., and Scheier, M.F. (2000). Scaling back goals and recalibration of the affect system are processes in normal adaptive self-regulation: Understanding—Response shift phenomena. *Soc. Sci. Med.*, *50*, 1715–1722.

Cronbach, L., and Furby, L. (1970). How we should measure—Change—Or should we?. *Psychol. Bull.*, *74*, 68–80.

Daltroy, L.H., Larson, M.G., Eaton, H.M., Phillips, C.B., and Liang, M.H. (1999). Discrepancies between self—Reported and observed physical function in the elderly: The influence of response shift and other factors. *Soc. Sci. Med.*, *48*, 1549–1561.

Elliott, B.A., Gessert, C.E., Larson, P.M., and Russ, T.E. (2014). Shifting responses in quality of life: People living with dialysis. *Qual. Life Res.*, *23*, 1497–1504. DOI:10.1007/s11136-013-0600-9

Eton, D.T. (2010). Why we need response shift: An appeal to functionalism. *Qual. Life Res.*, *19*, 929–930. DOI:10.1007/s11136-010-9684-7

Fayers, P.M., and Machin, D. (2007). *Quality of Life: The Assessment, Analysis, and Interpretation of Patient- Reported Outcomes* (2nd Edition). Chichester, UK/ Hoboken, NJ: J. Wiley.

Finkelstein, J.A., Razmjou, H., and Schwartz, C.E. (2009). Response shift and outcome assessment in orthopedic surgery: Is there a difference between complete and partial treatment?. *J. Clin. Epidemiol.*, *62*, 1189–1190. DOI:10.1016/j.jclinepi.2009.03.022

Fokkema, M., Smits, N., Kelderman, H., and Cuijpers, P. (2013). Response shifts in mental health interventions: An illustration of longitudinal measurement invariance. *Psychol. Assess.*, *25*, 520–531. DOI:10.1037/a0031669

Gandhi, P.K., Ried, L.D., Huang, I-C., Kimberlin, C.L., and Kauf, T.L. (2013a). Assessment of response shift using two structural equation modeling techniques. *Qual. Life Res.*, *22*, 461–471. DOI:10.1007/s11136-012-0171-1

Gandhi, P.K., Ried, L.D., Kimberlin, C.L., Kauf, T.L., and Huang, I-C. (2013b). Influence of explanatory and confounding variables on HRQoL after controlling for measurement bias and response shift in measurement. *Expert. Rev. Pharmacoecon. Outcomes Res.*, *13*, 841–851. DOI:10.1586/14737167.2013.852959

Golembiewski, R.T. (1976). Measuring change and persistence in human affairs: Types of change generated by OD designs. *J. Appl. Behav. Sci.*, *12*, 133–157. DOI:10.1177/002188637601200201

Guilleux, A., Blanchin, M., Vanier, A., Guillemin, F., Falissard, B., Schwartz, C.E., et al. (2015). RespOnse Shift ALgorithm in Item response theory (ROSALI) for response shift detection with missing data in longitudinal patient-reported outcome studies. *Qual. Life Res.*, *24*, 553–564. DOI:10.1007/s11136-014-0876-4

Hagedoorn, M., Sneeuw, K.C.A., and Aaronson, N.K. (2002). Changes in physical functioning and quality of life in patients with cancer: Response shift and relative evaluation of one's condition. *J. Clin. Epidemiol.*, *55*, 176–183.

Helson, H. (1964). *Adaptation Level Theory*. New-York: Harper and Row.

Howard, G.S., and Dailey, P.R. (1979). Response-shift bias: A source of contamination of self-report measures. *J. Appl. Psychol.*, *64*, 144–150. DOI:10.1037/0021-9010.64.2.144

Howard, G.S., Ralph, K.M., Gulanick, N.A., Maxwell, S.E., Nance, D.W., and Gerber, S.K. (1979). Internal invalidity in pretest-posttest self-report evaluations and a re-evaluation of retrospective pretests. *Appl. Psychol. Meas.*, *3*, 1–23. DOI:10.1177/014662167900300101

Jansen, S.J., Stiggelbout, A.M., Nooij, M.A., Noordijk, E.M., and Kievit, J. (2000). Response shift in quality of life measurement in early-stage breast cancer patients undergoing radiotherapy. *Qual. Life Res.*, *9*, 603–615.

Joore, M.A., Potjewijd, J., Timmerman, A.A., and Anteunis, L.J.C. (2002). Response shift in the measurement of quality of life in hearing impaired adults after hearing aid fitting. *Qual. Life Res.*, *11*, 299–307.

King-Kallimanis, B.L., Oort, F.J., Nolte, S., Schwartz, C.E., and Sprangers, M.A.G. (2011). Using structural equation modeling to detect response shift in performance and health-related quality of life scores of multiple sclerosis patients. *Qual. Life Res.*, *20*, 1527–1540. DOI:10.1007/s11136-010- 9844-9

King-Kallimanis, B.L., Oort, F.J., Visser, M.R.M., and Sprangers, M.A.G. (2009). Structural equation modeling of health-related quality-of-life data illustrates the measurement and conceptual perspectives on response shift. *J. Clin. Epidemiol.*, *62*, 1157–1164. DOI:10.1016/j.jclinepi.2009.04.004

Korfage, I.J., de Koning, H.J., and Essink-Bot, M.-L. (2007). Response shift due to diagnosis and primary treatment of localized prostate cancer: A then-test and a vignette study. *Qual. Life Res.*, *16*, 1627–1634. DOI:10.1007/s11136-007-9265-6

Korfage, I.J., Hak, T., de Koning, H.J., and Essink-Bot, M.-L. (2006). Patients' perceptions of the side-effects of prostate cancer treatment—A qualitative interview study. *Soc. Sci. Med.*, *63*, 911–919. DOI:10.1016/j.socscimed.2006.01.027

Lazarus, R., and Folkman, S. (1984). *Stress, Apraisal, and Coping*. New-York, NY: Springer.

Leplège, A., and Hunt, S. (1997). The problem of quality of life in medicine. *JAMA*, *278*, 47–50.

Li, Y., and Rapkin, B. (2009). Classification and regression tree uncovered hierarchy of psychosocial determinants underlying quality-of-life response shift in HIV/AIDS. *J. Clin. Epidemiol.*, *62*, 1138–1147. DOI:10.1016/j.jclinepi.2009.03.021

Li, Y., and Schwartz, C.E. (2011). Data mining for response shift patterns in multiple sclerosis patients using recursive partitioning tree analysis. *Qual. Life Res.*, *20*, 1543–1553. DOI:10.1007/s11136-011-0004-7

Lix, L.M., Sajobi, T.T., Sawatzky, R., Liu, J., Mayo, N.E., Huang, Y, et al. (2012). Relative importance measures for reprioritization response shift. *Qual. Life Res.*, *22*, 695–703. DOI:10.1007/s11136-012-0198-3

Mayo, N.E., Scott, S.C., Dendukuri, N., Ahmed, S., and Wood-Dauphinee, S. (2008). Identifying response shift statistically at the individual level. *Qual. Life Res.*, *17*, 627–639. DOI:10.1007/s11136-008- 9329-2

McClimans, L. (2010). A theoretical framework for patient-reported outcome measures. *Theor. Med. Bioeth.*, *31*, 225–240. DOI:10.1007/s11017-010-9142-0

McClimans, L., Bickenbach, J., Westerman, M., Carlson, L., Wasserman, D., and Schwartz, C. (2013). Philosophical perspectives on response shift. *Qual. Life Res.*, *22*, 1871–1878. DOI:10.1007/s11136-012-0300-x

Mishel, M. (1988). Uncertainty in illness. *J. Nurs. Scolarsh.*, *20*, 225–232.

Nagl, M., and Farin, E. (2012). Response shift in quality of life assessment in patients with chronic back pain and chronic ischaemic heart disease. *Disabil. Rehabil.*, *34*, 671–680. DOI:10.3109/09638288.2011.619616

Nolte, S., Elsworth, G.R., Sinclair, A.J., and Osborne, R.H. (2009). Tests of measurement invariance failed to support the application of the—Then-test. *J. Clin. Epidemiol.*, *62*, 1173–1180. DOI:10.1016/j.jclinepi.2009.01.021

Norman, G. (2003). Hi! How are you? Response shift, implicit theories and differing epistemologies. *Qual. Life Res.*, *12*, 239–249.

O'Boyle, C.A., McGee, H.M., Browne, J.P. (2000). Measuring response shift using the Schedule for Evaluation of Individual Quality of Life. In Schwartz, C.E., Sprangers, M.A.G. (eds.), *Adaptation to Changing Health: Response Shift in Quality-of-Life Research* (pp. 123–136). Washington, DC: American Psychological Association, xvi, 227 pp.

Oort, F.J. (2005a). Towards a formal definition of response shift (in reply to G.W. Donaldson). *Qual. Life Res.*, *14*, 2353–2355. DOI:10.1007/s11136-005-3978-1

Oort, F.J. (2005b). Using structural equation modeling to detect response shifts and true change. *Qual. Life Res.*, *14*, 587–598.

Oort, F.J., Visser, M.R.M., and Sprangers, M.A.G. (2005). An application of structural equation modeling to detect response shifts and true change in quality of life data from cancer patients undergoing invasive surgery. *Qual. Life Res.*, *14*, 599–609.

Oort, F.J., Visser, M.R.M., and Sprangers, M.A.G. (2009). Formal definitions of measurement bias and explanation bias clarify measurement and conceptual perspectives on response shift. *J. Clin. Epidemiol.*, *62*, 1126–1137. DOI:10.1016/j.jclinepi.2009.03.013

Osborne, R.H., Hawkins, M., and Sprangers, M.A.G. (2006). Change of perspective: A measurable and desired outcome of chronic disease self-management intervention programs that violates the premise of preintervention/postintervention assessment. *Arthritis Rheum., 55*, 458–465. DOI:10.1002/art.21982

Postulart, D., and Adang, E.M. (2000). Response shift and adaptation in chronically ill patients. *Med. Decis. Making., 20*, 186–193.

Rapkin, B.D., and Schwartz, C.E. (2004). Toward a theoretical model of quality-of-life appraisal: Implications of findings from studies of response shift. *Health Qual. Life Outcomes, 2*, 14. DOI:10.1186/1477-7525-2-14

Razmjou, H., Schwartz, C.E., and Holtby, R. (2010). The impact of response shift on perceived disability two years following rotator cuff surgery. *J. Bone Joint Surg. Am., 92*, 2178–2786. DOI:10.2106/JBJS.I.00990

Razmjou, H., Schwartz, C.E., Yee, A., and Finkelstein, J.A. (2009). Traditional assessment of health outcome following total knee arthroplasty was confounded by response shift phenomenon. *J. Clin. Epidemiol., 62*, 91–96. DOI:10.1016/j.jclinepi.2008.08.004

Reeve, B.B. (2010). An opportunity to refine our understanding of—Response shift and to educate researchers on designing quality research studies: Response to Ubel, Peeters, and Smith. *Qual. Life Res., 19*, 473–475. DOI:10.1007/s11136-010-9612-x

Ring, L., Höfer, S., Heuston, F., Harris, D., and O'Boyle, C.A. (2005). Response shift masks the treatment impact on patient reported outcomes (PROs): The example of individual quality of life in edentulous patients. *Health Qual. Life Outcomes, 3*, 55.

Schmitt, N. (1982). The use of analysis of covariance structures to assess beta and gamma change. *Multivar. Behav. Res., 17*, 343–358. DOI:10.1207/s15327906mbr1703_3

Schwartz, C.E. (1999). Teaching coping skills enhances quality of life more than peer support: Results of a randomized trial with multiple sclerosis patients. *Health Psychol., 18*, 211–220.

Schwartz, C.E., Ahmed, S., Sawatzky, R., Sajobi, T., Mayo, N., Finkelstein, J, et al. (2013). Guidelines for secondary analysis in search of response shift. *Qual. Life Res., 22*, 2663–2673. DOI:10.1007/s11136-013-0402-0

Schwartz, C.E., Bode, R., Repucci, N., Becker, J., Sprangers, M.A.G., and Fayers, P.M. (2006). The clinical significance of adaptation to changing health: A meta-analysis of response shift. *Qual. Life Res., 15*, 1533–1550. DOI:10.1007/s11136-006-0025-9 Schwartz, C.E., and Rapkin, B.D. (2004). Reconsidering the psychometrics of quality of life assessment in light of response shift and appraisal. *Health Qual Life Outcomes, 2*, 16.

Schwartz, C.E., and Sendor, R.M. (1999). Helping others helps oneself: Response shift effects in peer support. *Soc. Sci. Med., 48*, 1563–1575.

Schwartz, C.E., and Sprangers, M.A.G. (1999). Methodological approaches for assessing response shift in longitudinal health-related quality-of-life research. *Soc. Sci. Med., 48*, 1531–1548.

Schwartz, C.E., and Sprangers, M.A.G. (2010). Guidelines for improving the stringency of response shift research using the then-test. *Qual. Life Res., 19*, 455–464. DOI:10.1007/s11136-010- 9585-9

Schwartz, C.E., Sajobi, T.T., Lix, L.M., Quaranto, B.R., and Finkelstein, J.A. (2013). Changing values, changing outcomes: The influence of reprioritization response shift on outcome assessment after spine surgery. *Qual. Life Res., 22*, 2255–2264. DOI:10.1007/s11136-013-0377-x

Schwartz, C.E., Sprangers, M.A., and Fayers, P.M. (2005). Response shift: You know it's there, but how do you capture it? Challenges fo the next phase of research. In: *Assessing quality of life in clinical trials* (2nd Edition). Oxford; New-York, NY: Oxford University Press.

Schwartz, C.E., Sprangers, M.A.G., Carey, A., and Reed, G. (2004). Exploring response shift in longitudinal data. *Psychol. Health, 19*, 51–69. DOI:10.1080/0887044031000118456

Schwartz, C.E., Sprangers, M.A.G., Oort, F.J., Ahmed, S., Bode, R., Li, Y, et al. (2011). Response shift in patients with multiple sclerosis: An application of three statistical techniques. *Qual. Life Res.*, *20*, 1561–1572. DOI:10.1007/s11136-011-0056-8

Sprangers, M.A. (1996). Response-shift bias: A challenge to the assessment of patients' quality of life in cancer clinical trials. *Cancer Treat Rev.*, *22*(Suppl. A), 55–62.

Sprangers, M.A.G., and Schwartz, C.E. (1999). Integrating response shift into health-related quality of life research: A theoretical model. *Soc. Sci. Med.*, *48*, 1507–1515.

Sprangers, M.A.G., and Schwartz, C.E. (2010). Do not throw out the baby with the bath water: Build on current approaches to realize conceptual clarity. Response to Ubel, Peeters, and Smith. *Qual. Life Res.*, *19*, 477–479. DOI:10.1007/s11136-010-9611-y

Stanton, A.L., Revenson, T.A., and Tennen, H. (2007). Health psychology: Psychological adjustment to chronic disease. *Annu. Rev. Psychol.*, *58*, 565–592. DOI:10.1146/annurev.psych.58.110405.085615

Timmerman, A.A., Anteunis, L.J.C., and Meesters, C.M.G. (2003). Response-shift bias and parent-reported quality of life in children with otitis media. *Arch. Otolaryngol. Head Neck Surg.*, *129*, 987–991. DOI:10.1001/archotol.129.9.987

Ubel, P.A., Peeters, Y., and Smith, D. (2010). Abandoning the language of—Response shift: A plea for conceptual clarity in distinguishing scale recalibration from true changes in quality of life. *Qual. Life Res.*, *19*, 465–471. DOI:10.1007/s11136-010-9592-x

Ubel, P.A., and Smith, D.M. (2010). Why should changing the bathwater have to harm the baby?. *Qual. Life Res.*, *19*, 481–482. DOI:10.1007/s11136-010-9613-9

Vanier, A., Leplège, A., Hardouin, J-B., Sébille, V., and Falissard, B. (2015a). Semantic primes theory may be helpful in designing questionnaires such as to prevent response shift. *J. Clin. Epidemiol.*, *68*, 646–654. DOI:10.1016/j.jclinepi.2015.01.023

Vanier, A., Sébille, V., Blanchin, M., Guilleux, A., and Hardouin, J-B. (2015b). Overall performance of Oort's procedure for response shift detection at item level: A pilot simulation study. *Qual. Life Res.*, *24*, 1799–1807. DOI:10.1007/s11136-015-0938-2

Visser, M.R.M., Oort, F.J., and Sprangers, M.A.G. (2005). Methods to detect response shift in quality of life data: A convergent validity study. *Qual. Life Res.*, *14*, 629–639.

Visser, M.R.M., Oort, F.J., Lanschot, J.J.B., Velden, J., Kloek, J.J., Gouma, D.J, et al. (2012). The role of recalibration response shift in explaining bodily pain in cancer patients undergoing invasive surgery: An empirical investigation of the Sprangers and Schwartz model. *Psychooncology*, *22*, 515–522. DOI:10.1002/pon.2114

Wang, W., and Chyi, I. (2004). Gain score in item response theory as an effect size measure. *Edu. Psychol. Meas.*, *64*, 758–780.

Wilson, I.B., and Cleary, P.D. (1995). Linking clinical variables with health-related quality of life. A conceptual model of patient outcomes. *JAMA*, *273*, 59–65.

16 Interpretation of perceived health data in specific disorders

Anne-Christine Rat and Jacques Pouchot

Health-related quality of life (HRQoL) assessments are widely used as outcome measures. However, one of the main issues they raise relates to the interpretation of their results for health data collected for the general population as well as for specific disorders. Because statistical significance does not guarantee that observed differences are meaningful to patients, we need to document what level or what level of change in a perceived health measure is important to patients. Being able to translate changes or differences in scores into clinically meaningful terms is crucial to the interpretation of the results of interventions or to the description of the evolution of a disease over time. Therefore, an essential aspect of research into perceived health data outcomes is to determine what a high/good or low/poor score represents and what is a meaningful difference or change in the score. We need to have comparisons or reference thresholds to describe health states in any specific disease.

We discuss the issue of interpreting the result of a single measure of a health measure typically obtained in a cross-sectional study involving general population references, between-group comparisons, definition of a good or poor state, and finally variables associated with health state.

We then describe various methods to interpret a meaningful change in score in longitudinal studies. Different approaches have been used to define responders at an individual level by threshold values for change, by final state, or both. At the group level, identifying the minimum important difference in mean change from baseline between treatments is also important.

Here, we discuss the interpretation of perceived health data outcomes in specific diseases, with illustrations from osteoarthritis (OA) and rheumatoid arthritis (RA) in terms of major causes of disability and impaired HRQoL (Vos et al., 2012; Cross et al., 2014). Moreover, these conditions allow for mentioning several specific difficulties in interpreting perceived health data: how to interpret longitudinal patterns of symptomatic change in joints in rheumatology because joint disease is rarely monosymptomatic; how to consider the different dimensions of perceived health instruments in interpreting the global outcome of patients; and how a response shift can modify the measure of change.

Data from the Knee and Hip Osteoarthritis Long-Term Assessment (KHOALA) cohort (Guillemin et al., 2012) and Nancy thermal study (Rat et al., submitted) are used as examples. The KHOALA cohort included 878 subjects recruited from a multiregional prevalence survey of OA performed in France from 2007 to 2009 (Guillemin et al., 2011). The subjects were of both genders, from 40 to 75 years old, with confirmed uni- or bilateral symptomatic hip and/or knee OA. The KHOALA cohort is representative of the prevalent cases of OA in the general French population. Subjects were followed once a year. The Nancy thermal clinical trial compared two programs of spa therapy for knee OA. Patients in both studies completed the Western Ontario and McMaster Universities Osteoarthritis Index (WOMAC), Medical Outcomes Survey Short Form 36 (SF-36), and OA Knee and Hip Quality of Life (OAKHQOL) survey. References on interpretability are available for the WOMAC and SF-36, which are extensively used, but not the OAKHQOL (Rat et al., 2005), which was more recently developed.

We also briefly present data from RA patients to illustrate a method that could be used to understand and calibrate the measured changes in health status measurements (i.e., fatigue instruments) (Pouchot et al., 2008).

Assessment of the health status measure as a state

To answer self-reported questionnaires, people must consider what QoL means to them and what and how their experiences have changed their QoL. They must structure and combine appraisals to arrive at a QoL rating (Rapkin and Schwartz, 2004). Therefore, people use their own frame of reference, comparing their actual state with predisease status, with peers or with themselves at a younger age, which leads to different interpretations and answers (Fayers et al., 2007).

Moreover, self-reported health status questionnaires measure what patients think they can do or the degree of difficulty patients perceive. This perception is affected by many factors such as self-efficacy, optimism, expectations, needs, and mood. Different contextual features of a simple task can have a great effect on self-reported mobility (e.g., the height of a chair can make standing up from a chair more or less difficult) (Marsh et al., 2011). In this way, cross-sectional data are challenging to interpret.

Comparison with other populations

Many generic questionnaires can be used to compare patients with different diseases. For example, cancer survivors report better levels of HRQoL than does the general population. After renal and neurologic diseases, musculoskeletal diseases have the greatest detrimental impact on QoL (Sprangers et al., 2000).

The SF-36, a generic HRQoL with eight dimensions (physical functioning, role physical, bodily pain, general health, social functioning, mental health, role emotional, and vitality), has been used to compare patients with various musculoskeletal diseases (Picavet and Hoeymans, 2004). Results were first presented with scores between 0 and 100 (Table 16.1) but more appropriately with a standardized difference score (Figure 16.1), that is, the difference

Table 16.1 Short form 36 (SF-36) scores for patients with musculoskeletal diseases (Dutch population-based musculoskeletal complaints and consequences cohort [DMC3] study)

	No.	Physical functioning	Role, physical	Bodily pain	General health	Vitality	Social functioning	Role, emotional	Mental health
Herniated disc	368	73.2 (1.1)	65.8 (2.0)	67.3 (1.3)	62.9 (1.1)	61.4 (1.1)	77.7 (1.2)	82.6 (1.7)	73.2 (0.9)
Gout	138	75.6 (2.0)	68.1 (3.6)	70.2 (2.2)	64.7 (1.9)	60.8 (1.9)	79.1 (2.2)	78.7 (3.0)	73.2 (1.7)
Knee OA	547	67.6 (1.0)	61.0 (1.9)	62.7 (1.1)	60.1 (1.0)	58.8 (1.0)	75.7 (1.1)	80.4 (1.6)	72.0 (0.9)
Hip OA	354	62.4 (1.4)	52.8 (2.5)	59.1 (1.5)	60.0 (1.3)	56.8 (1.3)	73.2 (1.5)	80.5 (2.1)	73.5 (1.2)
RA	156	62.3 (2.0)	49.0 (3.5)	58.0 (2.2)	52.1 (1.8)	52.2 (1.9)	70.3 (2.1)	72.3 (3.0)	69.2 (1.6)
Fibromyalgia	43	55.0 (3.2)	41.4 (5.8)	48.2 (3.6)	50.1 (3.0)	39.9 (3.1)	60.3 (3.4)	81.5 (4.8)	64.1 (2.6)

OA, osteoarthritis; RA, rheumatoid arthritis.
Source: Picavet, H.S., and Hoeymans, N. *Ann. Rheum. Dis.*, 63, 723–729, 2004.
Note: Data are mean (standard error of the mean [SEM]).

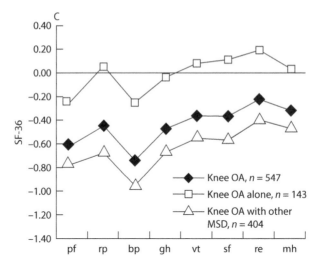

Figure 16.1 Patterns of health-related quality of life (HRQoL) findings for knee OA compared with the general population. Short form 36 (SF-36) scores are expressed as number of standard deviations (SDs) from the population mean. bp, bodily pain; gh, general health; mh, mental health; pf, physical functioning; re, role–emotional; rp, role–physical; sf, social functioning; vt, vitality; MSD, musculoskeletal diseases; OA, osteoarthritis.

between the subject's score and the weighted score of the general population divided by the standard deviation (SD) of the unweighted score of the general population. This standardized score (the z value or normal score) is a rescaled score with a population mean of 0 and a SD of 1.

Patients with fibromyalgia showed the greatest impairment of perceived health, although clinical or imaging examination results for this disease are usually poor, which illustrates the concept and importance of perceived health (Picavet and Hoeymans, 2004).

In the same study (Picavet and Hoeymans, 2004), for knee OA, HRQoL patterns expressed as standardized scores showed impaired scores for all dimensions, especially for bodily pain and physical functioning dimensions. When knee OA was the only condition, impairment was much less important than when it was associated with coexistent musculoskeletal disorders, which is a frequent situation and highlights the role of comorbidities (Figure 16.1).

Similarly, in the KHOALA cohort, standardized scores for the SF-36 were low, especially for bodily pain and physical functioning dimensions. Patterns were similar for knee or hip OA, with the highest HRQoL impairment in patients with both knee and hip OA (Figure 16.2).

Comparison to a reference population is of great importance for interpreting the level of impaired HRQoL in patients with a specific disease. However, such comparisons of course are only available with generic instruments, only for a few of them and not for all countries. In France, SF-36 data have been collected from the general population. Such data should be used in a population with comparable structure, including age categories, gender, and education level

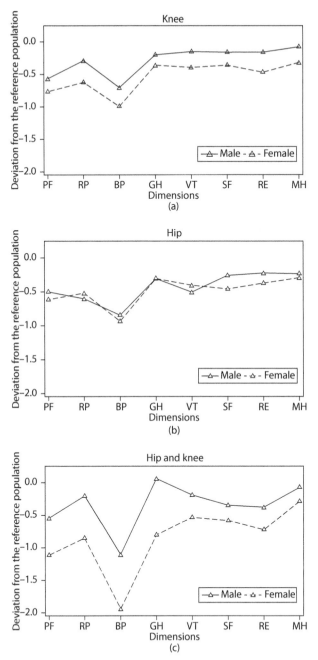

Figure 16.2   (a)–(c) Patterns of HRQoL findings for knee or hip OA compared with the general population. SF-36 scores are expressed as number of SDs from the population mean. bp, bodily pain; gh, general health; mh, mental health; pf, physical functioning; re, role–emotional; rp, role–physical; sf, social functioning; vt, vitality; MSD, musculoskeletal diseases; OA, osteoarthritis. Scores expected from the population reference are set to 0.

(Leplège and Coste, 1999). Comparison of HRQoL between patients with different chronic diseases is also very useful, in particular for allocating resources.

Standardized scores also allow for comparing different studies of the same disease. Clinical and perceived health data from different cohorts can be compared with inform results by better understanding the differences in populations included.

Although the Cohort Hip and Cohort Knee (CHECK) and Osteoarthritis Initiative (OAI) studies focused on the early phase of OA, patients differed significantly in perceived health and structural (radiographic) characteristics. Scores for the WOMAC (functioning, pain, stiffness subscales) and the SF-36 physical component summary score were worse for CHECK than for OAI patients, with no difference in the mental component summary score. Fewer individuals in CHECK had radiography-defined knee OA at baseline as compared with OAI patients. Therefore, the CHECK could represent patients in an even earlier phase of disease (Wesseling et al., 2009). However, in this example, the use of the component summary scales of the SF-36 could be debated, particularly because the weights needed were established in a US population, whereas the CHECK is a Dutch cohort.

Between-group comparisons

Group comparisons within a given disorder are useful to understand perceived health data. The joint affected, presence of comorbidities, and severity of disease (radiographic grades of severity) can be compared in OA (Table 16.2).

In this example, only the visual analog scale (VAS) for pain and physical activities dimension of the OAKHQOL were significantly more impaired for patients with knee than hip OA. In contrast, for most of the dimensions, severe OA according to x-ray grading (Kellgren–Lawrence grade) was associated with impaired perceived health.

Assessment by using various health state definitions

A cross-sectional method proposed by Jacobson et al. (1999) is based on the principle that a patient should be in the normal range of functioning after a clinical intervention. Thus, dysfunctional and functional populations serve as anchors for determining recovery status. The authors proposed three alternatives for determining recovery status, with the patient's score after clinical intervention being (Vos et al., 2012) two SDs or more from the mean of the dysfunctional population in the functional direction (Cross et al., 2014) within two SDs of the mean of the functional population, or (Guillemin et al., 2012) closer to the mean of the functional than dysfunctional population. These methods can be used in observational studies to interpret cross-sectional data.

Another way to interpret patient-reported outcomes (PROs) is the patient-acceptable symptom state (PASS), defined as the value beyond which patients consider themselves well. The minimal clinically important improvement

Table 16.2 HRQoL scores for the KHOALA cohort

	Hip		Knee		p-value	Radiographic grade (Kellgren–Laurence)					
						2		3		4	p-value
	n = 222		n = 607			n = 297		n = 197		n = 167	
OAKHQOL											
Physical activities	68.2	(19.7)	65.9	(22.1)	.04	68.4	(22.1)	65.0	(22.1)	60.0	(22.3)	.004
Pain	61.4	(22.5)	60.5	(24.9)	.66	63.5	(23.2)	58.9	(26.7)	55.8	(24.7)	.02
Mental health	75.9	(19.8)	74.2	(21.6)	.15	74.6	(21.3)	73.7	(22.5)	72.0	(22.6)	.64
Social functioning	72.9	(27.4)	74	(27.6)	.31	75.0	(27.9)	70.5	(29.4)	74.1	(25.8)	.31
Social support	58.5	(25.3)	57.2	(26.1)	.59	57.4	(26.9)	57.0	(24.5)	58.5	(25.5)	.99
SF-36											
Physical functioning	67.2	(21.8)	63	(23.7)	.05	66.2	(23.8)	61.4	(22.6)	58.1	(23.6)	.01
Bodily pain	51.8	(19.5)	51.2	(20.3)	.03	53.0	(21)	49.0	(20.5)	48.1	(18.3)	.04
Mental health	62.2	(18.5)	62.2	(19.5)	.89	61.6	(19.6)	63.4	(19.7)	62.3	(19.2)	.05
Social functioning	71.2	(21.9)	72.8	(22.8)	.38	72.5	(22.8)	74.9	(22.8)	69.7	(22.6)	.03
Vitality	50.7	(17.9)	52.4	(17.6)	.45	52.0	(18.2)	51.8	(17.2)	53.0	(17.3)	.06

(Continued)

Table 16.2 HRQoL scores for the KHOALA cohort (Continued)

	Hip (n = 222)		p-value	Knee (n = 607)		p-value	Radiographic grade (Kellgren–Lawrence)						p-value
							2 (n = 297)		3 (n = 197)		4 (n = 167)		
WOMAC													
Function	33.5	(20.5)	.12	33.7	(22.4)		30.9	(21.9)	35.0	(22.1)	39.6	(22.9)	.00
Pain	31.6	(18.9)	.14	32.8	(19.3)		30.0	(18.0)	33.2	(20.4)	39.3	(19.5)	<.0001
Stiffness	42.6	(20.9)	.53	40.9	(22.6)		39.1	(22.5)	41.5	(23.0)	44.6	(21.6)	.06
VAS pain	34.4	(24.2)	.01	36.8	(25.3)		32.9	(23.6)	37.1	(26.3)	46.6	(24.9)	<.0001

HRQoL, health-related quality of life; KHOALA, Knee and Hip Osteoarthritis Long-Term Assessment; OAKHQOL, OA Knee Health-related Quality of Life; SF-36, short form 36; VAS, visual analog scale; WOMAC, Western Ontario and McMaster Universities Osteoarthritis Index.
Note: Data are mean (SD). OAKHQOL and SF-36: 100 = best; WOMAC and VAS pain: best = 0.

(MCII) deals with the concept of improvement (feeling better), whereas the PASS deals with the concept of well-being or remission/improvement of symptoms (feeling good) (Tubach et al., 2006). Interestingly, the MCII was shown to be the change required to achieve the PASS, whatever the baseline level of symptoms, outcome (pain or function), or type of condition (chronic or acute). This acceptable state for pain was higher with chronic than acute conditions (27.0–36.4 vs. 16.7–24.1 on a scale of 0–100 across the baseline score) (Tubach et al., 2006).

In one study of OA, the PASS varied by tertiles of baseline scores (with knee OA, the PASS estimate for the WOMAC function scale was higher for more disabled than less disabled patients [43.1 vs. 20.4]) but not by age, disease duration, or gender (Tubach et al., 2005). In another study of knee and hip OA, the PASS was higher for patients with more than less pain, obese than nonobese patients, females than males, and patients >75 than ≤75 years old (Perrot and Bertin, 2013). In the different studies, PASS estimates for self-reported outcomes were estimated by an anchoring method based on patient opinion and targeting the 75th percentile of the cumulative distribution (Tables 16.3 and 16.4).

The PASS values were comparable with two different anchors in the Nancy_thermal cohort and was a little higher in the KHOALA cohort, which suggests that in observational studies, patients accept a higher level of QoL impairment and consider their state satisfactory with this higher level of impairment. The published PASS estimates were slightly lower for the WOMAC functional disability than in the Nancy_thermal cohort, but patients were recruited by their rheumatologist and not from the general population. The anchor also differed.

In a sample of patients with five rheumatic diseases treated with a nonsteroidal anti-inflammatory drug, the PASS estimates for pain and physical function measured with specific instruments were consistent across diseases and across countries when sample sizes were sufficient (Tubach et al., 2012). The study found a PASS value of 40 on a scale of 0–100 that could reasonably be used. For each PRO measure (PROm), patients with hip or knee OA who had the highest baseline scores had the highest PASS estimate. However, patients receiving effective treatment may have different expectations of treatment efficacy, which may affect PASS estimates.

So far, the PASS has been mainly determined in interventional studies to inform the efficacy of treatment. In observational studies, the PASS can be used to determine the evolution at the individual level, but the thresholds could be different.

Factors associated with perceived health

In a healthy or ill population, numerous factors affecting perceived health measures, such as sociodemographic characteristics (age and gender, deprivation), personality (optimism, self-confidence, etc.), or cultural factors should be taken into account in interpreting data.

Table 16.3 Published patient-acceptable symptom state (PASS) for hip or knee osteoarthritis (OA)

Scale	Location (reference)	PASS values	
VAS (0–100)			
Pain	Knee	32.3	Tubach et al. (2005)
	Hip	35.0	Tubach et al. (2005)
	Knee and hip	46.0	Tubach et al. (2012)
Pain at rest	Knee and hip	40.0	Perrot and Bertin (2013)
Pain on movement	Knee and hip	50.0	Perrot and Bertin (2013)
Patient global assessment	Knee	32.0	Tubach et al. (2005)
	Hip	34.6	Tubach et al. (2005)
	Knee and hip	47.0	Tubach et al. (2012)
WOMAC functional disability	Knee	31.0	Tubach et al. (2005)
(0–100)	Hip	34.4	Tubach et al. (2005)
	Knee and hip	46.0	Tubach et al. (2012)
	Knee and hip	48.0	Bellamy et al. (2015)
WOMAC pain (0–100)	Knee and hip	39.0	Bellamy et al. (2015)

VAS, visual analog scale; WOMAC, Western Ontario and McMaster Universities Osteoarthritis Index.

For ill patients, the presence of comorbidities is an important issue. Patient QoL is much impaired with the presence of several chronic diseases (Loza et al., 2008; Rijken et al., 2005; Michelson et al., 2000), particularly for physical dimensions of QoL (Michelson et al., 2000). However, interesting questions are the relative impact of each disease on QoL, whether the most serious disease is responsible for the greatest impact on QoL, and whether the effects of different diseases on QoL are additive or whether a synergy or an interaction exists.

Some effect modifiers have been highlighted. Rijken et al. (2005) and Fortin et al. (2007) reported a synergistic negative effect of the association of diabetes, cardiovascular disease, and chronic respiratory disease and QoL. Patients with these disease associations were at greater risk of physical disability than was expected from the separate effects. Other additive or synergistic rather than subtractive interactions have been described (Oldridge et al., 2001; Ettinger et al., 1994; Wee et al., 2005).

Table 16.4 PASS in the KHOALA and Nancy_thermal studies

	KHOALA SF-36[a]	Nancy_thermal SF-36[a]	Nancy_thermal Global assessment[b]
OAKHQOL			
Physical activities	47.5	50.6	46.0
Pain	60.0	50.0	47.5
Mental health	39.2	38.0	35.4
Social functioning	56.7	40.0	36.7
Social support	67.5	58.8	55.0
SF-36			
Physical functioning	55.0	55.0	50.0
Bodily pain	68.0	59.0	59.0
Mental health	52.0	44.0	40.0
Social functioning	50.0	37.5	37.5
Vitality	60.0	55.0	50.0
WOMAC			
Function	48.4	42.6	41.2
Pain	45.0	45.0	40.0
Stiffness	57.0	48.0	45.0

SF-36, short form 36; KHOALA, Knee and Hip Osteoarthritis Long-term Assessment; WOMAC, Western Ontario and McMaster Universities Osteoarthritis Index; OAKHQOL, OA Knee and Hip Quality Of Life; PASS, patient-acceptable symptom state.
a   SF-36 global health state item.
b   Taking into account all the activities you have during your daily life, your level of pain, and also your functional impairment, do you consider that your current state is satisfactory?

Among patients with multimorbidity, those with a musculoskeletal disease, mainly OA, showed the greatest impaired function and QoL over those without (Bellamy et al., 2015). In patients with hip OA in the KHOALA cohort, increased body mass index (BMI) and being socially disadvantaged but not the presence of a cardiovascular comorbidity were independently associated with reduced HRQoL. The relationship between BMI and HRQoL was not modified by social disadvantage or cardiovascular disease. In contrast, Sowers et al. (2009) showed that the presence of cardiometabolic diseases exacerbated the effect of BMI on pain and physical functioning dimensions of HRQoL in women with knee OA. Self-reported comorbidities seem to be better associated with QoL scores than diagnoses reported in medical charts or other indices of comorbidities (ten Klooster et al., 2006). Other factors that can affect changes in HRQoL include treatment factors, patient expectations, and increased social support and self-monitoring that occur during treatment.

Assessment of health data as a change

HRQoL measures are commonly used to assess the result of a medical intervention or to analyze the natural disease course, and despite their widespread use, data are lacking on whether the observed changes are clinically meaningful as opposed to statistically significant. In interpreting longitudinal data, the meaningful difference or change in score needs to be defined. Estimates of change in health state can be analyzed at the individual or group level.

Methods to interpret a perceived health change at an individual level: Definition of "responder"

At the individual level, interpreting longitudinal data supposes previous determination of "responders" or patients in different groups defined by evolution of disease, such as worsened, stable, or improved. To determine these groups, one can use change in scores or minimal important difference (MID), final health state such as the PASS, or comparison to the healthy population or both (Tubach et al., 2005; Crosby et al., 2003; Beaton et al., 2002).

A composite definition of a responder, the OsteoArthritis Research Society International—Outcome Measures in Rheumatology (OARSI-OMERACT) set of criteria, was first used in clinical trials of OA. This definition was based on expert opinion and combined pain and functional disability measures and patient global assessment. Thresholds of 20% or 50% improvement or 10 or 20 absolute units of change were used as responder criteria (Pham et al., 2004). Other definitions based on arbitrary thresholds included an improvement of 20% or 50% in criteria such as pain or WOMAC scores (Bellamy et al., 1988, 2005).

Patients reaching the PASS or the MID of a PROm are another way to interpret changes in scores that otherwise are expressed as units of an abstract scale that are not directly meaningful.

Definition of responder based on change: MID

The MID has been defined as the smallest change in a PROm that is perceived by patients as beneficial or would result in a clinician considering a change in treatment (Guyatt et al., 2002; Jaeschke et al., 1989). In the 2009 release of the US Food and Drug Administration Guidance for Industry Patient-Reported Outcomes (US FDA guidelines for PROs), the definition for response is "a score change in a measure, experienced by an individual patient over a predetermined time period that has been demonstrated in the target population to have a significant treatment benefit" (FDA, 2006). With OA-specific scales, MIDs have been defined for the VAS for pain, the WOMAC index, particularly the physical function score, and QoL scores. However, when using a predefined MID value, the sources of variations in this MID should be known to interpret the results.

Perspectives of the MID: Individual versus group

The interpretation of change in score can be based on different perspectives: whether the analysis is at the individual or group level (computation of the answers of responders or difference of the mean between groups), the scores to compare (change in a group over time, cross-sectional difference between groups, difference in changes over time between groups), and the kind of change assessed (minimum potentially detectable, observed change detectable given the measurement error of the instrument, or observed changes in patients with an important change according to an external standard) (Beaton et al., 2001).

An MID estimated as a group mean change for patients with sufficient improvement according to an external standard is not an appropriate threshold for individual change. Group change and individual change have different standard errors, and thus group-level estimates should not be used to define responders. In the 2009 release of the US FDA guidelines for PROs, the concept of "mean effect" (differences between group means) is clearly differentiated from a responder effect (change in an individual patient that would be considered important).

Methods to define an MID

Many authors recommend anchor-based methods because they compare observed score differences with external criteria that have clinical relevance. Distribution-based methods provide an alternative when an appropriate anchor is not available but do not directly reflect patient preferences or assessments of meaningful change (FDA, 2006). However, one of the advantages of distribution-based methods is that they can establish change beyond some level of random variation.

Numerous anchor- or distribution-based approach methods have been used (Crosby et al., 2003; Terwee et al., 2010; Copay et al., 2007; Revicki et al., 2008; Beaton et al., 2011; Rouquette et al., 2014; McLeod et al., 2011; Schunemann et al., 2006), each with specific shortcomings. A few authors found similarities in different threshold methods (Wyrwich et al., 1999), most concluding on wide variability (Beaton et al., 2002, 2011; Terwee et al., 2010; Turner et al., 2010). The MID for questionnaires has recently been determined as an interval scale, the trait level scale, with item response theory (IRT) models (Rouquette et al., 2014).

In OA, examples of these differences have been published for VAS pain, WOMAC, and SF-36 scores. OAKHQOL MIDs were also determined to illustrate the variability with a newly developed instrument (Tables 16.5 and 16.6).

The MID for improvement always differed from the MID for worsening, most of the time smaller for improvement than for worsening.

Table 16.5 Variations in MID estimations by VAS pain, WOMAC, and SF-36 scores in OA

Scale	Domain	Location	MID		MCII	Study
			Worsening	Improvement	improvement %	
VAS (0–100)	Pain	Knee			19.9 (40.8)	(Tubach et al., 2005)
		Hip			15.3 (32.0)	
	Pain (17)				10.0	(Perrot and Bertin, 2013)
	Patient global (47)	Knee			18.3 (39.0)	(Tubach et al., 2005)
		Hip			15.2 (32.6)	
WOMAC (0–100)	Function	Knee			29.1 (26.0)	(Tubach et al., 2005)
		Hip			27.9 (21.1)	
	Function	Hip/knee			12.0 (20.0)	(Tubach et al., 2012)
	Function		13.3	6.7		(Angst et al., 2001)
	Function		9.3			(Ehrich et al., 2000)
	Pain		11.0	7.5		(Angst et al., 2001)
	Pain		9.7			(Ehrich et al., 2000)
	Stiffness		5.1	7.2		(Angst et al., 2001)
	Stiffness		10.0			(Ehrich et al., 2000)

(Continued)

Table 16.5 Variations in MID estimations by VAS pain, WOMAC, and SF-36 scores in OA (*Continued*)

Scale	Domain	Location	MID Worsening	MID Improvement	MCII improvement %	Study
SF-36	Bodily pain		7.2	7.8		(Angst et al., 2001)
(0–100)	Physical function		5.3	3.3		(Angst et al., 2001)
	PCS score		2		2	(Angst et al., 2001)

WOMAC, Western Ontario and McMaster Universities Osteoarthritis Index; VAS, visual analog scale; SF-36, short form 36; OA, osteoarthritis; PCS, physical component summary; MID, minimal important difference; MCII, minimal clinically important improvement.

Table 16.6 Variations in MID estimations of the WOMAC, SF-36, and OAKHQOL scores in OA from the KHOALA cohort and Nancy_thermal study

Sample	KHOALA	KHOALA	Nancy_thermal	Nancy_thermal	KHOALA	KHOALA	Nancy_thermal	Nancy_thermal	KHOALA	KHOALA
Anchor	SF-36	SF-36	SF-36	VAS	Flexion	SF-36	SF-36	VAS	0.5 SD	SEM
Method	MID	MID	MID	MID	MID	MCII	MCII	MCII		
Direction	Impairment	Improvement	Improvement	Improvement	Improvement					
	n = 155	n = 66	n = 32	n = 64	n = 262	n = 66	n = 32	n = 64		
OAKHQOL										
Physical activities	5.8	6.3	16.2	6.7	10.7	12.5	26.5	14.7	10.8	8.9
Pain	6.9	4.5	21.7	9.3	14.3	17.5	35.0	22.5	12.1	11.9
Mental health	6.3	3.5	13.9	3.4	6.7	9.2	21.5	10.8	10.7	9.5
Social functioning	−0.6	4.0	5.6	1.5	6.2	13.3	21.7	10.0	13.9	18.7
Social support	−4.1	−0.5	1.6	2.4	1.4	17.5	16.3	12.5	12.9	21.0
SF-36										
Physical functioning	4.4	11.6	15.5	5.8	5.9	20.0	25.5	20.0	11.6	11.7
Bodily pain	6.5	8.7	22.4	0.9	15.6	21.0	33.0	20.0	10.0	11.8

(Continued)

Table 16.6 Variations in MID estimations of the WOMAC, SF-36, and OAKHQOL scores in OA from the KHOALA cohort and Nancy_thermal study (*Continued*)

Sample	KHOALA		Nancy_thermal			KHOALA	Nancy_thermal		KHOALA	
Anchor	SF-36		SF-36	VAS	Flexion	SF-36	SF-36	VAS	0.5 SD	SEM
Method	MID	MID	MID	MID	MID	MCII	MCII	MCII		
Direction	Impairment	Improvement	Improvement	Improvement	Improvement					
	$n=155$	$n=66$	$n=32$	$n=64$	$n=262$	$n=66$	$n=32$	$n=64$		
OAKHQOL										
Mental health	1.2	5.6	13.9	2.4	5.7	16.0	16.0	16.0	9.6	9.8
Social functioning	5.3	7.1	9.8	5.2	10.8	25.0	18.8	12.5	11.3	13.1
Vitality	3.3	5.4	11.4	4.2	8.0	15.0	17.5	10.0	8.8	9.3
WOMAC										
Function	1.1	9.6	20.4	11.0	12.1	16.3	29.4	17.2	11.0	9.2
Pain	7.0	5.4	17.6	13.3	15.0	15.0	23.8	17.2	9.6	9.0

WOMAC, Western Ontario and McMaster Universities Osteoarthritis Index; SF-36, short form 36; OA, osteoarthritis; KHOALA, Knee and Hip Osteoarthritis Long-term Assessment; OAKHQOL, OA Knee and Hip Quality of Life; MID, minimal important difference; MCII, minimal clinically important improvement; SEM, standard error of the mean.
Note: For all scales, 100 = best.
Differences exist between the KHOALA and Nancy_thermal cohorts, which illustrates the impact of the sample on MID determination. Different anchors also result in different MID values: in the Nancy_thermal, the MID for the SF-36 was the lowest. The MCII was higher than the MID, and the SEM in the KHOALA cohort was between the MID and MCII.

As another example, a cross-sectional study design based on interindividual comparisons was used to estimate the MID of seven measures of fatigue in 61 patients with RA. After completing the fatigue questionnaires, subjects had several one-on-one conversations with different people in the group to discuss their fatigue. After each conversation, each patient compared their fatigue to their partner's by a global rating. The ratings were compared with the scores of the fatigue measures to estimate the MID. Both nonparametric and linear regression analyses were used (Figure 16.3) (Pouchot et al., 2008). Indeed, both usual anchor-based cross-sectional and longitudinal designs provide group-based MID estimates. The estimates are obtained by relating mean values for clinical assessments for different subjective comparison ratings to measurements of the underlying concept taken as the independent variable. To derive the individual-based MID, models for predicting values of the measured concept from the measured health state values were used. In regression-based estimates, the individual-based MID is mathematically equal to the group-based MID times the ratio of the variance of both estimates (the variance larger for the individual-based estimate reflecting the additional uncertainty in individual observations on patients). The more sensitive an instrument, the larger the group-based MID and the smaller the individual-based MID (Pouchot et al., 2008).

Anchors used to define an MID

With the anchor-based approach, potential retrospective anchors can be patient ratings, clinician ratings, and direct clinical anchors. They should be adapted to each disease and to the different subscales (Wyrwich et al., 2013).

The most common anchor is the patient global rating of change. The change scores for patients reporting "minimal" or "small" changes are averaged to calculate the MID. For patients reporting moderate and large changes, an important difference threshold can be defined to determine the definition of response with important improvement expected from a treatment as, for example, with total hip replacement surgery. One must establish the amount of change in the anchor that is a reasonable indicator of the minimal change before determining an MID and when one wants to use a specific threshold.

Patient global rating of change may not be appropriate for diseases of which symptoms vary during short periods of time. Change in the number of "symptom-free days" has been studied in patients with asthma and could provide meaningful data in OA.

Other examples of anchors are patient ratings of satisfaction with the results of an intervention, a clinical anchor, amount of ingested pain medication (Farrar et al., 2000), combined patient and clinician ratings of improvement (Stratford et al., 1998), experience of future events such as mortality or medical care use, or social comparison, whereby patients compare themselves to other patients (Copay et al., 2007). The anchor item might refer globally to change in HRQoL but might be worded more specifically, such as physical functioning, pain, and

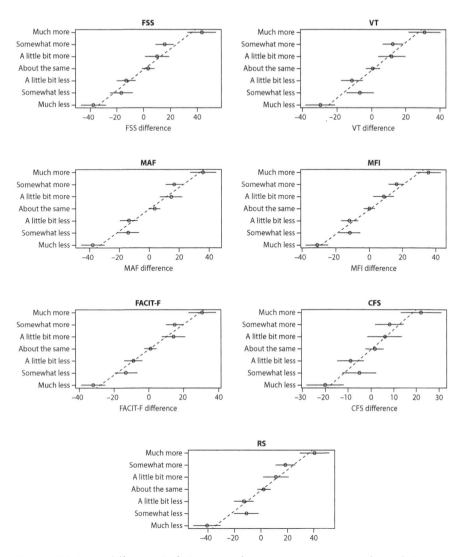

Figure 16.3 Mean differences in fatigue score for seven measurement tools in relation to pairwise contrasts for 61 patients with rheumatoid arthritis. The results are presented as normalized fatigue scores from 0 to 100 with mean differences in fatigue score and 95% confidence intervals for all seven contrast categories and regression lines. The plotted lines represent the regression of differences against integer scores (i.e., inverse regression). FSS, Fatigue Severity Scale; VT, Vitality Scale of the Medical Outcomes Study Short Form 36 items (MOS-SF36) questionnaire; MAF, Multidimensional Assessment of Fatigue; MFI, Multidimensional Fatigue Inventory; FACIT–F, Functional Assessment of Chronic Illness Therapy–Fatigue Scale; CFS, Chalder Fatigue Scale; RS, global assessment of fatigue by a 10-point numerical rating scale. (From Pouchot, J. et al., *J. Clin. Epidemiol.*, 61, 705–713, 2008.)

psychological state. The choice of words and the number of response categories of the anchor may also affect the value of the MID (Copay et al., 2007).

In interpreting results with an MID, some characteristics of the anchor should be checked. The anchor validity should be established and correlated with the PRO. The anchor correlation with the actual change score should be at least 0.30–0.35 (using Cohen's rules of thumb), although alternative thresholds may be acceptable with supplementary information (Revicki et al., 2008). In our example, correlations between QoL scores and our anchor (SF-36 general health items) were moderate, between 0.22 and 0.38, except for the social support score (low correlation).

Improvement versus deterioration in determining an MID

MIDs for improvement or deterioration are not symmetrical. A smaller change may be needed to be considered clinically important when a patient's condition is improving rather than worsening. For example, for the general health dimension of the SF-36, the threshold was smaller for improvement than deterioration (1.58 vs. –7.91 points) (Rouquette et al., 2014).

Impact of baseline impairment in MID determination

The MID is largely affected by baseline PROm level (Rouquette et al., 2014; Stratford et al., 1998; Terwee et al., 2010; de Vet et al., 2007; Crosby et al., 2004; ten Klooster et al., 2006). In a study determining a meaningful change in HRQoL in response to weight loss treatment, HRQoL change was more strongly associated with baseline HRQoL severity than with the weight lost. HRQoL change was greater with more severe baseline HRQoL impairment. Furthermore, a significant interaction between weight loss and baseline HRQoL impairment suggested that the effect of weight change on HRQoL change was minimal with no baseline HRQoL impairment but was substantial with severe impairment (Crosby et al., 2004).

In OA, baseline scores affect the MCII, that is, the 75th percentile of the change in score for patients who considered they had a slightly or moderately important improvement in WOMAC function scale and VAS pain. Patients with more severe symptoms at baseline need to have more improved scores than do those with less severe symptoms so that they feel improved (Tubach et al., 2005). Interestingly, the MCII was also shown to be the change required to achieve the PASS, whatever the baseline level of symptom, outcome (pain or function), or type of condition (chronic or acute). Patients considered that they experienced an important improvement only if this improvement allowed them to achieve a state they considered satisfactory (Tubach et al., 2006).

Several potential reasons explain the association of baseline scores and change scores: the regression to the mean (RTM), floor and ceiling effect, and noninterval scales (Copay et al., 2007; Rouquette et al., 2014). The RTM suggests that patients with extreme scores should show a greater change for a clinically meaningful change than those with less extreme scores. The RTM is established by showing a significant correlation between baseline distance from the mean (typically a normative mean) and pre-to-post change. In the KHOALA cohort, correlations between the baseline distance from the mean of the SF-36 scores in a reference population and pre-to-post change varied from 0.38 (bodily pain) to 0.48 (social functioning dimension). Not correcting for the RTM may result in a less conservative MID, particularly for patients with severe HRQoL impairment at baseline. Several methods have been proposed to correct for RTM: use of the percentage of change rather than raw change scores or define a range of minimal clinically important difference (MCID) rather than an absolute MCID (Copay et al., 2007), Edwards–Nunnally method (Crosby et al., 2004), or use of the linking equation (unaffected by r): MID = Anchor Change × (standard deviation target/standard deviation anchor) (Fayers and Hayes, 2014).

Another reason for the association between baseline scores and change scores could be that the scale level of the score does not necessarily have interval scale properties. The MID derived from IRT models that express the results in terms of an interval scale could provide fewer misclassifications of patients experiencing "at least a minimally important change" versus "no change" over time than with the MID determined by the score scale. However, one study showed that determining the MID for the SF-36 general health subscale with IRT models did not greatly enhance its sensitivity, specificity, and predictive values as compared with determination by the score scale (Rouquette et al., 2014).

Floor or ceiling effects of a PROm can limit its change. Patients with baseline scores close to the ends of the scale are not able to show a great improvement because such a change would exceed the span of the scale. On the reverse, a PROm would not be able to detect an impairment if patients are far above the best values at baseline. The KHOALA cohort showed no floor effect (<3% of all PROm scores were 0). A ceiling effect existed for the social activities score, which suggests that many patients are not limited in their social activities and cannot improve their score. However, in an observational study, the absence of a ceiling effect is probably less important.

Impact of sampling

The demographic, clinical, natural history of the disease, and other characteristics could influence the MID. In OA, the MCII of the WOMAC function score and VAS for pain were not affected by age, sex, joint, or disease duration in one study (Tubach et al., 2005) but were affected by level of pain at baseline and BMI in another (Perrot and Bertin, 2013). However, in a sample of five rheumatic diseases, the MCII estimates were consistent across diseases and countries when the samples were sufficient. An MCII of 15/100 for absolute improvement and 20% for relative improvement in reporting the results of trials with the outcome criteria of pain, patient global assessment, functional disability, or physician global assessment seemed appropriate for any of the five involved rheumatic diseases (Tubach et al., 2012). In OA, differences exist between the KHOALA and Nancy_thermal cohorts; however, sample sizes were small.

Impact of response shift

Memory bias and response shift can affect the MID. Patient perceptions of the concept assessed by the questionnaire and changes in patient values may occur between two assessments and thus modify the MID. To avoid this bias, the determination of the MID would be ideally preceded by a verification of the absence of a response shift.

Recommendations

Recommendations are to estimate the MID with several anchor-based methods involving relevant clinical or patient-based indicators, examine various distribution-based estimates, and then triangulate on a single value or small range of values for the MID (Yost et al., 2005; Purcell et al., 2010). The US FDA guidelines for PROs recommend the use of empirical evidence derived from anchor-based methods. Distribution-based methods are considered supportive in determining clinical significance but are not appropriate as the sole definition of response (FDA, 2006).

Several examples exist of attempts made to combine different information to determine an MID. In a few studies, a patient's condition was considered improved (or deteriorated) only when anchor- and distribution-based criteria were met for establishing a clinically meaningful change (Crosby et al., 2004; Cella et al., 2002). For some authors, the smallest detectable change is considered a complement toward establishing the MID when anchor-based methods or different populations yield different MID values. In these cases, the knowledge that one value is below the smallest detectable change could aid in the decision to select the other value (Turner et al., 2010).

Definition of responder based on final state

The PASS estimate and comparison to a reference population described above can help define a response.

Impact of various definitions of responders

The impact of various methods in defining response is not negligible. In comparing different combinations of approaches, Bauer et al. found responses of 24%–46% and moderate agreement (Bauer et al., 2004). Beaton et al. (2011) found a large variability in the proportion of patients considered responders (39%–89%). Final-state approaches and combined approaches had similar sensitivity and specificity in defining response according to an external anchor of meeting treatment goals. The MID-only approaches tended to be sensitive but lacked specificity, so numerous patients are falsely considered responders when they are not. In the KHOALA cohort, the proportion of patients with improved scores varied (Table 16.7).

Table 16.7 Proportion of patients with improved and impaired difference scores in the KHOALA and Nancy_thermal (N_thermal) cohorts

Scale	Improved patients					Impaired patients
	KHOALA Low MID	High MID	N_thermal MID	KHOALA PASS	N_thermal PASS	MID
OAKHQOL						
Physical activities	21.7	12.4	3.0	21.1	19.7	33.6
Pain	36.0	12.9	3.1	46.6	31.8	36.9
Mental health	35.6	18.3	5.7	7.5	6.4	29.9
Social functioning	33.5	16.5	13.7	26.6	13.3	59.7
Social support	56.8	21.0	–	63.1	47.9	54.9
SF-36						
Physical functioning	20.2	11.8	6.4	35.1	30.0	38.9
Bodily pain	30.6	9.7	3.7	46.6	31.8	39.4
Mental health	31.7	14.9	–	32.3	16.0	41.8
Social functioning	32.6	16.6	–	25.5	11.5	34.3
Vitality	25.3	14.9	8.0	73.3	51.6	43.9
WOMAC						
Function	27.5	13.3	3.8	73.2	63.7	35.6
Pain	23.1	13.3	4.4	75.3	68.6	29.8

WOMAC, Western Ontario and McMaster Universities Osteoarthritis Index; SF-36, short form 36; KHOALA, Knee and Hip Osteoarthritis Long-term Assessment; OAKHQOL, OA Knee and Hip Quality of Life; MID, minimal important difference; PASS, patient-acceptable symptom state.

The proportion of responders differed by more than 10% according to the MID method used and was often higher when using the PASS definition. The proportion was always higher for impaired than improved scores.

For clinical trials, two publications found that although the MID or PASS or combinations of thresholds differed, the relative differences in responders between two groups were similar (Tubach et al., 2009; Lemieux et al., 2007).

Thus, data now suggest that researchers and clinicians should work with a range of MID values and consider both the final state, the combinations of the final state, and the change (Beaton et al., 2011).

Because a range of MID estimates often varies across patient populations and clinical study contexts, an analysis of the cumulative distribution of responses (i.e., the proportion of patients who experience every magnitude of change) could allow the researcher to select a response threshold appropriate for the particular application (Figure 16.4). This approach avoids the need to define a unique threshold for a response (FDA, 2006; McLeod et al., 2011; Wyrwich et al., 2013). The percentage of responders at each value of the PRO change score is provided, if that value is considered the responder threshold (McLeod et al., 2011).

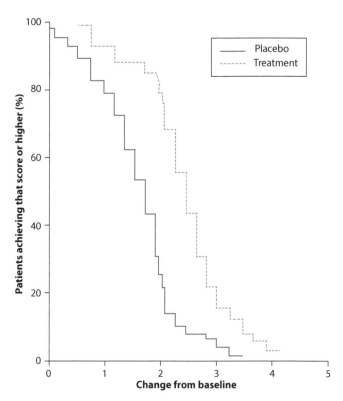

Figure 16.4 Sample cumulative distribution function. *y*-axis represents the proportion of patients who are considered responders at a particular threshold value (i.e., the proportion of patients who experience a score change of X points or more): when higher change scores indicate improvement, the curves will most often be shown as decreasing from left to right because as change scores increase, fewer patients achieve improvement at that value or higher. (From McLeod, L.D. et al., *Expert Rev. Pharmacoecon. Outcomes Res.*, 11, 163–169, 2011. The data used to draw this figure were generated for illustration purposes.)

Methods to interpret a perceived health change at a group level

When planning clinical trials involving PRO assessment, identifying the minimum difference in mean change from baseline between treatment groups that can be interpreted as an MID remains an important threshold to consider because the MID value will affect sample size calculation. The evolution of PROm should be depicted by graphs comparing different groups (e.g., by joint, as in the KHOALA cohort) (Figure 16.5).

At the group level, over only the first 4 years, evolution was fairly stable, with HRQoL lower for patients with knee and hip OA than knee or hip OA alone.

Evolution over time is not simple to model because in chronic diseases, patterns of evolution are numerous (Figure 16.6).

Statistical measures have been proposed for identifying longitudinal patterns of change in quantitative health indicators (Leffondre et al., 2004).

Elements to interpret a change of a score

Response shift

Response shift, originally studied in the context of cancer, refers to the fact that the meaning of a PRO changes over time. According to the Sprangers and Schwartz model, response shift refers to a change in the meaning of one's self-evaluation of a target construct as a result of recalibration (change in the respondent's internal standards of measurement), reprioritization (change in the respondent's values), and reconceptualization (redefinition of the target construct) (Sprangers et al., 1999; Oort et al., 2009; Rapkin et al., 2004). Changes

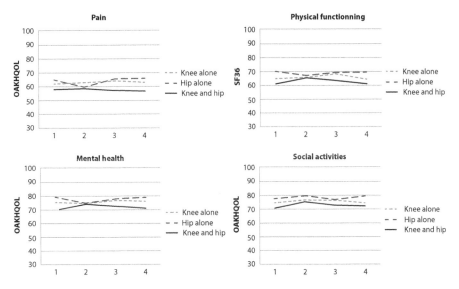

Figure 16.5 PRO evolution in knee alone, hip alone, or hip and knee OA in the KHOALA cohort. KHOALA, Knee and Hip Osteoarthritis Long-term Assessment; PRO, patient-reported outcome; OA, osteoarthritis.

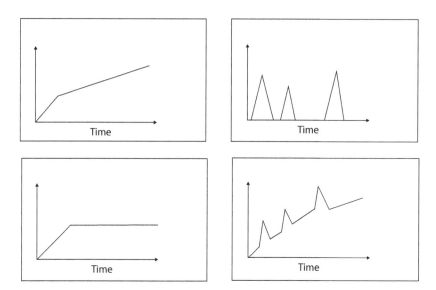

Figure 16.6 Examples of patterns of change.

in health, coping mechanisms, and the subject's characteristics and personality may induce a response shift that can hide or overestimate an accurate measurement of improved self-assessment of QoL. In contrast, the evaluation of response shift helps to capture dynamic changes in the illness experience. In rheumatology, few studies have been published on this phenomenon, mainly after total joint replacement surgery but never during the natural evolution of OA.

In randomized studies, the conceptualization of QoL or other PROm will be balanced between the groups and response shift will probably be similar among the groups except if the results of treatments differ greatly or if the intervention includes psychosocial, behavioral components, or support, as, for example, in therapeutic education or self-management programs. In these cases, the difference between two treatments could be reduced by a differential response shift: patients with health state impairments could lower their standards and patients with health state improvement could increase their standards. In observational studies, response shift can alter the comparison of repeated measurements and treatment effect changes.

Combination of health dimensions

Reporting the results of different dimensions of PROm results is important. Patients with chronic pain can perceive their level of pain as unchanged but with a clear improvement in their functional ability or psychological state.

Longitudinal patterns of change in symptomatic joints

In OA, as in most of the rheumatic diseases, one difficulty in interpreting longitudinal data is the variability in pain and also pain of the symptomatic joint. After total hip or knee replacement surgery, increased painful locations other than the arthroplasty location were associated with impaired QoL (Rat et al., 2010). Therefore, results of interventions or evolution of perceived health are complex to interpret. However, follow-up of the painful joints can also enlighten the patient evolution.

In the KHOALA cohort, the number of painful joints increases over time, so the number of patients with involvement of both hip and knee pain and bilateral pain increases (Table 16.8).

However, more detailed examination of the data showed a high variability in evolution because of no cumulative number of painful joints but sometimes disappearance of pain in one side instead of the other.

In terms of the agreement between the number of painful joints at baseline and at 3 years, data are more numerous in the right part of Table 16.9, which indicates increasing number of painful joints. However, the number of patients who are less symptomatic at follow-up is not negligible.

Table 16.8 Evolution of symptomatic joints in the KHOALA cohort

Criterion	Year			
	0	*1*	*2*	*3*
	n = 878	*n = 795*	*n = 727*	*n = 747*
	n (%)	*n (%)*	*n (%)*	*n (%)*
No. of painful joints				
VAS pain <20/100	300 (34.2)	311 (43.4)	257 (43.1)	212 (28.4)
1	307 (35.0)	171 (23.9)	137 (23.0)	200 (26.8)
2	185 (21.1)	161 (22.5)	137 (23.0)	224 (30.0)
3	51 (5.8)	36 (5.0)	35 (5.9)	65 (8.7)
4	33 (3.8)	37 (5.2)	30 (5.0)	45 (6.0)
Painful joint				
Knee alone	338 (58.7)	208 (51.4)	170 (50.1)	268 (50.2)
Hip alone	107 (18.6)	74 (18.3)	68 (20.1)	82 (15.4)
Knee and hip	131 (22.7)	123 (30.4)	101 (29.8)	184 (34.5)
Painful side				
Right	180 (31.3)	107 (26.4)	91 (26.8)	136 (25.5)
Left	157 (27.3)	101 (24.9)	75 (22.1)	118 (22.1)
Right and left	239 (41.5)	197 (48.6)	173 (51.0)	280 (52.4)

KHOALA, Knee and Hip Osteoarthritis Long-term Assessment; VAS, visual analog scale.

Table 16.9 Agreement in number of painful joints between baseline and follow-up at 3 years in the KHOALA cohort

	No. of painful joints at follow-up (3 years)					Total
	VAS pain, <20/100	1	2	3	4	
	n = 165	n = 155	n = 336	n = 100	n = 122	n = 878
No. of painful joints at baseline						
VAS pain <20/100	20	14	8	10	3	55
1	42	70	84	17	22	235
2	64	45	176	32	34	351
3	7	11	26	13	19	76
4	32	15	42	28	44	161

KHOALA, Knee and Hip Osteoarthritis Long-term Assessment; VAS, visual analog scale.

Quality of data and standards for perceived health measures

Effect of missing data on results

Quality of data is important for the critical interpretation of PRO results. According to best practices and as highlighted by the recommendations, completion rates, analyses of drop-out rates, and number of assessments that did not fall within a specified time window should be detailed. If missing data are related to the outcome being measured, then the resulting estimate of the treatment effect may be biased. Depending on the mechanism of the missing data, an appropriate analytic approach must be used for estimating change in PRO.

Instrument properties

Interpretability, considered an important characteristic of a measurement instrument, should be described with measurement properties. A full disclosure of information on the development, psychometric characteristics, and performance of perceived health instruments is a prerequisite to interpreting perceived health data.

Conclusions

Perceived health data outcomes are increasingly being reported, but we still need a greater understanding of the analyses and interpretation of PROm. Sources of variability of the results should be discussed and researchers should be encouraged to report their work with a range of methods. Researchers need to determine what is considered a clinically meaningful difference for a perceived health measure and report it for all studies involving PROs. With recommendations and standardization of the interpretation of perceived health data, these data will be credible for regulatory agencies.

References

Angst, F., Aeschlimann, A., and Stucki, G. (2001). Smallest detectable and minimal clinically important differences of rehabilitation intervention with their implications for required sample sizes using WOMAC and SF-36 quality of life measurement instruments in patients with osteoarthritis of the lower extremities. *Arthritis Rheum.*, 45(4), 384–391.

Bauer, S., Lambert, M.J., and Nielsen, S.L. (2004). Clinical significance methods: A comparison of statistical techniques. *J. Pers. Assess.*, 82(1), 60–70.

Beaton, D.E., Boers, M., and Wells, G.A. (2002). Many faces of the minimal clinically important difference (MCID): A literature review and directions for future research. *Curr. Opin. Rheumatol.*, 14(2), 109–114.

Beaton, D.E., Bombardier, C., Katz, J.N., Wright, J.G., Wells, G., Boers, M., et al. (2001). Looking for important change/differences in studies of responsiveness. OMERACT MCID Working Group. Outcome Measures in Rheumatology. Minimal Clinically Important Difference. *J. Rheumatol.*, 28(2), 400–405.

Beaton, D.E., Van, E.D., Smith, P., van d, V., Cullen, K., Kennedy, C.A, et al. (2011). Minimal change is sensitive, less specific to recovery: A diagnostic testing approach to interpretability. *J. Clin. Epidemiol.*, 64(5), 487–496.

Beaton, D.E., Van, E.D., Smith, P., van d, V., Cullen, K., Kennedy, C.A, et al. (2011). Minimal change is sensitive, less specific to recovery: A diagnostic testing approach to interpretability. *J. Clin. Epidemiol.*, 64(5), 487–496.

Bellamy, N., Bell, M.J., Goldsmith, C.H., Pericak, D., Walker, V., Raynauld, J.P, et al. (2005). Evaluation of WOMAC 20, 50, 70 response criteria in patients treated with hylan G-F 20 for knee osteoarthritis. *Ann. Rheum. Dis.*, 64(6), 881–885.

Bellamy, N., Buchanan, W.W., Goldsmith, C.H., Campbell, J., and Stitt, L.W. (1988). Validation study of WOMAC: A health status instrument for measuring clinically important patient relevant outcomes to antirheumatic drug therapy in patients with osteoarthritis of the hip or knee. *J. Rheumatol.*, 15(12), 1833–1840.

Bellamy, N., Hochberg, M., Tubach, F., Martin-Mola, E., Awada, H., Bombardier, C., et al. (2015). Development of multinational definitions of minimal clinically important improvement and patient acceptable symptomatic state in osteoarthritis. *Arthritis Care Res.* (Hoboken), 67(7), 972–980.

Cella, D., Eton, D.T., Lai, J.S., Peterman, A.H., and Merkel, D.E. (2002). Combining anchor and distribution-based methods to derive minimal clinically important differences on the Functional Assessment of Cancer Therapy (FACT) anemia and fatigue scales. *J. Pain Symptom Manage.*, 24(6), 547–561.

Copay, A.G., Subach, B.R., Glassman, S.D., Polly, D.W., Jr., and Schuler, T.C. (2007). Understanding the minimum clinically important difference: A review of concepts and methods. *Spine J.*, 7(5), 541–546.

Crosby, R.D., Kolotkin, R.L., and Williams, G.R. (2003). Defining clinically meaningful change in health-related quality of life. *J. Clin. Epidemiol.*, 56(5), 395–407.

Crosby, R.D., Kolotkin, R.L., and Williams, G.R. (2004). An integrated method to determine meaningful changes in health-related quality of life. *J. Clin. Epidemiol.*, 57(11), 1153–1160.

Cross, M., Smith, E., Hoy, D., Nolte, S., Ackerman, I., Fransen, M., et al. (2014). The global burden of hip and knee osteoarthritis: Estimates from the Global Burden of Disease 2010 study. *Ann. Rheum. Dis.*, 73, 1323–1330.

de Vet, H.C., Ostelo, R.W., Terwee, C.B., van der Roer, N., Knol, D.L., Beckerman, H., et al. (2007). Minimally important change determined by a visual method integrating an anchor-based and a distribution-based approach. *Qual. Life Res.*, 16(1), 131–142.

Ehrich, E.W., Davies, G.M., Watson, D.J., Bolognese, J.A., Seidenberg, B.C., and Bellamy, N. (2000). Minimal perceptible clinical improvement with the Western Ontario and McMaster Universities osteoarthritis index questionnaire and global assessments in patients with osteoarthritis. *J. Rheumatol.*, 27(11), 2635–2641.

Ettinger, W.H., Davis, M.A., Neuhaus, J.M., and Mallon, K.P. (1994). Long-term physical functioning in persons with knee osteoarthritis from NHANES. I: Effects of comorbid medical conditions. *J. Clin. Epidemiol.*, 47(7), 809–815.

Farrar, J.T., Portenoy, R.K., Berlin, J.A., Kinman, J.L., and Strom, B.L. (2000). Defining the clinically important difference in pain outcome measures. *Pain*, 88(3), 287–294.

Fayers, P.M., and Hayes, R.D. (2014). Don't middle your MIDs: Regression to the mean shrinks estimates of minimally important differences. *Qual. Life Res.*, 23(1), 1–4.

Fayers, P.M., Langston, A.L., and Robertson, C. (2007). Implicit self-comparisons against others could bias quality of life assessments. *J. Clin. Epidemiol.*, 60(10), 1034–1039.

FDA. (2006). Guidance for Industry Patient-Reported Outcomes: Use in Medical Product development to Support Labeling Claims. [cited 1912 Sept.] Available at: www.fda.gov/cder/guidance/5460dft.pdf

Fortin, M., Dubois, M.F., Hudon, C., Soubhi, H., and Almirall, J. (2007). Multimorbidity and quality of life: A closer look. *Health Qual. Life Outcomes*, 5, 52.

Guillemin, F., Rat, A.C., Mazieres, B., Pouchot, J., Fautrel, B., Euller-Ziegler, L., et al. (2011). Prevalence of symptomatic hip and knee osteoarthritis: A two-phase population-based survey. *Osteoarthritis Cartilage*, 19(11), 1314–1322.

Guillemin, F., Rat, A.C., Roux, C.H., Fautrel, B., Mazieres, B., Chevalier, X., et al. (2012). The KHOALA cohort of knee and hip osteoarthritis in France. *Joint Bone Spine*, 79(6), 597–603.

Guyatt, G.H., Osoba, D., Wu, A.W., Wyrwich, K.W., and Norman, G.R. (2002). Methods to explain the clinical significance of health status measures. *Mayo Clin. Proc.*, 77(4), 371–383.

Jacobson, N.S., Roberts, L.J., Berns, S.B., and McGlinchey, J.B. (1999). Methods for defining and determining the clinical significance of treatment effects: Description, application, and alternatives. *J. Consult. Clin. Psychol.*, 67(3), 300–307.

Jaeschke, R., Singer, J., and Guyatt, G.H. (1989). Measurement of health status. Ascertaining the minimal clinically important difference. *Control. Clin. Trials*, 10(4), 407–415.

Leffondre, K., Abrahamowicz, M., Regeasse, A., Hawker, G.A., Badley, E.M., McCusker, J., et al. (2004). Statistical measures were proposed for identifying longitudinal patterns of change in quantitative health indicators. *J. Clin. Epidemiol.*, 57(10), 1049–1062.

Lemieux, J., Beaton, D.E., Hogg-Johnson, S., Bordeleau, L.J., and Goodwin, P.J. (2007). Three methods for minimally important difference: No relationship was found with the net proportion of patients improving. *J. Clin. Epidemiol.*, 60(5), 448–455.

Leplège, A., and Coste, J. (1999). *Mesure De la Santé Perceptuelle et de la Qualité de Vie-Méthodes et Applications*. Paris: Estem éditions.

Loza, E., Jover, J.A., Rodriguez, L., and Carmona, L. (2008). Multimorbidity: Prevalence, effect on quality of life and daily functioning, and variation of this effect when one condition is a rheumatic disease. *Semin. Arthritis Rheum.*, 38, 312–319.

Marsh, A.P., Ip, E.H., Barnard, R.T., Wong, Y.L., and Rejeski, W.J. (2011). Using video animation to assess mobility in older adults. *J. Gerontol. A Biol. Sci. Med. Sci.*, 66(2), 217–227.

McLeod, L.D., Coon, C.D., Martin, S.A., Fehnel, S.E., and Hays, R.D. (2011). Interpreting patient-reported outcome results: US FDA guidance and emerging methods. *Expert Rev. Pharmacoecon. Outcomes Res.*, 11(2), 163–169.

Michelson, H., Bolund, C., and Brandberg, Y. (2000). Multiple chronic health problems are negatively associated with health related quality of life (HRQoL) irrespective of age. *Qual. Life Res.*, 9(10), 1093–1104.

Oldridge, N.B., Stump, T.E., Nothwehr, F.K., and Clark, D.O. (2001). Prevalence and outcomes of comorbid metabolic and cardiovascular conditions in middle- and older-age adults. *J. Clin. Epidemiol.*, 54(9), 928–934.

Oort, F.J., Visser, M.R., and Sprangers, M.A. (2009). Formal definitions of measurement bias and explanation bias clarify measurement and conceptual perspectives on response shift. *J. Clin. Epidemiol.*, 62(11), 1126–1137.

Perrot, S., and Bertin, P. (2013). "Feeling better" or "feeling well" in usual care of hip and knee osteoarthritis pain: Determination of cutoff points for patient acceptable symptom state (PASS) and minimal clinically important improvement (MCII) at rest and on movement in a national multicenter cohort study of 2414 patients with painful osteoarthritis. *Pain*, 154(2), 248–256.

Pham, T., van der Heijde, D., Altman, R.D., Anderson, J.J., Bellamy, N., Hochberg, M., et al. (2004). OMERACT-OARSI initiative: Osteoarthritis Research Society International set of responder criteria for osteoarthritis clinical trials revisited. *Osteoarthritis Cartilage*, 12(5), 389–399.

Picavet, H.S., and Hoeymans, N. (2004). Health related quality of life in multiple musculoskeletal diseases: SF-36 and EQ-5D in the DMC3 study. *Ann. Rheum. Dis.*, 63(6), 723–729.

Pouchot, J., Kherani, R.B., Brant, R., Lacaille, D., Lehman, A.J., Ensworth, S., et al. (2008). Determination of the minimal clinically important difference for seven fatigue measures in rheumatoid arthritis. *J. Clin. Epidemiol.*, 61(7), 705–713.

Purcell, A., Fleming, J., Bennett, S., Burmeister, B., and Haines, T. (2010). Determining the minimal clinically important difference criteria for the Multidimensional Fatigue Inventory in a radiotherapy population. *Support Care Cancer*, 18(3), 307–315.

Rapkin, B.D., and Schwartz, C.E. (2004). Toward a theoretical model of quality-of-life appraisal: Implications of findings from studies of response shift. *Health Qual. Life Outcomes*, 2, 14.

Rat, A.C., Loeuille, D., Vallata, A., Bernard, L., Spitz, E., Desvignes, A., Boulanger, M., Paysant, J., Guillemin, F., Chary Valckenaere, I. Comparison of spa therapy with or without physical rehabilitation for knee osteoarthritis: the Nancy-Thermal randomized controlled trial. Submitted for Publication.

Rat, A.C., Coste, J., Pouchot, J., Baumann, M., Spitz, E., Retel-Rude, N., et al. (2005). OAKHQOL: A new instrument to measure quality of life in knee and hip osteoarthritis. *J. Clin. Epidemiol.*, 58(1), 47–55.

Rat, A.C., Guillemin, F., Osnowycz, G., Delagoutte, J.P., Cuny, C., Mainard, D., et al. (2010). Total hip or knee replacement for osteoarthritis: Mid- and long-term quality of life. *Arthritis Care Res. (Hoboken)*, 62(1), 54–62.

Revicki, D., Hays, R.D., Cella, D., and Sloan, J. (2008). Recommended methods for determining responsiveness and minimally important differences for patient-reported outcomes. *J. Clin. Epidemiol.*, 61(2), 102–109.

Rijken, M., van Kerkhof, M., Dekker, J., and Schellevis, F.G. (2005). Comorbidity of chronic diseases: Effects of disease pairs on physical and mental functioning. *Qual. Life Res.*, 14(1), 45–55.

Rouquette, A., Blanchin, M., Sebille, V., Guillemin, F., Cote, S.M., Falissard, B., et al. (2014). The minimal clinically important difference determined using item response theory models: An attempt to solve the issue of the association with baseline score. *J. Clin. Epidemiol.*, 67(4), 433–440.

Schunemann, H.J., Akl, E.A., and Guyatt, G.H. (2006). Interpreting the results of patient reported outcome measures in clinical trials: The clinician's perspective. *Health Qual. Life Outcomes*, 4, 62.

Sowers, M., Karvonen-Gutierrez, C.A., Palmieri-Smith, R., Jacobson, J.A., Jiang, Y., and Ashton-Miller, J.A. (2009). Knee osteoarthritis in obese women with cardiometabolic clustering. *Arthritis Rheum.*, 61(10), 1328–1336.

Sprangers, M.A., de Regt, E.B., Andries, F., van Agt, H.M., Bijl, R.V., de Boer, J.B, et al. (2000). Which chronic conditions are associated with better or poorer quality of life?. *J. Clin. Epidemiol.*, 53(9), 895–907.

Sprangers, M.A., and Schwartz, C.E. (1999). Integrating response shift into health-related quality of life research: A theoretical model. *Soc. Sci. Med.*, 48(11), 1507–1515.

Stratford, P.W., Binkley, J.M., Riddle, D.L., and Guyatt, G.H. (1998). Sensitivity to change of the Roland-Morris Back Pain Questionnaire: Part 1. *Phys. Ther.*, 78(11), 1186–1196.

ten Klooster, P.M., Drossaers-Bakker, K.W., Taal, E., and van de Laar, M.A. (2006). Patient-perceived satisfactory improvement (PPSI): Interpreting meaningful change in pain from the patient's perspective. *Pain*, 121(1–2), 151–157.

Terwee, C.B., Roorda, L.D., Dekker, J., Bierma-Zeinstra, S.M., Peat, G., Jordan, K.P, et al. (2010). Mind the MIC: Large variation among populations and methods. *J. Clin. Epidemiol.*, 63(5), 524–534.

Tubach, F., Dougados, M., Falissard, B., Baron, G., Logeart, I., and Ravaud, P. (2006). Feeling good rather than feeling better matters more to patients. *Arthritis Rheum.*, 55(4), 526–530.

Tubach, F., Giraudeau, B., and Ravaud, P. (2009). The variability in minimal clinically important difference and patient acceptable symptomatic state values did not have an impact on treatment effect estimates. *J. Clin. Epidemiol.*, 62(7), 725–728.

Tubach, F., Ravaud, P., Baron, G., Falissard, B., Logeart, I., Bellamy, N., et al. (2005). Evaluation of clinically relevant states in patient reported outcomes in knee and hip osteoarthritis: The patient acceptable symptom state. *Ann. Rheum. Dis.*, 64(1), 34–37.

Tubach, F., Ravaud, P., Baron, G., Falissard, B., Logeart, I., Bellamy, N., et al. (2005). Evaluation of clinically relevant changes in patient reported outcomes in knee and hip osteoarthritis: The minimal clinically important improvement. *Ann. Rheum. Dis.*, 64(1), 29–33.

Tubach, F., Ravaud, P., Martin-Mola, E., Awada, H., Bellamy, N., Bombardier, C., et al. (2012). Minimum clinically important improvement and patient acceptable symptom state in pain and function in rheumatoid arthritis, ankylosing spondylitis, chronic back pain, hand osteoarthritis, and hip and knee osteoarthritis: Results from a prospective multinational study. *Arthritis Care Res. (Hoboken)*, 64(11), 1699–1707.

Turner, D., Schunemann, H.J., Griffith, L.E., Beaton, D.E., Griffiths, A.M., Critch, J.N, et al. (2010). The minimal detectable change cannot reliably replace the minimal important difference. *J. Clin. Epidemiol.*, 63(1), 28–36.

Vos, T., Flaxman, A.D., Naghavi, M., Lozano. R., Michaud, C., Ezzati, M., et al. (2012). Years lived with disability (YLDs) for 1160 sequelae of 289 diseases and injuries 1990–2010: A systematic analysis for the Global Burden of Disease Study 2010. *Lancet*, 380(9859), 2163–2196.

Wee, H.L., Cheung, Y.B., Li, S.C., Fong, K.Y., and Thumboo, J. (2005). The impact of diabetes mellitus and other chronic medical conditions on health-related Quality of Life: Is the whole greater than the sum of its parts?. *Health Qual. Life Outcomes*, 3, 2.

Wesseling, J., Dekker, J., van den Berg, W.B., Bierma-Zeinstra, S.M., Boers, M., Cats, H.A., et al. (2009). CHECK (Cohort Hip and Cohort Knee): Similarities and differences with the Osteoarthritis Initiative. *Ann. Rheum. Dis.*, 68(9), 1413–1419.

Wyrwich, K.W., Nienaber, N.A., Tierney, W.M., and Wolinsky, F.D. (1999). Linking clinical relevance and statistical significance in evaluating intra-individual changes in health-related quality of life. *Med. Care*, 37(5), 469–478.

Wyrwich, K.W., Norquist, J.M., Lenderking, W.R., and Acaster, S. (2013). Methods for interpreting change over time in patient-reported outcome measures. *Qual. Life Res.*, 22(3), 475–483.

Yost, K.J., Sorensen, M.V., Hahn, E.A., Glendenning, G.A., Gnanasakthy, A., and Cella, D. (2005). Using multiple anchor- and distribution-based estimates to evaluate clinically meaningful change on the Functional Assessment of Cancer Therapy-Biologic Response Modifiers (FACT-BRM) instrument. *Value Health*, 8(2), 117–127. Analysis and substantive work on modern organizations for understanding the trajectory of institutional change in both western and eastern Europe.

Section 4
Knowledge and decision

17 Perceived individual freedom and collectively provided care

Emmanuel Picavet

Introduction

How are we expected to deal collectively with the subjective freedom of choice in the presence of functional losses, both physical and mental? The problem gains relevance at a time when an ever-increasing number of institutions—and indeed, institutional forms—adapt to chronic (sometimes degenerative) illnesses and long-term health care. Individual patients are free persons and attention should be paid to their ability to organize their life as they plan to do, using specific aptitudes for that (Bratman, 1987; Schick, 1997; Kolm, 1998). Although this topic does not rank high on the present-day agenda of research, empirical knowledge about perceived capacities for choice and intentional deliberative action is likely to be increasingly relevant in this respect. It could result in significantly more elaborate ways to deal collectively with individual freedom of choice.

Being a free person creates a number of expectations when it comes to evaluating the conduct of other people toward the person. However, the extent and modalities of the expected "respect" are under scrutiny and arguments in the field always involve the nature of freedom and the associated normative claims. When pressing security and caring issues must be addressed simultaneously in practice, these arguments occasionally support divergent practical guidelines. At a fundamental level, collectively dealing with individual freedom of choice is somehow complicated by the conceptual difficulties that surround the legitimate claims associated with a person's status as a free person (Berlin, 1969; Benn and Weinstein, 1971).

The domain of free choice and the full use of our specifically *action-related* abilities (or "agency" status in philosophical parlance) are potentially impacted by functional deficits and losses; medical data are of course relevant in this respect. Furthermore, these deficits and losses condition the kind of well-adapted collective care that can be conventionally framed as "good practices." The way we deal with the agency status of cared-for people is therefore *indirect* by and large: making use of available and relevant information is only possible through the elaborate and conventional norm-setting of social practices in given institutional settings.

Allowing that functional deficits and losses result in increased interdependence between beneficiaries and care-providing persons in institutional settings the available information on agency status should be interpreted in terms of antecedently defined individual prerogatives, to be equated with "side constraints" on medical practice and caring services (especially, prescriptions not to meddle with beneficiaries' intentions). For example, we could consider that the ability to walk without aid should result in the capacity to do so with no restriction. Or should we promote an alternative view? This choice matters when it comes to choosing the conventions which should make it possible, in principle, to use the potentially available information on the freedom of choice. If we take the beneficiaries' agency status into account in an appropriate way, should we let them have independent and potentially risky initiatives? I will focus on a particular dimension of this kind of investigation.

The connections between the norms of collective care and individual perceptions of one's freedom of choice must be investigated with a view to characterizing this tension between basic objectives (measurement). Then I will argue that collective health and social care for people with persistent disabilities should rely on conventions pertaining to a shared commitment to take perceived individual freedom into account.

The entanglement of agency-based respect and care

Quality-of-life measurement and individual freedom

Two main questions call for conceptual investigation in the field that we have just delineated:

1. How are we to develop a conception of measurable capacity for choice and intentional deliberative action?

For the reasons, I have explained, the focus here is rather on a second, distinct (and related) question:

2. How is freedom of choice evidence (provided it is meaningful and available) to be articulated with the consequentialist dimension in collective care provision (i.e., the dimension which centers on the optimal production of valuable results, subject to the constraint of impartiality)?

As health-related quality-of-life (QoL) measurement has long made patent, subjective data in health care allow practitioners, institutional decision makers, and patients as well to rely on a fine-grained picture of individual mental and physical functionings (i.e., personal experiences and "doings"), choice-based capacities, and subjectively described well-being (see, e.g., Fagot-Largeault 1991; Leplège, 1996). Accordingly, as perceptual measures of the medical and psychological condition of individuals develop, it is pretty obvious that they are able to give versatile information on matters of interest for evaluative purposes.

They provide data on psychological states and medical states of affairs, from the point of view of the patient. But they also provide information on personal abilities or functionings, as well as choice capacities. Conceptual clarifications are called for, at the very least for interpretative purposes, whenever a linkage is to be established between available data and actual practice (see Leplège and Marciniak, 1997 for such an attempt).

First of all, let us recall that classical QoL measurement is not unfamiliar to freedom-related information, even when freedom concepts do not figure prominently in the explicit categories. A distinctive feature of QoL measurement is its ability to incorporate information pertaining to functional capabilities (and the lack or loss of them). Medical QoL measurement is indeed remarkable on account of its treatment of objective functional capabilities as central, definitional components of welfare itself. For example, attention is typically given to the ability of individuals to perform ordinary tasks of everyday life in such a way that they can fulfill their own wishes. This approach is rooted in the objective capacities of persons in concrete environments. It stands in sharp contrast with the predominant vision of utility or welfare, which portrays it (in the continuity of Pareto's landmark contribution in economics) as purely subjective (the vision which is targeted in Fleurbaey, 1996; Sen, 1987, 1991 among other contributions). Standard utility theory focuses on welfare or preference-satisfaction associated with "results" or final individual and social states. Subjective utility theories—in normative economics and in some ethical contributions alike—therefore leave no room for abilities or capabilities as such. Following theories of this kind, it can be allowed that abilities or capabilities account for the structure of preferences, but preferences themselves are usually taken as given, or left undefined, given that the formal structure of preferences is the proper object of investigation.

In contrast, QoL measurement deals with capabilities and freedom of choice, and the relevant concept of freedom depends in turn crucially on individual preferences. QoL measurement draws some of its relevance from nonutility information, but nonutility values have a deep connection with preferences or utilities here, even though it is well-known (at a theoretical level) that dealing with the two kinds of values simultaneously is a complex task, which raises logical difficulties (Klemisch-Ahlert, 1993; Gravel, 1994).

In Sen's widely used "functioning-and-capability" approach to welfare and freedom (see Sen, 1985, 1992), living itself can be equated with a set of interrelated "functionings" (beings and doings) such as "being adequately nourished," "being happy" (or "experiencing pleasure"), and "surviving." A person's state is then understood as a vector of functionings and the set of all the feasible combinations of functionings in such vectors is the "capability set." The capability set reflects the relevant constraints of feasibility, be they connected with budget, technical possibilities, and so on. It epitomizes information about a person's ability to achieve well-being while living as a freedom-concerned entity, with goals, values, and a concern for the nature and details of the chosen actions. We may also say, following Sugden (1993), that it expresses the person's positive freedom—that is, freedom in terms of "freedom to ..." rather than "freedom from ... ." Quite clearly, the measurement procedures for perceptual personal states of affairs that are used in medicine deal with this kind of information, which is potentially significant for collective caring procedures and the associated norms.

Practical dilemmas

In care-providing institutional settings—such as hospitals or medically equipped retirement houses, and in medically equipped prisons—organizational choices are dependent on information about functionings, abilities, and agency status. Indeed, such information bears on matters of potential free choice on the part of the cared-for agents. These agents are not *only* patients, but also agents who interact with other agents in collective organizations. To be sure, "consequentialist" (result-based) information on the quality of subjectively perceived patient's condition has given rise to hopes of better caring procedures based on such information. Even "consequentialist" information must be considered with a view to the details of circumstances and human relations; such details must be taken into account and this makes contextual personal judgment all-important. Compared with information about good and bad consequences of caring procedures for individuals, the freedom-related informative material is even less mechanically interpretable and translatable into caring strategies. The investigation of practical dilemmas that raise problems of freedom is, therefore, instructive.

Among existing practical dilemmas, let us mention those dilemmas that stem from the implementation of autonomy-based principles (in France, e.g., the principles of respect for the free choice of patients which are expressed in such normative documents as *Code de déontologie médicale* [Code of medical deontology] or *Charte des droits et libertés de la personne âgée dépendante* [Charter of the rights and freedoms of the dependent elderly person]), when conciliation with the prevention of personal risks is necessary. As emphasized by Amyot and Villez (2001), managers of caring institutions know that administrative law calls for prudence (endangering nobody), even "precaution." The scope of "precaution," however, is quite indefinite and does not presuppose—they argue—"precise knowledge of specific risks." Furthermore, in the *Fondation de France* project "*Dignité des personnes âgées, droit au choix, droit au risque et responsabilité*" (Dignity of elderly people, right to choice, right to risk-taking and responsibility), field work involving 140 caring professionals and elderly people shows that security-oriented practices are not without risk; for example, preventing people from going out of a building might induce fragile elderly people to commit suicide (Amyot and Villez, 2001).

One step further, let us distinguish possible (or future dilemmas) from real-world dilemmas about the conciliation of respect for individually perceived freedom and collectively provided care. The first species of dilemmas commands attention partly because greater conceptual precision has been acquired along several axes: measures of functional losses (in connection with legal or administrative approaches to handicap or disability, impairment and functional losses, or old-age "dependence"); applications of the functioning-and-capability theoretical analyses to health- and social-care contexts (Picavet and Guibet Lafaye, 2011 develop an example); philosophical and economic attempts to characterize and measure individual freedom in social contexts.

As a result, it becomes possible to characterize individual freedom of choice and capacity for intentional, deliberative action more accurately than ever. This is all the more useful that real-word dilemmas with similar causes exemplify substantial tensions or conflicts of values that are otherwise under scrutiny—sometimes with greater accuracy—in the exploration of possible, conceptual problems. Real-world dilemmas may thus benefit from the conceptual exploration of the latter. This is the reason why I will discuss a stylized situation.

Taking freedom into account: Partly a matter of convention and shared commitment

A stylized dilemma

Let us consider a collective choice situation (a variant of the classical applications of Sen's (1970) "Impossibility of a Paretian Liberal" paradox, absent meddlesome preferences and with the important difference that a duality of "personal domains"—one for each of two individuals—is not brought into the picture) (Brunel-Petron, 1998).

Agent M is part of the medical staff. Agent P (the "patient") is a person with functional impairments that justify special attention and collective care. Agent M considers he or she has a special responsibility, given his or her particular training, with respect to the way collective care is provided to agent P (on the basis of available data about the objective and subjective health status and/or functional status of agent P). Agent P, symmetrically, is a free individual who is expected to act on his or her own will in certain domains of human activity. Providing care on his or her behalf should not prevent the caring staff from paying due attention to the concrete expression of his or her autonomy. Obviously, functional losses usually leave personal autonomy intact (even though changes in the ability to act independently are sometimes carelessly described in terms of autonomy losses).

On a superficial analysis, this kind of stylized situation could be approached in terms of meddlesome preferences or, more accurately, paternalistic preferences: Given that M knows better than P about the risks involved in P's situation, M considers he or she should have a say, in a predominant manner, concerning the ranking of a particular set of options in connection with P's personal situation. Looking at the problem with such glasses, however, leads us to miss the important point that P is in principle amenable to share M's viewpoint on his or her own situation (supposing that M follows good, well-justified collective care-providing practices). Paternalism is unlikely to be the final word. Even when collective care gives a role to subjective health or functioning data, one can deal with these data in a competent or incompetent way and knowing one's expertise provides reasons to claim privileges with respect to handling certain situations in a given way.

Consider, more precisely, the following interaction between these agents. There are three alternatives, subjectively described from P's point of view:

—*a*: staying quietly in one's room
—*b*: trying to go down the stairs and being prevented half-way to go any further by the care-providing staff
—*c*: getting out and going around in the park in a free and risky manner

In such a situation, the agents could unanimously agree that *a* is better than *b*.

In some cases, P could consider himself or herself to be legitimately decisive over the {*a, c*} pair of alternatives. If P considers himself or herself to be in a quite satisfactory mental and physical condition, with the required abilities to go along in the park, this pair of alternatives may look like a personal domain of choice ("private matters" for short). This, however, might be an occasion of disagreement with agent M who cares for P. Given his or her professional training and personal judgment, agent M might consider it a duty to interfere with P's attempts to get out and go around unaided.

In such circumstances, M should be considered decisive over the {*b,c*} pair of alternatives. Is it possible, then, collectively to determine a consistent attitude toward the existing options? If we insist that there should be no inconsistent collective judgment, the answer is no, because, socially speaking, we should have given their preferences and the recognized prerogatives:

b preferred to *c*
c preferred to *a*

and (as we already noticed) *a* could be recognized better than *b* unanimously. The outcomes of the actions of M and P are summarized in Table 17.1.

Note that, unlike the formally similar "liberal paradox," this conceptual difficulty is in substance a triadic conflict (between possible unanimous agreement, subjectively assessed freedom, and well-founded expertise) rather than a dyadic conflict (between subjective freedom and unanimous agreement).

Table 17.1 Outcomes of actions

	M	M
P	–	a
P	b	c

Plausibly (though not necessarily):
P prefers *c* to *a* and *a* to *b*.
M prefers *a* to *b* and *b* to *c*.

For the problem at hand, this suggests a way out (which is sadly lacking in the original liberal paradox).

It is *prima facie* implausible to look at agent M's prerogative as absolute. It is in effect very unlike some abstract and general prerogatives to do with rights and freedom (that were under scrutiny in Sen's problem). It can only be exercised on the basis of personal judgment in the circumstances, given the details about agent P's objective health indicators, physical, and mental functionings, functional status on the relevant scores, and subjective health data. Respecting agent M's prerogative has nothing to do with respecting an *a priori* delineated sphere of prerogative. Hence, there is a possibility to argue in favor of vague formulations of the relevant rules, so that case-based reasoning is made possible (regrettably with all the correlated disadvantages when it comes to assessing personal responsibility).

Looking at agent P's situation, it is apparent that his or her willingness to try to get out and walk around is not absolute either: The willingness to do so is manifest if we compare *a* and *c*, but the reverse holds if we compare *a* and *b*. In a strict sense, it cannot be said that the agent "wants" or "plans" to get out, irrespective of information about agent M's attitudes.

In such a stylized example, it is difficult to believe that the problem is adequately framed if we describe it as a conflict between safety matters and an otherwise absolute right. The fact of being cared for in an institutional context (be it insulated from the rest of society or not) gives relevance to rules and social roles that wait for interpretation in given contexts. It seems quite clear that this conventional dimension must be acknowledged in the development of value-based practices, that is to say, skills-based approaches to working with complex and conflicting values.[1]

Subjective views of one's domain of freedom and subjective interpretations of prudential rules (and institutional roles), provided they are not treated as absolute claims, should be harmonized somehow. Formulating them and taking them into account should be viewed as components of a social process. To be sure, respect for individual preferences is important, because it is part of one's agency capabilities to help the others act toward him or her in the way he or she deems appropriate, especially when this kind of judgment is formulated with a clear mind, whereas the person enjoys full deliberative aptitudes.[2] Accordingly, should we take as a benchmark the overlap of some well-articulated preferential judgments on the part of individuals? Following this path, we should pay attention to well-informed agreements among agents. On the side of the cared-for persons, this might involve the amalgamation of information from advance directives to make full use of well-considered preferences in caring contexts that are by no means end-of-life situations.

This account for the advantages of letting conversationally elaborated conventions about freedom of choice prevail over "brute" claims of free choice. Favoring debate about individual roles and the enforceable rules is an occasion to let mutual agreements emerge. Such agreements give a foundation for meaningful collective choices. They can reflect the available reasons in a sensible way, leading to collective choices that appear truly expressive of a benchmark collective preference. This can plausibly be part of the collective commitment to reflective ethics and the ethics of discussion, which is described by Parizeau (2012) as a major part of health-care ethics.

Filtering the aspirations to independence

The upshot of the preceding discussion is that we should not neglect the conventional elements in freedom of choice and independence losses. This provides a rationale for the kind of selection our arrangements operate on an everyday basis, when it comes to choosing relevant aspects of individual freedom, which should be paid special attention. The process involved illustrates the institutional trimming procedures, which play a role when the details of personal freedom are being determined, starting from general principles of freedom (Picavet, 2011). Indeed, such general principles are not always explicit with respect to detailed capacities, rights, duties, and so on. Their implementation gives a role to interpretation choices, which are often related to institutional operations.

It is commonplace to observe that matters of rights and freedom are often framed in a dichotomous way. In such a frame of mind, what does it mean to become aware of data that testify to a person's subjective certainty of being able to deliberate before acting, control one's action, make free choices, and, possibly, act with no aid? It could mean that the person should be left absolutely free to act on his or her own mind, within the limits set by the mutual compatibility of actions in a social setting. This, however, might cause problems when there are substantial risks for the person. Typically, these are risks about which the professionals or other care-providing persons are better informed. In the face of this perplexity, especially in situations of close interdependence, subjective data that document self-control and deliberative capacities should perhaps not lead to the absolute priority of independent action whenever it is possible.

For practical purposes, it is advisable to observe that the relevant facts about personal initiative or wishes can hardly be insulated from the process through which they are articulated, in some cases at least. For example, from the sixth appendix in Aymard (2015) about 2013 interviews with manager operating within the MAIA framework (Method of Action for the Integration of Assistance and care services in the field of Autonomy, France), it appears that a key component of the role of a contact person (*"referent"*) in practice is to look for an adequate formulation of personal wishes, for relevant information from the relatives or friends, and for the content of personal wishes so far as personal matters are involved (that implies that a trust relationship must be established).

At a conceptual level, we should come to terms with the possibility that individual freedom in a social (or institutional) setting has a conventional component; it cannot be reduced to side constraints imposed onto the institutional functionings. Starting from this, trying to identify consensual grounds for the balance of independent initiative and risk prevention seems a good strategy to follow, on the face of it. Indeed, autonomy and freedom can be expressed through agreements and shared commitments, not only by independent action.

Conclusion

Against the background of heightened attention paid to patients' rights and prerogatives, chronic diseases and functional impairments call for a second look at subjective perceptions of freedom status. Of special interest, of course, are the subjective perceptions of one's capacities to behave freely, in a voluntary way, in a tolerably peaceful state of mind, and in awareness of the basics of one's empirical situation. The realities of collective care make it difficult, however, to cut off personal, voluntary actions from the context created by collectively provided care. Any attempt to do so in *a priori* manner would result in potential harm. The harmfulness can be assessed by pointing to the shared preferences of both providers and beneficiaries of collectively organized care.

Indicators of subjectively perceived capacities for independent choices and functionings cannot be convincingly interpreted as if they were able to delineate the frontier of the beneficiaries' immunities with respect to intervention by care providers. The conventional part of the delineation process must be addressed in its own right and the contents of the conventional agreements call for continuing dialogue. This provides a rationale for the *de facto* predominant association of open-interpretation rules and case-based management in institutional long-term care.

This broad compatibility with observed practice should probably not leave us in too peaceful a state of mind. As perceptual data about a person's agency status will develop and grow in complexity, it is likely that paternalistic caring procedures will come under increased pressure for change. It is thus advisable to realize that paying attention to a person's agency status does not necessarily result in an effort to make the agent's prerogatives absolute. In circumstances of deep-rooted interdependence, the gradual build-up of conventional arrangements through conversational procedures is an important complement to the philosophy of free choice and should be considered an integral part of applied discussion ethics.

Notes

1 A process of values-based practice may count as a decision-support process in association with shared values and principles, thus taking rank within present-day investigations of the implementation of values or principles in applied ethics, generally speaking. More specifically, it may include such elements as learnable values-related skills, an enabling clinical environment, links with evidence-based practice and a foundation in partnership between stakeholders (Fulford et al., 2011, p. 148). The connection with values-based practices has been pointed out to me by Caroline Guibet Lafaye in her comments on the presentation from which this chapter has developed. For a very useful survey of values-based practices, see Fulford (2014).

2 This has been forcefully stressed in Caroline Guibet Lafaye's comments on the first version of this contribution, on the basis of relevant examples from the psychiatric field.

Acknowledgments

The author would like to thank Caroline Guibet Lafaye for her detailed and thoughtful comments on the first version of this chapter, in a panel discussion that was set up during APEMAC congress, Nancy, 6 June 2014. The author also would like to thank Alain Leplège for additional remarks.

References

Amyot, J-J., and Villez, A. (2001). *Risque, Responsabilité, Éthique Dans Les Pratiques Gérontologiques*. Paris: Dunod/Fondation de France.

Amyot, J-J., and Villez, A. (2012). Droit au choix, droit au risque [presentation], *REIACTIS* congress, "Le droit de vieillir," Dijon. Available at: http://gsite.univ-provence.fr/gsite/Local/agis/dir/documentsreference/JJAMYOTDroitauchoix,Droita urisque.pdf

Aymard, S. (2015). Les Principes De Solidarité et d'Autonomie à l'aune De la Dépendance Des Personnes Âgées. Ph.D. thesis (philosophy). Besançon, France: Université De Franche-Comté; LETS graduate school.

Benn, S., and Weinstein, W.L. (1971). Being free to act and being a free man. *Mind*, 80, 194–211.

Berlin, I. (1969). Two concepts of liberty. In: *Four Essays on Liberty*. Oxford: Oxford University Press.

Bratman, M.E. (1987). *Intention, Plans, and Practical Reason*. Cambridge, MA: Harvard University Press.

Brunel-Petron, A. (1998). Contribution à l'Analyse Des Droits en Théorie Du Choix Social. Ph.D. thesis (economics). Université de Caen (France).

Fagot-Largeault, A. (1991). Réflexions sur la notion de qualité de la vie. *Archives De Philosophie Du Droit*, 36, 135–153.

Fleurbaey, M. (1996). *Théories Économiques De La Justice*. Paris: Economica.

Fulford, K.W.M. (2014). Values-based practice: The facts. In: M. Laughlin (ed.), *Debates in Values-Based Practice. Arguments For and Against* (chap. 1, pp. 3–19). Cambridge: Cambridge University Press.

Fulford, K.W.M., Caroll, H., and Peile, E. (2011). Values-based practice: Linking science with people. *J. Contemp. Psychother.*, 41, 145–156.

Gravel, N. (1994). Can a ranking of opportunity sets attach an intrinsic importance to freedom of choice? *Am. Econ. Rev.*, 84, 454–458.

Klemisch-Ahlert, M. (1993). Freedom of choice: A comparison of different rankings of opportunity sets. *Soc. Choice Welfare*, 10, 189–207.

Kolm, S.-C. (1998). The values of liberty. In: J-F. Laslier, M. Fleurbaey, N. Gravel, A. Trannoy (eds.), *Freedom in Economics. New Perspectives in Normative Analysis*. London: Routledge.

Leplège, A. (1996). Mesurer la qualité de vie du point de vue des patients. *L'Enseignement philosophique*. March–April 46 (4), 23–37.

Leplège, A., and Marciniak, A. (1997). Qualité de vie ou santé subjective: Problèmes conceptuels. *Prévenir*, 33, 69–76.

Parizeau, M-H. (2012). Vers une démarche éthique dans la relation de soin. In: M. Le Sommer-Péré and M-H. Parizeau (eds.), *Ethique De La Relation De Soin. Récits Cliniques et Questions Pratiques* (Chap. 10). Paris: Editions Seli Arslan.

Picavet, E. (2011). *La Revendication des Droits*. Paris: Classiques Garnier.

Picavet, E., and Guibet Lafaye, C. (2011). Capacités et concepts d'autonomie dans la construction de la 'dépendance. In: G. Ferréol (ed.), *Autonomie et Dépendance* (chap. 17). Bruxelles: EME & Intercommunications.

Schick, F. (1997). *Making Choices*. Cambridge: Cambridge University Press.

Sen, A.K. (1970). *Collective Choice and Social Welfare*. Edinburgh: Oliver and Boyd; Amsterdam: North Holland.

Sen, A.K. (1985). *Commodities and Capabilities*. Amsterdam: North Holland.

Sen, A.K. (1987). *On Ethics and Economics*. Oxford: Basil Blackwell.

Sen, A.K. (1991). Welfare, preference and freedom. *J. Econometrics*, 50, 15–29.

Sen, A.K. (1992). *Inequality Reexamined*. Cambridge, MA: Harvard University Press.

Sugden, R. (1993). Welfare, resources, and capabilities: A review of *Inequality Reexamined* by Amartya Sen. *J. Econ. Lit.*, 31(4), 1947–1962.

18 Patient-reported outcome measures: Clinical applications in the field of chronic pain self-management

James Elander and Elisabeth Spitz

Introduction

Patient-reported outcomes are defined as "any report of the patient's health condition that comes directly from the patient, without interpretation of the patient's response by a clinician or anyone else" (U.S. Department of Health and Human Services Food and Drug Administration, 2006). Patient-reported outcome measures (PROMs) include validated questionnaire measures that assess the impact of disease and treatment from the perspective of the patient. PROMs were originally developed for group comparisons in clinical trials and population studies, and the results were used to support treatment recommendations or inform health policy, with no direct clinical benefit for the patients who reported the outcomes. However, as experience with PROMs increased, the clinical value of using individual PROM profiles in routine practice to identify and monitor symptoms, evaluate treatment outcomes, and support shared decision making became more apparent (Santana et al., 2015).

Using PROMs in this way could potentially improve the diagnosis of medical conditions and the recognition of problems, and improve patient–physician communication, but considerable work still needs to be done to ensure that PROMs are used systematically and consistently to achieve those benefits. The value of PROMs is increasingly recognized for patient-centered approaches to care, but more well-controlled trials are needed to inform the ways that clinicians use PROMs in clinical practice (Valderas, 2008). For example, identification of goals, selection of patients and measures, timing of assessments, interpretation of scores, development of strategies for responding to PROMs, and evaluation of the impact of PROM use were among the issues identified in the *User's Guide for Implementing Patient-Reported Outcomes Assessment in Clinical Practice* produced by the International Society for Quality of Life Research (Snyder et al., 2012).

In this chapter, we consider how PROMs could be used to improve clinical care and promote greater patient self-management in two chronic pain conditions: rheumatic disorders and hemophilia. We first introduce the use of PROMs in routine clinical practice and explain their importance in self-management programs. We then discuss more specifically the role of PROMs in self-management of chronic pain, focusing specifically on pain coping and acceptance as influences on patient-reported quality of life (QoL), and discuss the importance of improving the use of PROMs among people with chronic painful conditions.

Using PROMs in routine clinical practice

PROMs are especially important in the clinical management of chronic pain conditions, because pain is a uniquely subjective phenomenon and patient self-management has an important influence on chronic pain treatment outcomes. In other medical contexts, PROMs have been used for screening, promoting patient-centered care, aiding decision making, facilitating multidisciplinary communication, and monitoring the quality of patient care (Greenhalgh, 2009). Reviews of evidence about the use of PROMs concluded that they have been used more frequently and more effectively to detect and assess problems with patients' health-related quality of life (HRQoL) than for patient management or to influence patient outcomes (Greenhalgh, 2009; Greenhalgh and Meadows, 1999). However, few of those studies included people with chronic pain conditions, and none to our knowledge involved people with hemophilia, who are mostly treated in specialist centers. In one review of 38 trials evaluating PROMs in clinical practice, 25 involved primary rather than specialist care, and 13 involved mental health problems. Only four of the trials involved patients with chronic illnesses, and none focused specifically on rheumatic disorders or hemophilia (Marshall et al., 2006).

However, several studies of PROMs have included aspects of pain management. One study evaluated an intervention for primary care patients with diverse pain and psychosocial problems, in which doctors received feedback about patients' problems and concerns. A nurse–educator then telephoned patients to teach problem-solving strategies and basic pain management skills, which led to improved outcomes (Ahles et al., 2006). Another study showed that the use of patient health status assessment by primary care clinicians in a health maintenance organization led to improved patient ratings of the help they received with managing pain (Wasson et al., 1992).

Greenhalgh et al. (2005, p. 839) argued that for PROM-based interventions to be effective in routine clinical care, three implicit assumptions must be met: (1) patients want to talk about their health status with clinicians, (2) clinicians feel it is appropriate to discuss HRQoL issues with patients, and (3) clinicians see that information as sufficiently important to prompt changes in patients' treatment or management. Fung and Hays (2008) argued that making more use of PROMs, especially QoL measures, can improve the quality of patient care, but clinicians may not be motivated to make greater use of patient-reported measures and most HRQoL measures were developed for research rather than clinical practice.

Using PROMs in routine clinical practice for rheumatology

Rheumatic diseases affect the joints and muscles. Some, like osteoarthritis (OA), damage joint cartilage and, as the cartilage wears down, the joints hurt and become harder to move. OA "flares" are painful exacerbations of inflammatory activity in the affected joints (Bingham et al., 2009). OA affects large numbers of people in the world and is one of the most common causes of pain, accounting for around 50% of clinical consultations for pain (Brooks, 2006).

Over the last 10 years, PROMs have been developed to assess symptoms associated with specific rheumatic conditions such as OA, rheumatoid arthritis (RA), and ankylosing spondylitis, and specific patterns of symptoms, especially the "flare." This is important because although physicians are more likely to base treatment decision-making on objective changes, patients are more concerned about subjective changes such as pain, mood disturbance, or the need to seek help (Bingham et al., 2009). Organizations including the American College of Rheumatology, the European League against Rheumatism, and the Outcome Measures in Rheumatology (OMERACT) group recommended considering both perspectives because they provide different but often complementary information (Sanderson et al., 2010). For example, a recently developed tool integrates patient and physician perspectives to assess current or recent RA flares and is suitable for daily clinical practice to identify and monitor both transient and long-lasting increases in RA symptoms (Berthelot et al., 2012).

Several tools have been used to measure HRQoL among patients with OA of the lower limbs and those undergoing total hip or knee surgery. The Medical Outcomes Study Short-Form 36 (SF36) has been widely applied but, as a generic instrument, tends to be less responsive than specific instruments, particularly in the context of medical or rehabilitation intervention rather than joint replacement. Comparisons of the SF36 with the disease-specific Western Ontario and McMaster Universities Arthritis Index (WOMAC) for patients undergoing knee replacement surgery reported that they measured different aspects of health and should probably be used together (Hawker et al., 1995). The Arthritis Impact Measurement Scales (AIMS2) tool and its short form AIMS2-SF have been considered for use in OA but have a limited usefulness among patients with a high prevalence of lower limb disability (Guillemin et al., 1997; Ren et al., 1999). Also, combining the SF36 with the WOMAC or the Lequesne index (Rat et al., 2005) may not capture specific aspects of HRQoL experienced by patients with osteoarthritic knee and hip problems, whereas the knee and hip osteoarthritis quality of life questionnaire (OAKHQOL) is specifically designed for that purpose (Rat et al., 2005).

Recently, Golightly et al. (2015) developed a list of recommended PROMs that could feasibly be applied in common clinical settings for the management of hip and knee OA. Suitable PROMs were categorized across the four domains of pain, function, fatigue, and sleep. The PROMs were also ranked into three tiers: (1) very brief measures for initial use in clinical settings, (2) brief measures with more in-depth assessment, and (3) more detailed assessment. This three-tiered approach provides a basis for tools to systematically track outcomes, facilitate provider–patient dialogue, and guide treatment for hip or knee OA. First, tier 1 measures, particularly for pain, can be used to detect early joint symptoms within primary care settings. Second, the tiered PROMs provide a way to track symptoms over time and guide treatment among patients with established OA. For example, tier 2 PROMs could detect emerging or advancing sleep problems, triggering referral to a specialist for additional evaluation or management. Third, the tiered PROMs can be used to assess the effectiveness of new treatments. The recommended PROMs may serve as clinical tools to systematically screen for and monitor outcomes associated with knee or hip OA, promote and support provider–patient dialogue about OA-related outcomes, and guide OA treatment.

In other work, a review of patient-centered care for RA concluded that fatigue should be included as a routine patient-reported outcome because of its significance to patients and its responsiveness to treatment (Matcham et al., 2015). The psychological correlates of fatigue include affect, mental disorders, RA-related cognitions, non-RA related cognitions, personality traits, stress, coping, social support, and interpersonal relationships. Early identification and management may prevent acute fatigue from becoming chronic. There are a range of different patient-report measures of fatigue, which can be assessed when patients first present to primary and secondary care, and then continually monitored throughout the course of treatment (Matcham et al., 2015).

Personal factors such as self-efficacy, optimism, resilience, and coping strategies are also important in the life stories of people with RA, but only 55% of PROMS covered personal factors (Dür et al., 2015). Coping strategies and reflecting about one's life in an optimistic way were the personal factors covered most frequently, while job satisfaction was not covered by any PROM. Dür et al. (2015) concluded that when evaluating personal factors important to people with RA, health professionals should be alert to which PROMs can be used to assess which personal factors.

Using PROMs in routine clinical practice for hemophilia

Hemophilia is an inherited bleeding disorder caused by deficiencies of blood clotting factors. Hemophilia A (caused by factor VIII deficiency) and hemophilia B (caused by factor IX deficiency) are both sex-linked recessive disorders in which the classic pattern of transmission is from carrier mother to affected son. Hemophilia A affects about 1 in 5000 males and hemophilia B about 1 in 30,000 males (Kliegman, 2011). Prevalence rates vary considerably between countries and over time (Stonebraker et al., 2010), but in 2012 there were 6742 people identified with hemophilia in the United Kingdom, 6035 in France, 4660 in Germany, and 18,628 in the United States (World Federation of Hemophilia, 2013).

People with hemophilia are susceptible to hemarthroses (joint bleeds), which happen when small blood vessels in the joint are ruptured and the joint space fills with blood, causing severe acute pain. Recurrent joint bleeds damage the joints, leading to arthropathy and severe chronic pain (Acharya, 2012).

Bleeds and arthropathy can be prevented or minimized by early prophylactic (preventative) clotting factor treatment (Rodriguez-Merchan, 2012). A survey of over 5000 adults with hemophilia in Europe showed that 67% had arthropathy and 35% had chronic pain (Holstein et al., 2012), and one in the United States showed that 39% of people with hemophilia believed their pain was not well treated (Witkop et al., 2012).

In hemophilia, there has been considerable use of PROMs such as the SF36, which is a very widely used measure of HRQoL that meets most of the minimum standards criteria for PROM measures (Reeve et al., 2013). Studies have shown that people with hemophilia have poorer physical HRQoL than the general population (Fischer et al., 2003; Szende et al., 2003) and that physical HRQoL is poorer among people with hemophilia who have more joint damage or are not receiving prophylactic clotting factor treatment (Fischer et al., 2005; Royal et al., 2002; Solovieva, 2001). However, mental QoL is less affected by hemophilia and is less closely associated with joint status (Poon et al., 2012; Zhou et al., 2011).

Research with PROMs has influenced overall standards of care for hemophilia, for example, by demonstrating the value of prophylactic clotting factor treatment. This in turn led to more efforts to involve patients in self-management, for example, by self-administering clotting factor (Stover, 2000). More recently there have been efforts to use PROMs more directly to inform individual treatment and management. In one example, a doctor used a HRQoL PROM to help decide about treatment with prophylaxis (preventative treatment to avoid bleeding episodes): "You discuss the impact of hemophilia on his HRQoL and consider measuring his HRQoL over time using a generic measure of HRQoL to determine whether prophylaxis will reduce interruptions, pain, and lost time from work and improve his HRQoL" (Buchbinder and Ragni, 2013, p. 52).

The main emphasis in the use of patient-reported QoL measures so far has, therefore, been the prevention of joint bleeds and chronic joint pain, rather than the self-management of chronic pain, but there is now more emphasis on chronic pain management and self-management. Some analyses called for a more standardized approach to assessing and managing pain in hemophilia, based on good practice guidelines and recommendations (Riley et al., 2011). Others recommended more individualized, multimodal approaches, which would enable individual patient-reported information to inform treatment decisions and clinical management: "Ongoing psychosocial assessment is critical to identify those factors that may be contributing to the perpetuation of chronic pain or acting as barriers to effective management" (Young et al., 2013, p. 113).

However, that approach will probably require PROMs other than generic measures of HRQoL. One review of PROMs more generally concluded that generic measures like SF-36 may not be clinically relevant enough to prompt clinicians to make changes to patient management (Greenhalgh and Meadows, 1999), and the same conclusion has been reached in the context of hemophilia. One review concluded that generic measures such as SF-36 were not specific or responsive enough to changes in health status, and that a hemophilia-specific tool was needed to focus on specific features of hemophilia while also taking into account common comorbidities such as hepatitis and HIV, as well as arthropathy (Szende et al., 2003). Because arthropathy is so common in hemophilia, this might involve incorporating parts of arthritis-specific scales, although it would be important to recognize that arthropathy in hemophilia is different from primary arthritis; for example, it rarely affects the fingers and hands (Szende et al., 2003). Condition-specific QoL measures have been developed for hemophilia (Remor et al., 2004), but they are not widely used so far.

Using PROMs more effectively in routine clinical practice

For both rheumatic conditions and hemophilia, integrating PROMs in clinical practice has the potential to enhance patient-centered care and improve patients' self-management. However, a key issue limiting successful implementation may be clinicians' lack of knowledge on how to effectively utilize PROMs data in their clinical encounters (Santana et al., 2015). An analysis of consultations between oncologists and their patients suggested that the main obstacles for enhancing the use of PROMs for making changes in clinical care may be limitations in the collection and interpretation of PROM data. The study concluded that "explicit mention of PROM data in the consultation may strengthen opportunities for patients to elaborate on their problems, but that doctors may not always know how to do this" (Greenhalgh et al., 2013). A model for PROMs in clinical practice was proposed that combined standard questionnaires with disease-specific or treatment-specific items, plus a prompt list of items, to facilitate the discussion of individual-specific issues and minimize patient burden (Velikova et al., 2008). One review of 16 qualitative studies on the experiences of professionals PROMs concluded that the key ways to facilitate greater use of PROMs were to make the collection of PROM data part of normal work routines and to give the PROMs data meaning by using them to make changes to patient care (Boycel et al., 2014).

A model for implementing changes in clinical practice proposed combining several approaches, including experiential learning, producing evidence-based guidelines, adapting training for specific audiences, reviewing performance and giving feedback and reminders, supporting care providers and key opinion formers, and promoting organizational innovation (Grol, 1997). More recently, Santana et al. (2015) described the development and implementation of three programs for training clinicians to use PROM data effectively in routine practice, which aimed to identify the key components for successful clinician training. The programs were in diverse clinical areas (adult oncology, lung transplant, and pediatrics), and in three countries with different healthcare systems, providing a rare opportunity to extract common approaches while recognizing specific settings. The programs showed that clinicians with different professional backgrounds can be successfully trained to use PROMs effectively in clinical practice using brief training programs to help them interpret and act on PROM data (Santana et al., 2015).

Self-management programs and PROMs

Self-management is important in chronic illness because those affected must learn to live with and manage their condition. Self-management programs "usually consist of organized learning experiences designed to facilitate adoption of health-promoting behaviors" (Warsi et al., 2004, p. 1641). This can include the optimal use of drugs, exercise, nutrition, and other preventative and health behaviors, as well as communicating effectively with health professionals, family, and/or caregivers, and learning techniques to address both the physical and emotional challenges caused by chronic illness (Newman et al., 2004).

Evidence about the effectiveness of self-management interventions differs between conditions. There is evidence that these are beneficial for people with asthma, diabetes, or hypertension but have smaller effects for people with arthritis (Chodosh et al., 2005; Warsi et al., 2003, 2004). More recently, one review also concluded that people with rheumatoid arthritis receive only marginal benefits from participation in chronic disease self-management interventions, and that although the intervention program appeared to have worked in some cases, the data actually showed only small effects, which perhaps raises questions about the measures used in the evaluation of such programs (Nolte et al., 2013).

A wide variety of intervention programs have been developed to enable patients to become more independent in managing their disease and take appropriate decisions for a more active and fulfilling life (Nolte and Osborne, 2013) and PROM data can be useful at several stages of interventions. First, before the intervention begins, PROMs can be used to assess patients' resources and skills, so that the interventions can be made more effective and more focused by taking account of individual patient profiles. The World Health Organization (WHO) recommends developing psychoeducational diagnoses to define personalized self-management programs (WHO, 1998). PROMs can help to understand the different aspects of a patient's life, personality, goals, and needs, by making subjective assessments of the impact of life events and representations of the disease, as well as self-efficacy, coping strategies, motivation, and other factors, including respondents' perceptions of what it would take for them to change their behavior (Michie et al., 2014).

Second, PROMs can be used to monitor patients' progress during self-management interventions, and the results can inform possible adjustment or reframing of the intervention. For several years, researchers and clinicians worked to develop a taxonomy of behavior change techniques that could be applied to many different types of behavior change interventions across different disciplines and countries, including organizational and community interventions (Michie et al., 2005; 2013).

Third, at the end of the intervention, as the WHO recommends for therapeutic patient education, PROMs can be used to evaluate the overall effectiveness of the program, and assess changes in patients' skills and adaptation. Thus, at the different stages of self-management programs, there is value in enabling a standardized evaluation throughout the intervention.

PROMs can also be fully integrated into the intervention. The integration of PROMs and self-management for patients with inflammatory arthritis in a joint-fitness program succeeded in improving self-perceived health as well as disease activity (El Miedany et al., 2012). Integrating PROMs with patient education is also feasible in standard clinical practice, and empowering patients through education may allow them to be more proactive in seeking better evidence-based medical treatments at an earlier stage (Vermaak et al., 2015).

PROMs and chronic pain self-management

For assessment and evaluation of pain it may be useful to adopt or adapt patient-reported measures that have been employed in other chronic pain conditions (Humphries and Kessler, 2013). For chronic pain self-management, and to improve PROMs, it is also important to know about how people think and feel about their pain, and those aspects can be assessed using standardized self-report measures of knowledge, attitudes, beliefs, and behaviors, including pain coping, pain acceptance, and readiness to self-manage pain. For two decades, cognitive-behavioral therapy (CBT), more especially acceptance and commitment therapy (ACT; Hayes et al., 1999) and physical activity promotion have emerged as major tools in the treatment of patients with chronic pain. Harlacher et al. (2011) examined whether multidimensional pain inventory (MPI) subscale score changes could be used for monitoring pain rehabilitation programs, using the psychological general well-being (PGWB) index as a separate measure of rehabilitation outcome. They proposed combining the scores from four MPI subscales, and using pre-to-post differences in PGWB scores to indicate composite rehabilitation outcomes. One study also showed that patients' beliefs about the nature and treatment of their pain could change during participation in a multidisciplinary pain management program, and that modification of those beliefs may be associated with improvements in patients' perceptions of the level of their disability (Walsh and Radcliffe, 2002).

For managing chronic pain, it is necessary to evaluate the patient's beliefs. Most often, PROMs are used to identify cognitive errors in patients' thinking and to understand the relation between thoughts, emotion, and pain. Otis (2003) proposed using the ABC Worksheet to identify patients' beliefs and perceived consequences associated with pain. In the ABC Worksheet, A is for activating event (the stressful situation associated with). B is for beliefs (the things you tell yourself, and the thoughts you have about the pain situation). C is for consequences (reactions to pain, which can be emotional, physical, or behavioral, or all three). Patients may begin to see that negative thoughts make the experience of pain worse and learn to replace negative thoughts with more positive thoughts. This will help reduce negative emotions and can result in decreased pain. The assessment of cognitive distortions can be realized using Beck et al.'s (1991) dysfunctional attitudes scale (DAS).

To manage chronic pain it is also necessary to evaluate and regulate the emotional processes associated with pain. Emotional intelligence (EI), which refers to individual differences in the abilities to identify, assess, understand, express, regulate, and use emotional information, and can be applied separately to the emotions of oneself and others, has been found to be an important predictor of pain management and adaptation to environment (Mikolajczak et al., 2014). The profile of emotional competence (PEC) measures the skills required to identify, give meaning to and manage the emotions associated with pain (Brasseur et al., 2013). Through analysis of PROMs like the PEC, the multidisciplinary team can offer a targeted intervention to develop or strengthen the emotional competences of the chronic pain patient. Following this assessment of emotional skills, different types of interventions can be offered with the purpose of regulating the emotions associated with pain. For example, an integrative intervention (Positive Emotion Regulation program) was designed to help clinicians implement interventions and techniques that target different emotional processes (Weytens et al., 2014). The emotional processes involved are structured around a theoretical framework (Gross, 1998, 2013; Quoidbach et al., 2015). Other forms of intervention can be proposed that are based on emotion-focused therapy (EFT) (Greenberg, 2002; Greenberg and Pascual-Leone, 2006).

In hemophilia, it is vitally important to differentiate chronic joint pain from acute bleeding pain, for acute bleeding pain should be treated promptly with clotting factor. However, people with hemophilia may sometimes not make this distinction. In one study, people with hemophilia used similar descriptors for acute and chronic pain, and many reported using clotting factor to treat chronic pain, or failed to use factor treatment to treat acute pain (Witkop et al., 2011).

The key elements of chronic joint pain self-management for people with hemophilia are sometimes summarized as rest, ice, compression, and elevation (RICE). (Compression means applying pressure to the painful area, and elevation means raising the affected limb.) Those four things were in fact the most frequently used pain management strategies among a sample of people with hemophilia in United States (Witkop et al., 2012). Among people with hemophilia in the Netherlands, 36% of those with joint pain used analgesics (painkillers) (van Genderen et al., 2006). In Germany, 76% of the people with severe hemophilia took analgesics daily (Wallny et al., 2001). In the United Kingdom, 53% of the people with hemophilia used over-the-counter analgesics and 34% used prescription analgesics in the last month (Elander and Barry, 2003). Knowledge about analgesics is important because certain pain medications can cause complications for people with hemophilia (Holstein et al., 2012), but there is surprisingly little research evidence about patients' or practitioners' knowledge and beliefs about pain relief for people with hemophilia, or about how they can be improved to increase the quality of hemophilia-related joint pain management.

In other painful chronic conditions, self-management interventions in the form of small-group education sessions, often drawing on principles from cognitive-behavioral therapy, have been developed and evaluated (Moore et al., 2000; Von Korff et al., 1998; Barlow et al., 2000). Considerable attention has also focused on increasing motivation or "readiness" to self-manage pain, for self-management programs are limited by participants' readiness to self-manage. Readiness to self-manage chronic pain can be measured using a standardized patient-report questionnaire (Kerns et al., 1997). In the motivational model of pain self-management, a number of factors influence readiness to self-manage, and readiness to self-manage then influences self-management behaviors (Jensen et al., 2003).

One intervention to improve readiness to self-manage chronic joint pain among people with hemophilia comprised an information booklet and a digital video disc (DVD) (Elander et al., 2011). The booklet described the difference between acute bleeding pain and chronic arthritic joint pain, the impact of pain on emotions and other aspects of life, the benefits and risks of using pain medication, and the benefits of active self-management and exercise. The DVD was based very directly on patient-reported information; all the content was presented by five men with hemophilia who described their own experiences of living with joint pain, including its impact on their lives and how they had adjusted their life goals and values accordingly. The information was consistent with the motivational model of pain self-management, but the emphasis on direct patient reports was intended to increase viewers' motivation to self-manage their chronic joint pain (Elander et al., 2011).

The booklet and DVD were evaluated in a 6-month trial in which all the participants received the booklet and a randomly selected half also received the DVD. Compared with those who received only the booklet, patient-reported readiness to self-manage improved among those who received the DVD. Active pain coping also increased among participants generally, and active involvement in learning pain self-management strategies and incorporating those strategies in everyday life increased among those who reported reading or watching the materials (Elander et al., 2011). Evidence like this suggests that self-management can be improved by giving patients a role in communicating information about their experiences, and by incorporating patient-reported outcomes directly into the materials used in interventions.

Pain coping and acceptance as influences on patient-reported outcomes

Pain coping usually means the characteristic ways that people approach and respond to pain in order to control or avoid it, and is typically assessed using standardized patient-report questionnaires (Jensen et al., 1991). For people with hemophilia, a condition-specific patient-report measure of pain coping has been developed and evaluated (Barry and Elander, 2002; Elander and Robinson, 2008). The ways that people with hemophilia coped with pain were similar to people with other painful chronic conditions (Barry and Elander, 2002; Santavirta et al., 2001), and active pain coping (using active behavioral or cognitive strategies) was associated with greater readiness to self-manage pain, whereas negative thoughts about pain and passive pain coping were associated with less readiness to self-manage pain (Elander and Robinson, 2008). Negative thoughts about pain were associated with beliefs that chance factors were responsible for pain control and with concerns about drug use, whereas passive pain coping was associated with beliefs about doctors being responsible for pain control, more frequent visits to health-care professionals, and greater use of analgesic medication (Barry and Elander, 2002; Elander and Barry, 2003).

However, in much chronic pain research the emphasis has turned in recent years from pain coping to pain acceptance, because attempts to control or avoid pain can lead to negative outcomes when they are unsuccessful, as they may often be when pain is chronic. Pain acceptance means recognizing that pain cannot always be avoided or controlled and that pain should not prevent efforts to engage with other valued goals and activities (McCracken and Eccleston, 2003). Among people with more common chronic pain conditions, research often shows that acceptance rather than coping is a better predictor of outcomes, including patient-reported outcomes (McCracken and Eccleston, 2006).

We know about only two studies of patient-reported outcomes among people with hemophilia that included measures of both pain coping and pain acceptance, and both of these showed that pain intensity affected physical QoL and pain acceptance influenced mental QoL, whereas active coping did not influence either physical or mental QoL (Elander et al., 2009, 2013). This seems to suggest that improvements in patient-reported outcomes for people with hemophilia could be achieved by interventions that reduced pain intensity and increased pain acceptance.

Interventions to improve patient-reported outcomes for people with hemophilia-related joint pain could focus on reducing pain intensity and increasing pain acceptance, and both of those factors could be targeted by clinical practice and treatments that were informed by patient-reported outcomes. To reduce pain intensity, pain assessment could be improved by adapting patient-reported methods that are used in other chronic pain conditions (Humphries and Kessler, 2013), and by educating patients to differentiate acute bleeding pain from chronic arthritic pain, so that acute bleeding episodes can be promptly treated with clotting factor. Patients could also be informed and educated about analgesics and other pain management methods, including published guidance about pain management for people with hemophilia (Holstein et al., 2012).

To improve pain acceptance, existing programs designed for people with other chronic pain conditions could be refined and adapted for people with hemophilia. These typically involve small group exercises including exposure, habit reversal training, mindfulness meditation, and sensation focusing (McCracken et al., 2005), but pain acceptance must be interpreted differently in each context and medical condition (Risdon et al., 2003), so patient-reported outcomes could very usefully inform the development and adaptation of acceptance-based interventions for people with hemophilia. One technique that could be used to achieve this is the clinical pain acceptance Q-sort, which can be used to explore pain acceptance in clinical contexts and can be used as a therapeutic tool to discuss and promote pain acceptance in a sensitive, diplomatic way that takes into account patient-reported experiences and outcomes (La Cour, 2012).

A recent review suggested that there could be a conflict between the short-term goal of providing effective pain relief to reduce pain intensity and the longer-term goal of improving pain acceptance (Elander, 2014). The review recommended that interventions should be "very carefully designed to take into account the specific needs of the people for whom they are intended, and should take specific care not to reduce the importance that should be attached to prompt treatment of acute bleeding episodes with clotting factor" (Elander, 2014, p. 171).

Conclusions

Most of the research and reflective practice about PROMs generally are applicable to chronic pain conditions such as rheumatic disorders and hemophilia, so research and practice in those conditions might be expected to follow the more general direction of travel for improving PROM use. One challenge is to improve the PROMs themselves. Patients are increasingly committed to participating in the development and improvement of PROMs, and an international exploration of patient engagement in HRQL and PROM research highlighted that, in the absence of good practice guidelines, a framework or toolkit to help embed patient engagement within HRQoL and PROM research is required (Haywood, 2015). One issue is to ensure that PROMs are suitable for the wide range of people potentially affected by their use, including those with low literacy and members of minority cultural and ethnic groups (Petkovic et al., 2015). Another is to produce short forms of PROMS that preserve their psychometric properties but reduce the time needed to complete them (Guillemin, 2016; Goetz et al., 2013). The International Society for Quality of Life Research (ISOQOL) may have a key role in taking those ideas forward, by actively engaging with patient partners to shape a future ISOQOL patient engagement strategy (Haywood, 2015; Reeve et al., 2013).

A second challenge is to improve the ways PROMs are incorporated in the design and development of clinical interventions, to improve the quality and effectiveness of those interventions. To achieve this, health professionals may need to be better educated about PROM use. Increasing interest among clinicians in using PROMs in their clinical practice has led to the development of international registers and consortia that help to reach consensus among researchers and practitioners (Breckenridge et al., 2015). A reflection paper on the use of PROMs in oncology provides a useful update on design issues common to all trial research with PROM endpoints, and could serve as a model for using PROMs in other conditions (European Medicines Agency, 2014). Other areas that need to be investigated include the use of the Consolidated Standards of Reporting Trials (CONSORT) PROM extension to drive up standards of reporting, the value of "negative" PROM findings, the need for better information about historical labeling decisions, and the role of patients in PROM trial design and implementation (Kyte et al., 2016). All of these issues could be usefully applied to arthritis and hemophilia.

References

Acharya, S.S. (2012). Exploration of the pathogenesis of haemophilic joint arthropathy: Understanding implications for optimal clinical management. *Br. J. Haematol.*, *156*, 13–23. DOI:10.1111/j.1365-2141.2011.08919.x

Ahles, T.A., Wasson, J.H., Seville, J.L., Johnson, D.J., Cole, B.F., Hanscom, B., et al. (2006). A controlled trial of methods for managing pain in primary care patients with or without co-occurring psychosocial problems. *Ann. Fam. Med.*, *4*, 341–350. DOI:10.1370/afm.527

Barlow, J.H., Turner, A.P., and Wright, C.C. (2000). A randomized controlled study of the Arthritis Self-Management Programme in the UK. *Health Educ. Res.*, *15*, 665–680. DOI:10.1093/her/15.6.665

Barry, T., and Elander, J. (2002). Pain coping strategies among patients with haemophilia. *Psychol. Health Med.*, *7*, 271–281. DOI:10.1080/13548500220139430

Beck, A.T., Brown, G., Steer, R.A., and Weissman, A.N. (1991). Factor analysis of the dysfunctional attitude scale in a clinical population. *J. Consult. Clin. Psychol.*, *3*, 478–483.

Berthelot, J.M., De Bandt, M., Morel, J., Benatig, F., Constantin, A., Gaudin, P., et al. and the STPR group of French Society of Rheumatology. (2012). A tool to identify recent or present rheumatoid arthritis flare from both patient and physician perspectives: The 'FLARE' instrument. *Ann. Rheum. Dis.*, *71*(7), 1110–1116. DOI:10.1136/ard.2011.150656

Bingham, C.O., Pohl, C., Woodworth, T.G., Hewlett, S.E., May, J.E., Rahman, M.U., et al. (2009). Developing a standardized definition for disease "flare" in rheumatoid arthritis (OMERACT 9 Special Interest Group). *J. Rheumatol.*, *36*, 2335–2341.

Boycel, M.B., Browne J.P., and Greenhalgh J. (2014). The experiences of professionals with using information from patient-reported outcome measures to improve the quality of healthcare: A systematic review of qualitative research *BMJ Qual. Safety*, *23*, 508–518. DOI:10.1136/bmjqs-2013-002524

Brasseur, S., Grégoire, J., Bourdu, R., and Mikolajczak, M. (2013). The profile of emotional competence (PEC): Development and validation of a self-reported measure that fits dimensions of emotional competence theory. *PLOS One*, *8*(5), e62635. DOI:10.1371/journal.pone.0062635

Breckenridge, K., Bekker, H.L., Gibbons, E., van der Veer, S.N., Abbott, D., Briancon, S., et al. (2015). How to routinely collect data on patient-reported outcome and experience measures in renal registries in Europe: An expert consensus meeting. *Nephrol. Dial. Transplant.*, *30*(10), 1605–1614.

Brooks, P.M. (2006). The burden of musculoskeletal disease—A global perspective. *Clin. Rheumatol.*, *25*, 778–781.

Buchbinder, D., and Ragni, M.V. (2013). What is the role of prophylaxis in the improvement of health-related quality of life of patients with haemophilia? *Am. Soc. Hematol. Educ. Program Book*, *2013*(1), 52–55. DOI:10.1182/asheducation-2013.1.52

Chodosh, J., Morton, S.C., Mojica, W., Maglione, M., Suttorp, M.J., Hilton, L., et al. (2005). Meta-analysis: Chronic disease self-management programs for older adults. *Ann. Intern. Med.*, *143*, 427–438. DOI:10.7326/0003-4819-143-6-200509200-00007

Dür, M., Coenen, M., Stoffer, M.A., Fialka-Moser, V., Kautzky-Willer, A., Kjeken I., et al. (2015). Do patient-reported outcome measures cover personal factors important to people with rheumatoid arthritis? A mixed methods design using the International

Classification of Functioning, Disability and Health as frame of reference. *Health Qual. Life Outcomes*, 13, 27.

El Miedany, Y., El Gaafary, M., El Arousy, N., Ahmed, I., Youssef, S., and Palmer, D. (2012). Arthritis education: The integration of patient-reported outcome measures and patient self-management. *Clin. Exp. Rheumatol.*, 30, 899–904.

Elander, J. (2014). A review of evidence about behavioural and psychological aspects of chronic joint pain among people with haemophilia. *Haemophilia*, 20, 168–175. DOI:10.1111/hae.12291

Elander, J., and Barry, T. (2003). Analgesic use and pain coping among patients with haemophilia. *Haemophilia*, 9, 202–213. DOI:10.1046/j.1365-2516.2003.00723.x

Elander, J., Morris, J., and Robinson, G. (2013). Pain coping and acceptance as longitudinal predictors of health-related quality of life among people with hemophilia-related chronic joint pain. *Eur. J. Pain*, 1, 929–938. DOI:10.1002/j.1532-2149.2012.00258.x

Elander, J., and Robinson, G. (2008). A brief haemophilia pain coping questionnaire (HPCQ). *Haemophilia*, 14, 1039–1048. DOI:10.1111/j.1365-2516.2008.01822.x

Elander, J., Robinson, G., Mitchell, K., and Morris, J. (2009). An assessment of the relative influence of pain coping, negative thoughts about pain, and pain acceptance on health-related quality of life among people with hemophilia. *Pain*, 145, 169–175. DOI:10.1016/j.pain.2009.06.004

Elander, J., Robinson, G., and Morris, J. (2011). Randomized trial of a DVD intervention to improve readiness to self-manage joint pain. *Pain*, 152, 2333–2341. DOI:10.1016/j.pain.2011.06.026

European Medicines Agency (2014). Reflection paper on the use of patient reported outcome (PRO) measures in oncology studies. European Medicines Agency, Oncology Working Party; Doc. Ref. EMA/CHMP/292464/2014.

Fischer, K., Van der Bom, J.G., and Van den Berg, H.M. (2003). Health-related quality of life as outcome parameter in haemophilia treatment. *Haemophilia*, 9(Suppl. 1), 75–81. DOI:10.1046/j.1365-2516.9.s1.13.x

Fischer, K., Van der Bom, J.G., Mauser-Bunschoten, E.P., Roosendaal, G., and Van den Berg, H.M. (2005). Effects of haemophilic arthropathy on health-related quality of life and socio-economic parameters. *Haemophilia*, 11, 43–48. DOI:10.1111/j.1365-2516.2005.01065.x

Fung, C. H., and Hays, R. D. (2008). Prospects and challenges in using patient-reported outcomes in clinical practice. *Qual. Life Res.*, 17, 1297–1302.

Goetz, C., Coste, J., Lemetayer, F., Rat, A.C., Montel, S., Recchia, S., et al. (2013). Item reduction based on rigorous methodological guidelines is necessary to maintain validity when shortening composite measurement scales. *J. Clin. Epidemiol.*, 66, 710–718. DOI:10.1016/j.jclinepi.2012.12.015

Greenberg, L.S. (2002). *Emotion-focused Therapy. Coaching Clients to Work Through Their Feelings*. Washington, DC: American Psychological Association.

Greenberg, L.S., and Pascual-Leone, A. (2006). Emotion in psychotherapy: A practice-friendly research review. *J. Clin. Psychol.*, 62, 611–630.

Greenhalgh, J. (2009). The applications of PROs in clinical practice: What are they, do they work, and why? *Qual. Life Res.*, 18, 115–123. DOI:10.1007/s11136-008-9430-9436

Greenhalgh, J., and Meadows, K. (1999). The effectiveness of the use of patient-based measures of health in routine practice in improving the process and outcomes of patient care: A literature review. *J. Eval. Clin. Pract.*, 5, 401–416.

Greenhalgh, J., Abhyankar, P., McCluskey, S., Takeuchi, E., and Velikova, G. (2013). How do doctors refer to patient-reported outcome measures (PROMS) in oncology consultations? *Qual. Life Res.*, 22, 939–950.

Greenhalgh, J., Long, A.F., and Flynn, R. (2005). The use of patient reported outcome measures in routine clinical practice: Lack of impact or lack of theory? *Soc. Sci. Med.*, 60, 833–843. DOI:10.1016/j.socscimed.2004.06.022

Grol, R. (1997). Personal paper. Beliefs and evidence in changing clinical practice. *BMJ*, 315, 418–421.

Gross, J.J. (1998). The emerging field of emotion regulation: A integrative review. *Rev. Gen. Psychol.*, 2(3), 271–299.

Gross, J.J. (2013). Emotion regulation: Taking stock and moving forward. *Emotion*, 13(3), 359–365. DOI:10.1037/a0032135

Guillemin, F., Coste, J., Pouchot, J., Ghezail, M., Bregeon, C., and Sany, J. (1997). The AIMS2-SF: A short form of the arthritis impact measurement scales 2. French Quality of Life in Rheumatology Group. *Arthritis. Rheum.*, 40, 1267–1274.

Guillemin, F., Rat, A.C., Goetz, C., Spitz, E., Pouchot, J., and Coste, J. (2016). The Mini-OAKHQOL for knee and hip osteoarthritis quality of life was obtained following recent shortening guidelines. *J. Clin. Epidemiol.*, 69, 70–78.

Golightly, Y.M, Allen, K.D., Nyrop, K.A., Nelson, A.E., Callahan, L.F., and Jordan, J.M. (2015). Patient-reported outcomes to initiate a provider-patient dialog for the management of hip and knee osteoarthritis. *Semin. Arthritis. Rheum.*, 45(2), 123–131.

Harlacher, U., Persson, A.L., Rivano-Fischer, M., and Sjölund, B.H. (2011). Using data from Multidimensional Pain Inventory subscales to assess functioning in pain rehabilitation. *Int. J. Rehabil. Res.*, 34(1), 14–21. DOI:10.1097/MRR.0b013e3283440bda

Haywood, K., Brett, J., Salek, S., Marlett, N., Penman, C., Shklarov, S., et al. (2015). Patient and public engagement in health-related quality of life and patient-reported outcomes research: What is important and why should we care? Findings from the first ISOQOL patient engagement symposium. *Qual. Life Res.*, 24(5), 1069–1076. DOI:10.1007/s11136-014-0796-3

Hawker, G., Melfi, C., Paul, J., Green, R., and Bombardier, C. (1995). Comparison of a generic (SF-36) and a disease specific (WOMAC) (Western Ontario and McMaster Universities Osteoarthritis Index) instrument in the measurement of outcomes after knee replacement surgery. *J. Rheumatol.*, 22, 1193–1196.

Hayes, S.C., Strosahl, K., and Wilson, K.G. (1999). *Acceptance and Commitment Therapy*. New York, NY: Guilford Press.

Holstein, K., Klamroth, R., Richards, M., Carvalho, M., Perez-Garrido, R., and Gringeri, A. (2012). Pain management in patients with haemophilia: A European survey. *Haemophilia*, 18, 743–752. DOI:10.1111/j.1365-2516.2012.02808.x

Humphries, T.J., and Kessler, C.M. (2013). The challenge of pain evaluation in haemophilia: Can pain evaluation and quantification be improved by using pain instruments from other clinical situations? *Haemophilia*, 19, 181–187. DOI:10.1111/hae.12023

Jensen, M.P., Nielson, W.R., and Kerns, R.D. (2003). Towards the development of a motivational model of pain self-management. *J. Pain*, 4, 477–492. DOI:10.1067/S1526-5900(03)00779-X

Jensen, M.P., Turner, J.A., Romano, J.M., and Karoly, P. (1991). Coping with chronic pain—A critical review of the literature. *Pain*, 47, 249–283. DOI:10.1016/0304-3959(91)90216-K

Kerns, R.D., Rosenberg, R., Jamison, R.N., Caudill, M.A., and Haythornwaite, j. (1997). Readiness to adopt a self-management approach to chronic pain: The pain stages of change questionnaire (PSOCQ). *Pain*, 72, 227–234.

Kliegman, R. (2011). *Nelson Textbook of Pediatrics* (19th Edition). Philadelphia, PA: Saunders.

Kyte, D., Reeve, B.B., Efficace, F., Haywood, K., Mercieca-Bebber, R., King, M.T., et al. (2016). International Society for Quality of Life Research commentary on the draft European Medicines Agency reflection paper on the use of patient-reported outcome (PRO) measures in oncology studies. *Qual Life Res.*, 25, 359–362. DOI:10.1007/s11136-015-1099-z

La Cour, P. (2012). The clinical pain acceptance Q-sort: A tool for assessment and facilitation of pain acceptance. *Psychol Health Med.*, 17, 611–620. DOI:10.1080/13548 506.2011.648646

Marshall, S., Haywood, K., and Fitzpatrick, R. (2006). Impact of patient-reported outcome measures on routine practice: A structured review. *J Eval. Clin. Pract.*, 12, 559–568.

Matcham, F., Ali, S., Hotopf, M., and Chalder T. (2015). Psychological correlates of fatigue in rheumatoid arthritis: A systematic review. *Clin. Psychol. Rev.*, *39*, 16–29.

McCracken, L.M., and Eccleston, C. (2003). Coping or acceptance: What to do about chronic pain? *Pain*, *105*, 197–204. DOI:10.1016/S0304-3959(03)00202-1

McCracken, L.M., and Eccleston, C. (2006). A comparison of the relative utility of coping and acceptance-based measures in a sample of chronic pain sufferers. *Eur. J. Pain*, *10*, 23–29. DOI:10.1016/j.ejpain.2005.01.004

McCracken, L.M., Vowles, K.E., and Eccleston, C. (2005). Acceptance-based treatment for persons with long-standing chronic pain: A preliminary analysis of treatment outcome in comparison to a waiting phase. *Behav. Res. Ther.*, *43*, 1335–1346. DOI:10.1016/j.brat.2004.10.003

Michie, S., Johnston M., Abraham C., Lawton R., Parker D., and Walker A. (2005). Making psychological theory useful for implementing evidence based practice: A consensus approach. *Qual. Safety Health Care J.*, *14*(1), 26–33.

Michie S., Richardson, M., Johnston, M., Abraham, C., Francis, J., Hardeman, W., et al. (2013). The behavior change technique taxonomy (v1) of 93 hierarchically clustered techniques: Building an international consensus for the reporting of behavior change interventions. *Ann. Behav. Med.*, *46*, 81–95. DOI:10.1007/s12160-013-9486-6

Michie S., Atkins, L., and West R. (2014). *The Behavior Change Wheel. A Guide to Designing Interventions*. Silverback Publishing. Available at: http://www.silverback-publishing.org/

Mikolajczak, M., Brasseur, S., and Fantini-Hauwel, C. (2014). Measuring intrapersonal and interpersonal EQ: The short profile of emotional competence (S-PEC). *Pers. Individ. Dif.*, *65*, 42–46.

Moore, J.E., Von Korff, M., Cherkin, D., Saunders, K., and Lorig, K. (2000). A randomized trial of a cognitive-behavioral program for enhancing back pain self-care in a primary care setting. *Pain*, *88*, 145–153. DOI:10.1016/S0304-3959(00)00314-6

Newman, S., Steed, L., and Mulligan K. (2004). Self-management interventions for chronic illness. *Lancet*, *364*, 1523–1537.

Nolte, S., and Osborne, R.H. (2013). A systematic review of outcomes of chronic disease self-management interventions. *Qual. Life Res.*, *22*, 1805–1816.

Nolte, S., Elsworth, G.R., Newman S., and Osborne, R.H. (2013). Measurement issues in the evaluation of chronic disease self-management programs. *Qual. Life Res.*, *22*, 1655–1664.

Quoidbach, J., Mikolajczak, M., and Gross, J.J. (2015). Positive interventions: An emotion regulation perspective. *Psychol Bull.*, *141*, 655–693.

Otis, J.D. (2007). *Managing Chronic Pain. A Cognitive-Behavioral Therapy Approach*. New York, NY: Oxford University Press.

Petkovic, J., Epstein, J., Buchbinder, R., Welch, V., Rader, T., Lyddiatt, A., et al. (2015). Toward ensuring health equity: Readability and cultural equivalence of OMERACT patient-reported outcome measures. *J. Rheumatol.*, http://doi.org/10.3899/jrheum.141168

Poon, J.L., Zhou, Z.-Y., Doctor, J.N., Wu, J., Ullman, M.M., Ross, C., et al. (2012). Quality of life in haemophilia A: Hemophilia Utilization Group Study Va (HUGS-Va). *Haemophilia*, *18*, 699–707. DOI:10.1111/J.1365-2516.2012.02791.X

Rat, A.C., Coste, J., Pouchot, J., Baumann, M., Spitz, E., Retel-Rude, N., et al. (2005). OAKHQOL: A new instrument to measure quality of life in knee and hip osteoarthritis. *J. Clin. Epidemiol.*, *58*(1), 47–55.

Reeve, B.B., Wyrwich, K.W., Wu, A.W., Velikova, G., Terwee, C.B., Snyder, C.F., et al. (2013). ISOQOL recommends minimum standards for patient-reported outcome measures used in patient-centered outcomes and comparative effectiveness research. *Qual. Life Res.*, *22*, 1889–1905. DOI 10.1007/s11136-012-0344-y

Remor, E., Young, N.L., Von Mackensen, S., and Lopatinas, E.G. (2004). Disease-specific quality of life measurement tools for haemophilia patients. *Haemophilia*, *10*(Suppl. 4), 30–34.

Ren, X.S., Kazis, L., and Meenan, R.F. (1999). Short-form arthritis impact measurement scales 2: Tests of reliability and validity among patients with osteoarthritis. *Arthritis. Care Res.*, *12*, 163–171.

Riley, R.R., Witkop, M., Hellman, E., and Akins, S. (2011). Assessment and management of pain in haemophilia patients. *Haemophilia*, *17*, 839–845. DOI:10.1111/j.1365-2516.2011.02567.x

Risdon, A., Eccleston, C., Crombez, G., and Mccracken, L. (2003). How can we learn to live with pain? A Q-methodology analysis of the diverse understandings of acceptance of chronic pain. *Soc. Sci. Med.*, *56*, 375–386.

Rodriguez-Merchan, E.C. (2012). Prevention of the musculoskeletal complications of hemophilia. *Adv. Prev. Med.*, Epub 201271. DOI:10.1155/2012/201271

Royal, S., Schramm, W., Berntorp, E., Giangrande, P., Gringeri, A., Ludlam, C., et al. (2002). Quality of life differences between prophylactic and on-demand factor replacement therapy in European haemophilia patients. *Haemophilia*, *8*, 44–50. DOI:10.1046/j.1365-2516.2002.00581.x

Sanderson, T., Morris, M., Calnan, M., Richards, P., and Hewlett, S. (2010). Patient perspective of measuring treatment efficacy: The rheumatoid arthritis patient priorities for pharmacologic interventions outcomes. *Arthritis Care Res. (Hoboken)*, *62*(5):647–656. DOI:10.1002/acr.20151

Santana, M.J., Haverman, L., Absolom, K., Takeuchi, E., Feeny, D., Grootenhuis, M., et al. (2015). Training clinicians in how to use patient-reported outcome measures in routine clinical practice. *Qual. Life Res.*, *12*, 1707–1718. DOI:10.1007/s11136-014-0903-5

Santavirta, N., Bjorvell, H., Solovieva, S., Alaranta, H., Hurskainen, K., and Konttinen, Y.T. (2001). Coping strategies, pain, and disability in patients with hemophilia and related disorders. *Arthritis. Rheumatism-Arthritis Care Res.*, *45*, 48–55. DOI:10.1002/1529-0131(200102)45:1<48::AID-ANR83>3.0.CO;2-1

Snyder, C.F., Aaronson, N.K., Choucair, A.K., Elliott, T.E., Greenhalgh, J., Halyard, M.Y, et al. (2012). Implementing patient-reported outcomes assessment in clinical practice: A review of the options and considerations. *Qual. Life Res.*, *21*(8), 1305–1314. DOI 10.1007/s11136-011-0054-x

Solovieva, S. (2001). Clinical severity of disease, functional disability and health-related quality of life. Three-year follow-up study of 150 Finnish patients with coagulation disorders. *Haemophilia*, *7*, 53–63. DOI:10.1046/j.1365-2516.2001.00476.x

Stonebraker, J.S., Bolton-Maggs, P.H., Michael Soucie, J., Walker, I., and Brooker, M. (2010). A study of variations in the reported haemophilia A prevalence around the world. *Haemophili.*, *16*, 20–32.

Stover, B. (2000). Training the client in self-management of hemophilia. *J. Intraven. Nurs.*, *23*, 304–309.

Szende, A., Schramm, W., Flood, E., Larson, P., Gorina, E., Rentz, A.M., and Snyder, L. (2003). Health-related quality of life assessment in adult haemophilia patients: A systematic review and evaluation of instruments. *Haemophilia*, *9*, 678–687. DOI:10.1046/j.1351-8216.2003.00823.x

U.S. Department of Health and Human Services FDA Center for Drug Evaluation and Research, U.S. Department of Health and Human Services FDA Center for Biologics Evaluation and Research and U.S. Department of Health and Human Services FDA Center for Devices and Radiological Health (2006). Guidance for industry: Patient-reported outcome measures: Use in medical product development to support labeling claims: Draft guidance. *Health Qual. Life Outcomes*, *4*, 79 DOI:10.1186/1477-7525-4-79

Valderas, J.M., Kotzeva, A., Espallargues, M., Guyatt, G., Ferrans, C.E., Halyard, M.Y., et al. (2008). The impact of measuring patient-reported outcomes in clinical practice: A systematic review of the literature. *Qual. Life Res.*, *17*, 179–193. DOI 10.1007/s11136-007-9295-0 van Genderen, F.R., Fischer, K., Heijnen, L., de Kleijn, P., van den Berg, H.M., Helders, P.J.M., et al. (2006). Pain and functional limitations in patients with severe haemophilia. *Haemophilia, 12,* 147–153. DOI:10.1111/j.1365-2516.2006.01203.x

Velikova, G., Awad, N., Coles-Gale, R., Wright, E.P., Brown, J.M., and Selby, P.J. (2008). The clinical value of quality of life assessment in oncology practice-a qualitative study of patient and physician views. *Psycho-oncol., 17,* 690–698.

Vermaak, V., Briffa, N.K., Langlands, B., Inderjeeth, C., and McQuade, J. (2015) Evaluation of a disease specific rheumatoid arthritis self-management education program, a single group repeated measures study. *BMC Musculoskelet. Disord., 16,* 214. DOI 10.1186/s12891-015-0663-6

Von Korff, M., Moore, J.E., Lorig, K., Cherkin, D.C., Saunders, K., Gonzales, V.M., et al. (1998). A randomized controlled trial of a lay person-led self-management group intervention for back pain patients in primary care. *Spine, 23,* 2608–2615.

Walsh, D.A., and Radcliffe J.C. (2002). Pain beliefs and perceived physical disability of patients with chronic low back pain. *Pain, 97,* 23–31.

Warsi, A., LaValley, M.P., Wang, P.S., Avorn, J., and Solomon, D.H. (2003). Arthritis self-management education programs: A meta-analysis of the effect on pain and disability. *Arthritis. Rheum., 48,* 2207–2213.

Warsi, A., Wang, P.S., LaValley, M.P., Avorn, J., and Solomon, D.H. (2004). Self-management education programs in chronic disease: A systematic review and methodological critique of the literature. *Arch. Inter. Med., 164,* 1641–1649.

Wallny, T., Hess, L., Seuser, A., Zander, D., Brackmann, H.H., and Kraft, C.N. (2001). Pain status of patients with severe haemophilic arthropathy. *Haemophilia, 7,* 453–458. DOI:10.1046/j.1365-2516.2001.00540.x

Wasson, J., Hays, R., Rubenstein, L., Nelson, E., Leaning, J., Johnson, D., et al. (1992). The short-term effect of patient health status assessment in a health maintenance organization. *Qual. Life Res., 1,* 99–106. DOI:10.1007/BF00439717

Weytens, F., Luminet, O., Lesley, L. Verhofstadt, L.L., and Mikolajczak, M. (2014). An integrative theory-driven positive emotion regulation intervention. *PLoS On., 9*(4), e95677.

Witkop, M., Lambing, A., Divine, G., Kachalsky, E., Rushlow, D., and Dinnen, J. (2012). A national study of pain in the bleeding disorders community: A description of haemophilia pain. *Haemophilia, 18,* e115–e119. DOI:10.1111/j.1365-2516.2011.02709.x

Witkop, M., Lambing, A., Kachalsky, Divine, G., Rushlow, D., and Dinnen, J. (2011). Assessment of acute and persistent pain management in patients with haemophilia. *Haemophilia, 17,* 612–619. DOI:10.1111/j.1365-2516.2010.02479.x

World Federation of Hemophilia. (2013). Report on the Annual Global Survey 2012. World Federation of Hemophilia. Available at http://www1.wfh.org/publications/files/pdf-1574.pdf (accessed on 24 January 2017).

World Health Organization Regional Office for Europe Copenhagen. (1998) Therapeutic patient education, continuing education programmes for health care providers in the field of prevention of chronic diseases report of a WHO working group. Available at http://www.euro.who.int/__data/assets/pdf_file/0007/145294/E63674.pdf (accessed on 24 January 2017).

Young, G., Tachdjian, R., Baumann, K., and Panopoulos, G. (2013). Comprehensive management of chronic pain in haemophilia. *Haemophilia, 20,* e113–e120. DOI:10.1111/hae.12349

Zhou, Z.-Y., Wu, J., Baker, J., Curtis, R., Forsberg, A., Huszti, H., et al. (2011). Haemophilia Utilization Group Study—Part Va (HUGS Va): Design, methods and baseline data. *Haemophilia, 17,* 729–736. DOI:10.1111/j.1365-2516.2011.02595.x

19 Clinical decision based on evidence

Emmanuelle Busch and Marc Debouverie

Ever since patients' quality of life (QoL) has become an important health out-come, incorporating the measurement of patients' well-being into clinical trials and clinical care has opened up new perspectives in patient management and has brought emphasis on the implications of treatment adherence for patient outcomes in the course of their disease. Patient-reported outcomes (PROs) pro-mote treatment adherence and patient behavior change by giving attention to the patients' views on their health and health-related QoL.

Introduction

With a growing number of patients suffering from chronic diseases, clinicians have come to consider medical treatment through benefits, risks, and costs and through patients' subjective evaluations of their own treatment (Snoek, 2000). Patient-reported outcomes (PROs) thus aim to measure all possible aspects of a patient's health status by using standardized instruments (Valderas et al., 2008).

Some regulatory agencies, such as the French national Health Regulatory Authority (HAS), have rendered evaluation of QoL using the Short Form Health-Related Quality-of-Life Questionnaire (SF-36) mandatory in every clinical trial. Indeed, in the context of chronic disease, HAS requires QoL data before giving marketing authorization for new treatments. Clinical decision making and choice of treatment must take into consideration many aspects of the patients' well-being, such as health beliefs, and the impact on everyday life of the disease and of its treatment. Subjective well-being is multidimensional and does not necessarily meet the health-care professional's common view.

Chronic disease means that treatments may stabilize or slow down the dis-ease course but rarely ever cure. Considering this, it is important to work on the relationship with the patient, to understand how he or she feels and lives, and what his or her expectations on a multiple level are: *biological* (pain, phys-ical symptoms, side effects, fatigue), *psychological* (loss, guilt, despair, internal and external conflicts, perceived burden of treatment), and *social* (discontinued relationships, work loss, loneliness).

Long-term disease and treatment can mean satisfaction with the treatment but also possible weariness or too high expectations leading to disappointment and breach in confidence, leaving little room for improvement (Papadopoulou, 2015).

Using PROs may help work on the patient–clinician communication and relationship and enable both to establish common priorities and expectations. Studies (Snyder et al., 2012) have shown how important shared decision making in chronic disease is for treatment adherence; the use of appropriate PROs will indeed rigorously collect information from the patient's point of view and take into account the outcomes that are important to patients and support medical decision (Ahmed et al., 2012). Furthermore, the choice of treatment is now becoming more complex with a broad spectrum of possible treatments, which has an impact on the evolution in methodological and practical decisions in patient management.

Let us consider three possible applications of PROs in evidence-based practice: multiple sclerosis (MS), cancer, and diabetes; all three chronic diseases, with a high impact on many aspects of QoL, having several treatment options to choose from and for which specific PROs have been created over the years and the use thereof assessed in literature.

Fatigue in multiple sclerosis

Fatigue is a common and disabling symptom of multiple sclerosis (MS) at all stages of the disease for 50%–90% of patients. Fatigue negatively impacts daily living and QoL, as shown by the SF-36 outcomes. However, clinicians rely mostly on the more specific MS fatigue questionnaire, the Adapted French version of Fatigue Impact Scale (EMIF-SEP) to help patients describe this symptom. By taking fatigue into account with a specific PRO, there is better acceptance of the symptom: If asked about fatigue, it is normal to feel fatigue (Debouverie et al., 2008). Assessment formalizes the symptom, making it easier then to acknowledge by society. Indeed, from a psychological point of view, a major difficulty for patients comes from their family, friends, and professional colleagues who may be oblivious to this symptom and its consequences in everyday life. In any given medical context, PROs may help patients legitimize their symptoms, which are often misunderstood and invisible to others, but are disabling nonetheless.

In another study (Manceau et al., 2014), fatigue assessed using the EMIF-SEP has a positive predictive value in relation to interferon antibodies, which may appear when treated by interferon beta, one of several MS treatments. In this case, a relevant fatigue PRO provides the clinician with arguments to change the actual treatment line and consider treatment change. It also gives the clinician tangible arguments to discuss the relevance of treatment change with the patient.

Cancer pain assessment and management

Both acute and chronic pain have been well documented as one of the most frequent and distressing symptoms in cancer, present in 36%–61% of patients (Campbell, 2011) and has been shown to adversely affect QoL.

Cancer pain is multidimensional and comprehensive pain assessment is essential. The most frequently used standardized scales are the nonspecific Brief Pain Inventory (BPI), the Pain Treatment Acceptability Scale (PTA), and the Memorial Symptom Assessment Scale (MSAS). However, patients with complex pain syndromes often require more intensive therapeutic programs and more time to achieve stable pain control (Nekolaichuk et al., 2013). To be more specific to cancer, the Edmonton Classification System for Cancer Pain (ECS-CP) was developed by practitioners wishing to be able to foresee which patients will be more difficult or time consuming to manage and for whom increasing the opioid dosage is not a satisfactory outcome. The ECS-CP's goals may also be to help the practitioner decide whether a new therapy is preferable to a standard therapy, or determine whether a therapeutic regimen is better than supportive care only, considering the patients' survival time (Fainsinger and Nekolaichuk, 2008).

Using QoL measures in everyday practice may help to gain better understanding of the effects of pain in patients' everyday life. Depression and psychosocial distress must also be assessed because they can be strongly associated with cancer pain. This information may be used to develop treatment protocols and guidelines that minimize pain while maximizing patients' well-being (Ripamonti, 2011).

Diabetes and QoL

Diabetes remains a very demanding disease and the prevalence of depression in the diabetic population is 24% compared with 17% in the nondiabetic population (Testa, 2000). Although earlier treatment options were relatively limited, more recent technological and pharmacological advances have generated renewed interest in evaluating QoL outcomes as part of choosing the optimal therapeutic regimen (Goldney, 2004).

Evaluating the psychological and psychosocial aspects of the patients' life is therefore imperative, because depression or even distress will have an impact on QoL, which in turn will have effects on the patient's ability to adhere to often difficult and demanding treatment regimens. Depression will furthermore contribute to the high economic burden of health-care costs.

Clinicians working with diabetes patients have found the SF-36 to not be specific enough and have felt the need to develop the diabetes quality of life (DQoL) questionnaire, or more recently, the diabetes-specific QoL scale (DSQoLS), enabling more discriminate measures for which the usual SF-36 standards seem insufficient (Burroughs et al., 2004). The DQoL provides a total health-related QoL score that predicts self-reported diabetes care behaviors and satisfaction with diabetes control, as well as a screening process for patients' readiness to change and specific treatment-related concerns (Garratt et al., 2002). Use of DQoL and DSQoLS may help identify individual motivation or lack thereof and define individual treatment goals and strategies. One asset of these disease-specific PROs is to enable patients to express what really matters to them: studies have shown that physical health and well-being were consistently rated much lower than family and relationships in the general life questionnaire, and that feeling well was rated much lower than fear of complications and hypoglycemia in the DQoL, also recording a significantly better score during insulin pump therapy than during injection treatment (Pickup and Harris, 2007). More specifically, the DSQoLS focuses on the impacts of modern type 1 diabetes management (e.g., carbohydrate counting and flexible insulin dose adjustment) for adults (Cooke, 2013).

Discussion

When dealing with chronic diseases, the aim is to improve the QoL of patients. The three examples from cancer, MS, and diabetes have demonstrated how PRO outcomes, by focusing on the patient's health goals, may guide the clinician in his therapeutic decision making. Thus, they can be considered to have a positive impact on patient–provider interaction and are important for shared decision making in everyday clinical practice. PROs may also inspire change in therapeutic attitude when they encourage practitioners to complete the initial clinical assessment based on objective data. They may also be used to identify QoL issues that might not arise during the typical patient–provider encounter (Valderas et al., 2008).

Over the years, several studies investigating the use of PROs in clinical practice have been conducted in oncology, often showing more benefits in communication than in treatment and outcomes (Snyder, 2014): the intervention improved discussion of symptoms and demonstrated benefits in health-related QoL but did not necessarily change treatment (Bottomley et al., 2005; Kanatas et al., 2012). As such, three different approaches to the measurement of patient-reported health outcomes should be taken into account: generic instruments, disease-specific instruments, and situation-specific instruments (Mckenna, 2011).

Generic instruments will measure broad aspects of health and are therefore potentially suitable for a wide range of patient groups. They generate health state scores that can be used to compare QoL gained in different populations or to compare scores in a specific population with normative scores. Most importantly, generic measures distinguish themselves from condition-specific measures in that they will assess the impact of disease and treatment on overall functioning or pertaining to a broader range of health domains (Matza et al., 2007). However, being generic, they lack sensitivity in specific disease contexts and may overlook certain issues that are specific to a given disease. As a result, generic scales may lack the responsiveness needed in therapeutic decision making. Furthermore, asking patients to answer questions irrelevant to their situation may distract respondents and increase the risk of missing or inaccurate responses (Valderas et al., 2008).

In response to these generic PROs, and as we have seen for fatigue in MS, pain in cancer and QoL in diabetes, each field has developed more specific disease-related PROs to capture areas of concern and is of importance to specific patient populations. With these disease-specific PROs, patients will be asked questions that are relevant, meaningful, and acceptable to them (Mckenna, 2011). Consequently, with more accurate data, disease-specific instruments have greater potential for showing differences between different therapies and treatment options. However, self-assessment can be stressful, depending on the patients' motivation to minimize or maximize symptoms, hoping to appear less ill or, on the contrary, hoping for more attention and help. Stress may also ensue from items revealing symptoms otherwise unknown to a given patient, leaving him or her to ponder over the future and worsening his or her condition. Patients may also be simply reluctant to report what and how they feel. Finally, the restricted focus of disease-specific instruments may hinder detection of other side effects or non-health-related QoL issues.

Therefore, the use of disease-specific PROs may be combined with situation-specific instruments designed to measure knowledge, attitudes, and behavior (Mckenna, 2011), for example, a patients' frame of mind at a given time. Depression, for example, may be a frequently underdiagnosed symptom for which management and treatment may be difficult and interfere with current treatment or subjective well-being. Cognitive disorders, often associated with neurological diseases, are probably underestimated in that patients find ways to compensate. However, cognitive assessment is not systematic, making it difficult to know precisely which PRO outcomes we can use without knowing the patients cognitive status. As for patients with obvious cognitive disorders, how may the practitioner use PROs that could be useful for helping the patient and for better health management? When one is incapable of self-assessment or of answering questions, should asking the primary caregiver be considered?

Even apart from any downsides, the use of PROs carries a certain cost: time-consuming administration and data collection and time spent computing and reviewing PRO scores, especially when rapid data processing is needed.

Generic measures also tend to correlate well with condition-specific measures (Graue et al., 2003). Because generic and condition-specific measures have different strengths and are theoretically distinct, it is often recommended to administer both types of instruments as part of a complete assessment (Matza et al., 2007; Engstrom et al., 2001).

Health regulatory authorities are very fond of PROs, and PROs may be useful in clinical practice and evidence-based decision making, however, little changes in practice management after use of PRO have been shown to date (Marshall et al., 2006). The reasons relate to lack of adequate assessment and thus inadequate management (Greenhalgh, 2009); accurate assessment guides management, but poor assessment handicaps management. Clinicians and patients seem to prefer disease-specific measures, although policy makers prefer generic QoL measures. When aggregated, PROs can be used for many purposes, such as comparative effectiveness research, practice improvement, and to help inform policy makers of potential ways for implementing PROs in clinical practice (Van Der Wees et al., 2014). This explains the strong need for specific disease-related PROs, with relevance to context and population (the elderly and children population) and the need to know beforehand what clinical response is possible. Much work is still needed to develop and improve specific PROs that may help on a daily basis patients and practitioners (Van Der Wees et al., 2014).

In conclusion, PRO outcomes are unique indicators of the impact of a disease on the patients' QoL and health priorities. Generic PROs combined with disease-specific PROs remain helpful in enabling communication between patient and health-care providers, and in determining the efficacy of a given treatment, and are helpful in treatment decision making.

References

Ahmed, S., Berzon, R.A., Revicki, D.A., Lenderking, W.R., Moinpour, C.M., Basch, E., et al. (2012). The use of patient-reported outcomes (PRO) within comparative effectiveness research: Implications for clinical practice and health care policy. *Med. Care*, 50(12), 1060–1070.

Bottomley, A., Flechtner, H., Efficace, F., Vanvoorden, V., Coens, C., Therasse, P., et al. (2005). Health related quality of life outcomes in cancer clinical trials. *Eur. J. Cancer*, 41(12), 1697–1709.

Burroughs, T.E., Desikan, R., Waterman, B.M., Gilin, D., and McGill, J. (2004). Development and validation of the diabetes quality of life brief clinical inventory. *Diabetes Spectr.*, 17(1), 41–49.

Campbell, V. (2011). The challenges of cancer pain assessment and management. *Ulster Med. J.*, 80(2), 104–106.

Cooke, D., O'Hara, M.C., Beinart, N., Heller, S., La Marca, R., Byrne, M., et al. (2013). Linguistic and psychometric validation of the Diabetes-Specific Quality-of-Life Scale in U.K. English for adults with type-1 diabetes. *Diabetes Care*, 36(5), 1117–1125.

Debouverie, M., Pittion-Vouyovitch, S., Brissart, H., and Guillemin, F. (2008) Physical dimension of fatigue correlated with disability change over time in patients with multiple sclerosis. *J. Neurol.*, 255, 633–636.

Engstrom, C.P., Persson, L.O., Larsson, S., and Sullivan, M. (2001) Health-related quality of life in COPD: Why both disease-specific and generic measures should be used. *Eur. Respir. J.*, 18, 69–76.

Fainsinger, R.L., and Nekolaichuk, C.L. (2008). A "TNM" classification for cancer pain: The Edmonton Classification System for Cancer Pain (ECS-CP). *Support. Care Cancer*, 6(6), 547–555.

Garratt, A.M., Schmidt, L., and Fitzpatrick, R. (2002). Patient-reported health outcome measures for diabetes: A structured review. *Diabetic Med.*, 19, 1–11.

Goldney, R.D. (2004). Diabetes, depression, and quality of life. *Diabetes Care*, 27(5), 1066–1070.

Graue, M., Wentzel-Larsen, T., Hanestad, B.R., Båtsvik, B., and Søvik, O. (2003). Measuring self-reported, health-related, quality of life in adolescents with type 1 diabetes using both generic and disease-specific instruments. *Acta Paediatr.*, 92, 1190–1196.

Greenhalgh, J. (2009). The applications of PROs in clinical practice: What are they, do they work, and why? *Qual. Life Res.*, 18, 115–123.

Kanatas, A., Velikova, G., Roe, B., Horgan, K., Ghazali, N., Shaw, R.J., et al. (2012) Patient-reported outcomes in breast oncology: A review of validated outcome instruments, *Tumori*, 98(6), 678–688.

Manceau, P., Latarche, C., Pittion, S., Edan, G., De Sèze, J., Massart, C., et al. (2014) Neutralizing antibodies and fatigue as predictors of low response to interferon-beta treatment in patients with multiple sclerosis. *BMC Neurol.*, 14, 215.

Marshall, S., Haywood, K., and Fitzpatrick, R. (2006) Impact of patient-reported outcome measures on routine practice: A structured review. *J. Evol. Clin. Pract.*, *12*(5), 559–568.

Matza, L.S., Boye, K.S., and Yurgin, N. (2007). Validation of two generic patient-reported outcome measures in patients with type 2 diabetes. *Health Qual. Life Outcomes*, *5*, 47.

Mckenna, S.P. (2011). Measuring patient-reported outcomes: Moving beyond misplaced common sense to hard science. *BMC Med.*, *9*, 86.

Nekolaichuk, C.L., Fainsinger, R.L., Aass, N., Hjermstad, M.J., Knudsen, A.K., Klepstad, P., et al. (2013). The Edmonton classification system for cancer pain: Comparison of pain classification features and pain intensity across diverse palliative care settings in eight countries. *J. Palliat. Med.*, *16*(5), 516–523.

Papadopoulou, L. (2015). Depression and quality of life in patients with diabetes. *Am. J. Nurs. Sci.*, *4*(2–1), 88–91.

Pickup, J.C., and Harris, A. (2007) Assessing quality of life for new diabetes treatments and technologies: A simple patient-centered score. *J Diabetes Sci Technol*, *1*(3): 394–399.

Ripamonti, C.I. (2011) Management of cancer pain: ESMO clinical practice guidelines. *Ann. Oncol.*, *22*(6), 69–77.

Snoek, F.J. (2000). Quality of life: A closer look at measuring patients' well-being. *Diab. Spectr.*, *13*(1), 24–29.

Snyder, C.F. (2014). Using patient-reported outcomes in clinical practice: A promising approach? *J. Clin. Oncol.*, *32*(11), 1099–1100.

Snyder, C.F., Aaronson, N.K., Choucair, A.K., Elliott, T.E., Greenhalgh, J., Halyard, M.Y., et al. (2012). Implementing patient-reported outcomes assessment in clinical practice: A review of the options and considerations. *Qual. Life Res.*, *21*, 8, 1305–1314.

Testa, M.A. (2000). Quality-of-life assessment in diabetes research: Interpreting the magnitude and meaning of treatment effects. *Diab. Spectr.*, *13*(1), 29–34.

Valderas, J.M., Alonso, J., and Guyatt, G.H. (2008). Measuring patient-reported outcomes: Moving from clinical trials to clinical practice. *Med. J. Aust.*, *189*(2), 93–94.

Valderas, J.M., Kotzeva, A., Espallargues, M., Guyatt, G., Ferrans, C.E., Halyard, M.Y., et al. (2008). The impact of measuring patient-reported outcomes in clinical practice: A systematic review of the literature. *Qual. Life Res.*, *17*, 179–193.

Van Der Wees, P.J., Nijhuis-Van Der Sanden, M.W., Ayanian, J.Z., Black, N., Westert, G.P., and Schneider, E.C. (2014). Integrating the use of patient-reported outcomes for both clinical practice and performance measurement: Views of experts from 3 countries. *Milbank Q.*, *92*(4), 754–775.

20 Perceived health indicators, decision making, and public health

Serge Briançon

Prevention of premature death, disease, and disability is the main goal of public health policies, and decision makers expect to be provided with efficient indicators covering these fields as being easily interpretable and actionable for setting policy objectives. The epidemiological transition raised the prevention of chronic diseases and health promotion, while mortality and morbidity rates appeared as being not sufficient to monitor population health. Thus, the United Nations Convention on the Rights of Persons with Disabilities (2006) stated in its Article 31 named "Statistics and data collection," "… to collect appropriate information, including statistical and research data, to enable [nations] to formulate and implement policies … to identify and address the barriers faced by persons with disabilities in exercising their rights" (United Nations, 2006).

The perceived health measures, as well, could be used for public health decision in several ways including by

- Promoting enhancement of quality of life (QoL)
- Contributing to the appreciation of the results of public health policies and programs
- Allowing the identification of population groups with poor health-related QoL level and targeting interventions
- Enabling monitoring of the effectiveness of public health programs with broader goals
- Providing an endpoint for the QoL years in the elderly
- Assessing the population impact of disease and disability
- Identifying health needs and their disparity
- Contributing to cost-effective approaches
- Constituting a resource allocation criterion
- Serving as an endpoint in prevention research

The use of perceived health measures appears to be justified by their direct link with the general objectives of improving health status of populations defined at the national and international levels. Perceived health incorporates the broad definition of multidimensional health including mental and physical well-being. It determines the behavior of people toward the health-care system. It is a reflection of demographic and socioeconomic disparities and of the impact of the burden of physical and mental illness and disability.

Its use remains patchy in many health systems; the inherent constraints are to be found in its integration into a real surveillance system with the need for repeated transversal measures with the issue of the permanence, the repetition, and the continuity of the implementation, with the ability to obtain representative samples of the general population and patients—such as suffering from cancer, cardiovascular disease, chronic renal failure, diabetes, hemophilia, with the selection and maintenance of measure instruments and the concomitant collection of key determinants and eventually with the crucial choice of the level of territorial geographical granularity.

The main reasons for such a situation are then illustrated through the examples of French, European, American, and World Health Organization (WHO) experiences.

In France, the 2004 Public Health Policy Act (Loi no. 2004-806, 2004), as a primary promulgation, included five strategic plans to be implemented during 2004–2008. They were health and environment, cancer, rare diseases, violence, abuse, risk, and addictive behavior and last but not the least improvement of QoL in persons suffering from chronic disease. The then Director General of Health introducing this plan stated that making QoL an object of health policy is anything but a duty. It is clearly something not usual and a true paradigm shift in health practices. Then he declared that, "with this act and plan, we were living the concretisation of a major movement, of another approach of disease that not just takes in account the professional point of view but also that of the patient, which renewed the description framework of illness and evidenced its uniqueness regardless of medical categories. It's not so simple to plan, implement and monitor such an approach. In the model of strictly medical thinking, disease is seen as the cause of a malfunction of the individual requiring medical care provided in the form of individual treatment by professionals" (Dab, 2004). The act provided 100 achievable targets defined by a specific national task force after several months of literature review and dialogue with patients' and professionals' organizations. Of them, a few explicitly referred to QoL: (1) To decrease functional limitations and activity limitations due to Chronic Obstructive Pulmonary Disease (COPD) and their impact on QoL, (2) to decrease the impact of benign breast anomalies on health and QoL, (3) to improve QoL of people suffering from osteoarthritis, (4) to decrease the impact of inflammatory bowel disease on QoL, (5) to decrease mortality and to improve QoL of people with sickle cell disease, and (6) to decrease the impact of end-stage renal failure on QoL, especially for people undergoing dialysis. At the implementation phase of the plan most of the actors were unable to explain why these indicators had been chosen and thus to defend the need for obtaining indicators and actions. Thus, the first three objectives have been abandoned completely; the fourth and fifth were followed using only proxies such as medical complications, number of days in hospital, and number of blood transfusions. Only the sixth benefited from QoL measured in a specific survey in 2005 (dialysis) (Boini et al., 2009), 2007 (transplanted patients), and 2011 (Beauger et al., 2015) for both with of generic (short form 36 [SF-36]) and specific (Kidney Disease Quality of Life [KDQoL], Renal Transplant recipients Quality of Life questionnaire [ReTransQoL]) measures. Beyond the quantification of perceived health deterioration suffered by patients with end-stage renal disease (ESRD) on dialysis and of the improvement after transplantation, results were translated into recommendations to promote methods and place for dialysis that enhance patient autonomy, to control nutritional status (albuminemia >35 g/L), to take care of comorbidities, especially cardiovascular by multidisciplinary collaborations, to pay a greater attention to pain relieve at all time, not only at the end of life.

Globally, the plan recommended building up a national coordination for epidemiology and research on the QoL of patients suffering from a chronic condition, including all institutions and agencies producing data, representatives of experts, researchers, health professionals, and patients. The missions were to ensure consistent and coordinated use of quality measurement tools in institutional investigations, to make recommendations on the selection and use of measuring instruments, to participate in the monitoring of metrological research launched under the plan, and to prepare tenders for dissemination of analyses of QoL data from national surveys.

The national coordination never emerged. In 2013, the High Council for Public Health French (Haut Conseil de la Santé Publique—HCSP) committed an evaluation report on the plan (Haut Conseil de la Santé Publique, 2013); it concluded that it was an important step forward in the care of people with a chronic condition but that its impact was likely limited against the ambitions on improving the QoL of these patients. The HCSP considered that "improving the QoL of people with chronic diseases is an important but complex issue that allows setting a strong goal of development for the health system. A reflection and preliminary work on the concept of QoL and its determinants would have allowed measuring the impact of the plan beyond evaluating the implementation of measures. Improving the QoL, highly attractive and unifying theme has to go over the step of being a very general purpose to become an operational and measurable goal." In others words, other than politically correct, perceived health and QoL are neither useful nor operational for public policies.

Nevertheless national institutions developed large health surveys before and after the plan. Insee and Drees implemented the health interview surveys in general population in 1992 and 2002 (Bouvier, 2011) using perceived health, reported chronic diseases, and limitations with 40,000 persons (F. Jusot et al. (2017) paper relies on this survey data), and the health and disability surveys in 1998 and 2008 using SF-12 and reported limitations, chronic diseases, and deficiencies among 39,000 persons. The French Institute for Research and Documentation in Health Economics (IRDES) developed health interview surveys since 1988 (Lengagne et al., 2015), every other year, on 20,000 persons using perceived health, reported limitations and diseases, and access to health care (similar to European Statistics of Income and Living Condition [EU-SILC]). The French National Institute of Prevention and Health Education

(INPES) implemented the "health barometers" on a large sample (n = 28,000) of the general population over 15 year olds using a telephone interview (such as Behavioral Risk Factor Surveillance System [BRFSS]) using successively the Duke Health Profile (Parkerson et al., 1981; Guillemin et al., 1997; Baumann et al., 2011), the WHOQoL-Bref (The WHOQoL Group Development of the World Health Organization, 1998; Baumann et al., 2010), and the Centers for Disease Control and Prevention (CDC) Healthy days (Moriarty et al., 2003). It is repeated every 5 years.

The EU-SILC survey (Lancee and Van de Werfhorst, 2012) contains a small module on health, composed of three variables on health status and four variables on unmet needs for health care.

The variables on health status represent the so-called Minimum European Health Module (MEHM), and measure three different concepts of health namely, self-perceived health, self-reported chronic morbidity (long-standing illness or health problem), and activity limitation—disability (self-perceived long-standing limitations in usual activities due to health problems). The variables on unmet needs for health care target medical care and dental care and assess whether the person needs the respective type of examination or treatment but does not have it and if so what is the main reason of not having it. Summary measures of population health indicate the quality of the remaining years that a person is expected to live (i.e., free of chronic disease, free of disability, and in good perceived health). Implemented in 31 countries, users' satisfaction has been comprehensively evaluated and has been reported as good, but no use for decision making has been explicitly reported. Moreover, reported use by member states of the European Core Health Indicators (ECHI) (Verschuuren et al., 2013) with a particular focus on perceived health has been reported in 2013. Demographic, socioeconomic, life-style related mortality, disease-specific morbidity, and self-assessed general health are declared to be widely used, but "perceived disability and impact of disease on QoL are seen as somewhat more problematic in certain countries due to the subjectivity of the assessment." Forty percent of the interviewees strongly agree with the statement that "self-perceived health status is intrinsically unreliable for cross-country benchmarking because of cultural biases." More than 20% were neutral.

In the United States, the CDC National Center for Chronic Disease Prevention and Health Promotion tended to stimulate the development of health surveillance for tracking health-related quality of life (HRQoL) and health status data at the state and local levels and to encourage the use of these data for public health planning. It developed the CDC Healthy Days, comprising only four questions to be included in the 1993 BRFSS (Zullig et al., 2004; Pierannunzi et al., 2013), which uses telephone surveys to monitor health risk behaviors among adults. The information provided is believed to be interpretable in terms of health-care needs and of the health risk behaviors and sociodemographic conditions associated with these needs. "The BRFSS HRQOL measures thus provide a basis for projecting the demand for health services, developing targeted intervention programs, allocating resources, and evaluating intervention effects." Beyond this declaration, no comprehensive evaluation of the real utilization of perceived health indicators is available, despite a large diffusion of spatiotemporal data.

The WHO initiated the quality of life (WHOQoL) project in 1991 with the aim to develop an international cross-culturally comparable QoL assessment instrument and provided the WHOQoL-BREF, a shorter version of the original instrument that may be more convenient for use in large research studies or clinical trials. Nevertheless, the gold standard indicator at WHO remains the WHO global burden of disease based on the disability-adjusted-life-year (DALY), which reflects more on a societal perspective of disability burden than an individual perception of health.

Conclusion

Perceived health indicators are needed at the population level and are effectively in use in many health systems, near or in complement of so-called more objective measurement of health or as a whole. They are also used as predictors of subsequent mortality. They are often considered as health outcomes per se and analyzed in terms of their determinants.

Use for health policy is patchy or at least rarely explicitly mentioned. Possible reasons for nonuse are to be found among the followings: results might not be immediately actionable for policy-making purposes because deemed exceedingly influenced by cultural factors, policy makers could rely on more convincing sources of information for setting their targets, and policy makers would feel less confident to defend their policy near health professionals. In other words, health systems are encompassed in the biomedical model that is nowadays difficult to overcome.

Acknowledgments

I am grateful to Mrs. Catherine Le Galès (Cermes3, Inserm, Cnrs, Ehess, University of Paris Descartes) and Dr. Juliette Bloch for their fruitful contribution to the roundtable during the 3-4th of June 2014 APEMAC conference.

References

Baumann, C., Erpelding, M.L., Perret-Guillaume, C., Gautier, A., Régat, S., Collin, J.F., et al. (2011). Health-related quality of life in French adolescents and adults: Norms for the DUKE Health Profile. *BMC Public Health*, *11*, 401.

Baumann, C., Erpelding, M.L., Régat, S., Collin, J.F., and Briançon, S. (2010). The WHOQOL-BREF questionnaire: French adult population norms for the physical health, psychological health and social relationship dimensions. *Rev. Epidemiol. Sante Publique.*, *58*(1), 33–39.

Beauger, D., Gentile, S., Jacquelinet, C., Dussol, B., and Briançon, S. (2015). Comparison of two national quality of life surveys for patients with end stage renal disease between 2005–2007 and 2011: Indicators slightly decreased. *Nephrol. Ther.*, *11*(2), 88–96.

Boini, S., Bloch, J., and Briançon, S. (2009). Monitoring the quality of life of end-stage renal disease patients. Quality of life report—REIN—Dialysis 2005. *Nephrol. Ther.*, 5(Suppl 3), S177–S237.

Bouvier, G. (2011). L'enquête handicap-santé. Présentation générale. Insee; Paris, 2011 October; p. 61.

Dab, W. (2004). Intervention du Directeur Général de la Santé. in Santé publique, qualité de vie et maladies chroniques: Attentes des patients et des professionnels. DGS, Paris, 2004, December. Available at 2016 July at social-sante.gouv.fr/IMG/pdf/plan_actes2005-2.pdf

Guillemin, F., Paul-Dauphin, A., Virion, J.M., Bouchet, C., and Briançon, S. (1997). The DUKE health profile: A generic instrument to measure the quality of life tied to health. *Sante Publique.*, 9(1), 35–44.

Haut Conseil de la Santé Publique. (2013). Evaluation du plan pour l'amélioration de la qualité de vie des personnes atteintes de maladie chronique 2007–2011. Paris, 2013 October; p. 133.

Jusot, F., Tubeuf, S., Devaux, M., Sermet, C. (2017). Social heterogeneity in self-reported health status and the measurement of inequalities in health. In: Guillemin, F., Leplège, V., Briançon, S., Spitz, E., Coste, J. (eds.), *Perceived Health and Adaptation in Chronic Disease*. New York: Routledge, 175–195.

Lancee, B., and Van de Werfhorst, H.G. (2012). Income inequality and participation: A comparison of 24 European countries. *Soc. Sci. Res.*, 41(5), 1166–1178.

Lengagne, P., Penneau, A., Pichetti, S., and Sermet, C. (2015). L'accès aux soins courants et préventifs des personnes en situation de handicap en France tome 1. IRDES, Paris, 2015; N°560, p. 134.

Loi no. 2004-806 du 9 août 2004 relative à la politique de santé publique. JORF, n°185, 11 août 2004, p. 14277

Moriarty, D.G., Zack, M.M., and Kobau, R. (2003). The centers for disease control and prevention's Healthy days measures—Population tracking of perceived physical and mental health over time. *Health2 Qual. Life Outcomes.*, 1, 37.

Parkerson, G.R., Jr., Gehlbach, S.H., Wagner, E.H., James, S.A., Clapp, N.E., and Muhlbaier, L.H. (1981). The Duke-UNC health profile: An adult health status instrument for primary care. *Med. Care*, 19(8), 806–828.

Pierannunzi, C., Sean, Hu S., and Balluz, L. (2013). A systematic review of publications assessing reliability and validity of the Behavioral Risk Factor Surveillance System (BRFSS), 2004–2011. *BMC Med. Res. Methodol.*, 13, 49.

United Nations. (2006). Final report of the Ad Hoc Committee on a Comprehensive and Integral International Convention on the Protection and Promotion of the Rights and Dignity of Persons with Disabilities. Department of Public Information, United Nations, 2006, A/61/611.

Verschuuren, M., Gissler, M., Kilpeläinen, K., Tuomi-Nikula, A., Sihvonen, A.P., Thelen, J., et al. (2013). Public health indicators for the EU: The joint action for ECHIM (European Community Health Indicators & Monitoring). *Arch. Public Health*, 71(1), 12.

The WHOQOL Group Development of the World Health Organization. (1998). WHOQOL-BREF quality of life assessment. *Psychol. Med.*, 28(3), 551–558.

Zullig, K.J., Valois, R.F., Huebner, E.S., and Drane, J.W. (2004). Evaluating the performance of the Centers for Disease Control and Prevention core Health-Related Quality of Life scale with adolescents. *Public Health Rep.*, 119(6), 577–584.

Appendix A: Set of activities of the Animated Activity Questionnaire with levels of execution

1   **Ascending stairs (4)**
    Setting: Stairs with banister
    1. Without any problem, touching the banister but not leaning
    2. With slower speed, and pulling up at the banister
    3. One stair step at the time and pulling up at the banister
    4. One stair step at the time and pulling up at the banister and using one crutch and rest in between
    5. Unable to perform

2   **Descending stairs (5)**
    Setting: Stairs with banister
    1. Without any problem, touching the banister but not leaning
    2. With slower speed, a little bit leaning on the banister
    3. One stair step at the time and with more support of the bannister
    4. One stair step at the time and leaning on the banister and using one crutch
    5. One stair step at the time but going backwards and holding on to the banister
    6. Unable to perform

3   **Walking outside on a flat surface (5)**
    Setting: Outside on the sidewalk
    1. Without any problems
    2. With slower speed and shorter stand phase of the affected leg
    3. Shorter stand phase and longer sway phase injured leg and a Duchenne gait
    4. With help from a stick or crutch
    5. Shorter stand phase and longer sway phase injured leg and a walker
    6. Unable to perform

4   **Walking outside on an even terrain (4)**
    Settings: A forest
    1. Without any problems
    2. With slower speed and shorter stand phase of the affected leg
    3. Shorter stand phase and longer sway phase injured leg and a Duchenne gait
    4. With help from a stick or crutch
    5. Unable to perform

5   **Walking inside: Start walking after at least 15 minutes sitting (4)**
        Setting: Living room with ordinary chair
        1. Without any problem
        2. First making some steps on the place and then starting slowly with shorter stand phase and later normal stand phase
        3. With slower speed and starting with smaller steps
        4. With slower speed, starting in a more bending position and slowly stretching up the body during the first meters and walking with a Duchenne gait
        5. Unable to perform

6   **Ascending a bridge or small slope (4)**
        Setting: Small bridge and water
        1. Without any problems
        2. With slower speed and shorter stand phase of the affected leg
        3. With help from a stick or crutch
        4. Shorter stand phase and longer sway phase injured leg and a walker
        5. Unable to perform

7   **Descending a bridge or small slope (4)**
        Setting: Small bridge and water
        1. Without any problems
        2. With slower speed and shorter stand phase of the affected leg
        3. With help from a stick or crutch
        4. Shorter stand phase and longer sway phase injured leg and a walker
        5. Unable to perform

8   **Picking up an object from the floor (4)**
        1. Without any problem with bending knees
        2. With slower speed supported by leaning with the forearm on the thigh, legs somewhat spread
        3. Bending with lower back and little flexion in knees and spread legs and more support on good leg; index leg aside
        4. Leaning on chair or other object, spread legs with more weight on good leg and index leg aside
        5. Unable to perform

9   **Rising from the floor (3)**
        Setting: Room with table/chair
        1. Turning to the belly side and get into hands/knees position; subsequently lifting the good leg and leaning on the foot and lifting up oneself by pushing with hands on the knee
        2. Turning to the belly side and get into hands/knees position, spreading the legs; subsequently coming to hands/feet position and "walking" with hands toward feet, leaning first with one hand and then with two hands on the legs and pushing oneself to a standing position
        3. Turning to the belly side and getting into hands/knees position; subsequently standing up with the help of a chair or small cabinet to standing position, while leaning with the hands or forearms
        4. Unable to perform

10   **Rising from a chair (4)**
      Setting: Room with table/chair
      1. Without any problem
      2. With lower speed, leaning with hands on arm rest and with more weight on the good leg
      3. Leaning on both hands, bending forward and pushing oneself upwards, stretching legs first and secondly stretching up the upper body
      4. Scrolling forward on the chair, moving forward/backward with the upper body to make some speed to get up; when getting up pushing oneself with the hands on the arm rests, first stretching the legs with the upper body in bending position and subsequently erect the whole body
      5. Unable to perform

11   **Sitting down on a chair (4)**
      Setting: Room with table/chair
      1. Without any problem
      2. With slower speed, leaning with the hands on the arm rests and more weight on the good leg
      3. Leaning on both hands, bending forward and letting down oneself, leaning on the hands and with the affected leg more in forward and stretched position
      4. The same as above but with plopping down in the chair during the last phase of the movement
      5. Unable to perform

12   **Rising from a sofa (4)**
      Setting: Room with table/sofa
      1. Without any problem
      2. With lower speed, leaning with one hand on arm rest and with the other on the sofa and with more weight on the good leg
      3. The same as above but now also bending forward and pushing oneself upwards, stretching legs first and secondly stretching up the upper body
      4. Scrolling forward and moving forward/backward with the upper body to make some speed to get up; when getting up pushing oneself with the hands on the sofa, first stretching the legs with the upper body in bending position and subsequently erect the whole body
      5. Unable to perform

13   **Sitting down on a sofa (4)**
      Setting: Room with table/chair
      1. Without any problem
      2. With slower speed, leaning with one hand on the arm rest and the other on the sofa and more weight on the good leg
      3. Leaning on both hands, bending forward and letting down oneself, leaning on the hands and with the affected leg more in forward and stretched position
      4. The same as above but with plopping down on the sofa during the last phase of the movement
      5. Unable to perform

14   **Rising from a toilet (4)**
Setting: Toilet with a small fountain and holder for toilet paper
1. Without any problem
2. With support of leaning on the toilet on which they are sitting and good bending forward with the upper body
3. Rise with support of pulling oneself up at the small fountain, slower speed, and taking some time to find balance
4. Moving forward/backward with the upper body to make some speed to get up; rise with support of pulling oneself up at the small fountain
5. Unable to perform

15   **Sitting down on a toilet (4)**
Setting: Toilet with a small fountain and holder for toilet paper
1. Without any problem
2. With support of leaning on the toilet and bending forward while getting to be seated
3. The same but with some hanging on the small fountain
4. Slowly while hanging a bit on the small fountain and plopping down during the last phase of the movement
5. Unable to perform

16   **Putting on shoes (4)**
Setting: Bedroom with bed and night cabinet
1. Doing it while sitting and pulling up one leg
2. Doing it while sitting and leaning with one leg (ankle) on the other leg (knee)
3. Doing it sitting bending forward and leave the feet on the ground
4. With help from an assistive device
5. Unable to perform

17   **Taking off shoes (3)**
Setting: Bedroom with bed and night cabinet
1. Doing it standing taking of shoe with the help of the other foot
2. While sitting, pulling up the leg/foot, loosening laces and then taking of shoe with the help of the other foot
3. While sitting, bending forward, keeping the foot on the floor, loosening laces and taking of the shoe with the other foot
4. Unable to perform

Index